I0060875

Phytotherapy in the Management of Diabetes and Hypertension

Editor

Mohamed Eddouks

Moulay Ismail University
BP 21, Errachidia, 52000
Morocco

Co-Editor

Debprasad Chattopadhyay

ICMR Virus Unit, ID & BG Hospital
GB-4, First Floor, 57 Dr Suresh C Banerjee Road
Beliaghata, Kolkata 700 010
India

Phytotherapy in the Management of Diabetes and Hypertension

Volume: 1

Editor: Mohamed Edouks

Co-Editor: Debprasad Chattopadhyay

ISSN: 2452-3232 (Online)

ISSN: 2452-3224 (Print)

eISBN: 978-1-60805-014-7

ISBN: 978-1-60805-567-8

© 2012, Bentham eBooks imprint.

Published by Bentham Science Publishers –

Sharjah, UAE. All Rights Reserved.

CONTENTS

ABOUT THE EDITORS

Mohamed Eddouks is the Professor at Moulay Ismail University, Morocco. He is a researcher in Physiology and Pharmacology with a Master Degree in Metabolic and Molecular Endocrinology from University of Paris vi, a specialized certificate in Endocrine Pharmacology from University of Paris vii and PhD degrees in Physiology and Pharmacology from University of Liege, Belgium and Sidi Mohammed Ben Abdellah University, Fez, Morocco. After his post-doctoral fellowship at Department of Physiology, Faculty of Medicine of Montreal, Canada, he is working for the last 12 years on medicinal plants. His work on antidiabetic and antihypertensive plants is well recognized globally. His research focuses on ethnobiological as well as pharmacological issues in the use of Moroccan medicinal plants for the treatment of diabetes mellitus, obesity and hypertension.

His contribution to this field includes two international books and more than 70 peer-reviewed articles and book chapters of international repute. He is Guest Editor of American Journal of Pharmacology and Toxicology, Lead Guest Editor of Evidence-Based and Complementary Alternative Medicine, Regional Editor of the Following journals: American Journal of Food Technology, Journal of Applied Sciences, Trends in Applied Sciences Research and Singapore Journal of Scientific research, Member of Editorial Board of the following international journals: International Journal of Pharmacy and Pharmaceutical Sciences, Asian Journal of Pharmaceutical and Clinical Research, Metabolic and Functional Research on Diabetes, Pharmacology and Pharmacy, Research Journal of Pharmacology. He is also member of panel of experts of several international journals including Journal of Cardiovascular Pharmacology, Journal of Pharmacy and Pharmacology, Journal of Food Biochemistry, Plant Foods for Human Nutrition, Diabetes Research and Clinical Investigation, Journal of Herbal Pharmacotherapy, Evidence Based Complementary and alternative Medicine, Journal of Herbs Spices and Medicinal Plants, Life Sciences, Biophysica Biochemica Acta, Phytotherapy Research, Journal of Ethnopharmacology and Journal of Medicinal Plants Research. He is also Invited member of some prestigious international Associations including American Diabetes Association,

American Stroke Association, the Scientific Council for High Blood Pressure Research and European Institute for the Ambulatory Study of Obesity and Diabetes. He has been honoured with the first and the second Prizes of Scientific Research in 2008 by the Moroccan Association of Research and Development. He has been the Dean of Polydisciplinary School of Errachidia from 2008 to 2012.

Debprasad Chattopadhyay is the Assistant Director (Scientist) in the ICMR Virus Unit, Kolkata. After his Masters in Botany with Microbiology and Ph.D. in Pharmaceutical Microbiology, he received post doctoral training from the London Hospital Medical College, London, and the Statens Serum Institute, Copenhagen. His work on antimicrobial and related pharmacological potential of ethnomedicinal plants of different Indian tribes is well recognized globally. His in depth studies on ethnomedicinal practices of the Onge, Nicobarese, and Shompen tribes of Andaman and Nicobar Island by establishing personal relationship, help in recording the endemic, threatened and rare flowering plants of Bay Islands. Utilizing the tribal Knowledge-base, he has investigated the scientific basis of several medicaments and identified four herbal drugs with antimicrobial, anti-inflammatory, antipyretic, antipsychotic and sperm motility-inhibiting activities, which is under patenting. His group has also purified and characterized a phytophore that inhibit the *in vitro* proliferation of *Plasmodium falciparum*, highly effective against the chloroquine-resistant strain. He has also demonstrated the antibacterial activity of a tricyclic phenothiazine, methdilazine that produce synergism with aminoglycoside antibiotics and can reverse bacterial resistance by altering membrane permeability of resistant bacteria that facilitate the entry of other antibiotics.

He has contributed 55 original scientific papers in peer reviewed Journals of repute, 5 book chapters and 5 Review in Journals like Mini Review in Medicinal Chemistry, Biotechnology Annual Review, New Biotechnology *etc.*, along with four patents and 45 popular science articles. He is the Guest Editor of International Journal of Biomedical and Pharmaceutical Sciences, and the Research Signpost. He is the Editorial Board Member of three International Journals and Annual Reviews of Phytomedicine; and is the reviewer of several Journals including International Journal of Medical Sciences, Journal of Ethnopharmacology, Drug Discovery Today, Journal of Diabetes and

Complications, Journal of Pharmacy and Pharmaceutical Sciences, Methods and Findings in Experimental and Clinical Pharmacology, Biotechnology Journal, Journal of Medicinal Plant Research, International Journal of Antimicrobial Agents, Plant Foods for Human Nutrition, Journal of Antimicrobial Chemotherapy *etc.* He has conducted several research projects of national importance funded by ICMR, DBT, DST and National Innovation Foundation. He has honoured with awards from Indian Association of Medical Microbiologists, International Society of Chemotherapy, British Society for Antimicrobial Chemotherapy, Indian Association for the Study of Sexually transmitted Diseases & AIDS, World Conference on Dosing of Antiinfectives, Indian Dietetic Association, Indian Science Congress Association and DST, and is the guest faculty of several Universities.

FOREWORD

Diabetes and hypertension are two of the most prevalent chronic diseases in the world. It is predicted that by 2030, India, China and the United States will have the largest number of people with diabetes. Concerning the pattern in developing countries, Prof. Mohamed Eddouks and Dr. Debprasad Chattopadhyay have crafted a book entitled "Phytotherapy in the Management of Diabetes and Hypertension", bringing out a timely volume with contributors spread across three countries. Various aspects of these two prevalent diseases among the places are discussed. A number of topics are covered, including cellular nutrition and nutritional medicine in diabetes and related complications, as well as the relationship between diabetes and hypertension. As control of these diseases is critical to prevent their complications, phytotherapy in the management of diabetes and hypertension are also introduced.

This is an eBook different from the traditional concept of hard or soft cover book. This approach will make the book more easily accessible to a wider section of readers. It is a great pleasure on my part to pen a foreword for this nice, multi-authored, international publication on a topic very close to my heart. I wish the editors great success and will look forward to see a regular series culminating from this beginning. I also extend my sincere thanks to all the contributors for their excellent efforts in making this book a success.

William C.S. Cho

Department of Clinical Oncology, Queen Elizabeth Hospital, Hong Kong
RCMP, FHKSMDS, FHKIMLS, FIBMS (UK), Chartered Scientist (UK)
Guest Professor of Southern Medical University
Nanjing Medical University, Ningxia University
China

PREFACE

The serious health risks posed by hyperglycemia and hypertension need important elaboration. This book paves the way to success in the management of diabetes and hypertension through plant-based therapeutic and dietary intervention, systematically addressing the issues facing by the community, particularly the clinicians through a safe and effective way. Scientists demonstrate the potentials of naturaceuticals and lifestyle management in controlling the dreaded diseases diabetes and hypertension through studies and experiments are reported through this book. The result is a valuable source of information unavailable elsewhere. In this timely and original eBook plant pharmacologists from around the world demonstrate the potentials and pitfalls involved in turning traditionally used medicinal plants into safe and effective drugs in addition to a valuable source of otherwise unpublished information.

The eBook adds valuable data to the existing knowledge of hyperglycemia and diabetes and their management. The eBook emphasizes the basic biochemistry for diabetes mellitus and hypertension, and described every aspect of these lifestyle diseases and its control or remediation through a cost effective, safe, easy-going, easy-adaptable method through the age-old practice validated by scientific research. This eBook contains seven complementary chapters dealing with various aspects of these diseases and their Phytotherapy treatment and life style management. As the Phytotherapy can give long term benefit with less or no side effect, hence this eBook can be treated as authenticated alternative or complementary therapeutic compendium to the physicians and patients. This eBook will be useful to the students, teachers, researchers, scientists, clinicians and even the common people interested to know about the subject as health is a personal choice.

ACKNOWLEDGEMENTS

The Editors would like to express their deepest gratitude to all the contributors and Bentham Science Publishers.

Debprasad Chattopadhyay
ICMR Virus Unit, ID & BG Hospital
GB-4, First Floor, 57 Dr Suresh C Banerjee Road
Beliaghata, Kolkata 700 010
India

Mohamed Eddouks
Moulay Ismail University
BP 21, Errachidia, 52000
Morocco

List of Contributors

Adeneye A. Adewale

Department of Pharmacology, Faculty of Basic Medical Sciences, Lagos State University College of Medicine, Ikeja, Lagos State, Nigeria.

Adeyemi O. Olufunmilayo

Department of Pharmacology, College of Medicine of the University of Lagos, Idi-Araba, Lagos State, Nigeria.

Arpita Chakraborty

Department of Biochemistry, University of Calcutta, 35, Ballygunge Circular Road, Kolkata-700019, India.

Chitralekha Saha

Diabetic Clinic, Salt Lake City, Kolkata 700 064, India.

Hemanta Mukherjee

Student at ICMR Virus Unit, ID & BG Hospital, General Block 4, 57 Dr Suresh Chandra Banerjee Road, Kolkata 700010, India.

Maitree Bhattacharyya

Department of Biochemistry, University of Calcutta, 35, Ballygunge Circular Road, Kolkata-700019, India.

Naoufel Ali Zeggwagh

Moulay Ismail University, Morocco.

Paromita Bag

Student at ICMR Virus Unit, ID & BG Hospital, General Block 4, 57 Dr. Suresh Chandra Banerjee Road, Kolkata 700010, India.

Tapan Chatterjee

Pharmaceutical Technology Department, Jadavpur University, Kolkata 700 032, India.

Phytotherapy in the Management of Diabetes and Hypertension

2

CHAPTER 1

Cellular Nutrition and Nutritional Medicine in Diabetes and Related Complications: An Overview

Debprasad Chattopadhyay[1,*] and Mohamed Eddouks[2]

[1]ICMR Virus Unit, ID & BG Hospital, GB-4, First Floor, 57 Dr. Suresh C. Banerjee Road, Beliaghata, Kolkata 700010, India and [2]Moulay Ismail University, BP 21, Errachidia, 52000, Morocco

Abstract: Diabetes is a chronic condition of impaired glucose cycle that alters the whole metabolism leading to high blood glucose level. Diabetes occurs when the pancreatic beta cells are either unable to produce enough insulin, or the body cells were unable to use available insulin effectively. Insulin, a storage hormone produced in the pancreatic beta cells, helps to absorb glucose for the production of energy during cellular respiration. Thus, failure of absorbing glucose by body cells results in the accumulation of glucose in the blood, which is termed as hyperglycemia. Excess blood glucose causes serious damage to the major organ systems, leading to the heart disease, kidney failure (nephropathy), blindness (retinopathy), loss of sensation in the feet and hands and even an early death. Thus, diabetes is a chronic condition where the body's ability to convert food into energy is impaired. Prevalence of diabetes along with dyslipidaemia is increasing at an explosive rate throughout the globe. Though the exact cause is unknown, many factors are believed to play roles in this pathogenesis. Genetic predispositions, faulty dietary patterns, and sedentary life-styles are the key factors for the increased prevalence of type 2 diabetes. This progressive disease develops through many years, and pre-diabetic condition is known to be reversible. Though antidiabetic drugs are the first line of defence to control blood glucose level, conventional therapy is unable to cure it, nor can prevent the long term damage of the vital systems, but needs to be used lifelong. On the other hand, the benefit of nutritional medicine and dietary supplementation in diabetes is less explored scientifically. Therefore, the safer alternatives to prevent, or minimize the long term damage and control of diabetes need a combination of healthy eating, regular physical activity, monitoring of blood glucose level, dietary control and nutritional medicine. This review will cover not only the different aspects of diabetes, but also the role of complementary personalized therapy using nutrition and nutritional medicine in its management, highlighting a proper blend of conventional therapy with nutraceuticals, for effective diabetes management.

Keywords: Diabetes, pathophysiology, cellular mechanism, dyslipidaemia.

*Address correspondence to Debprasad Chattopadhyay: ICMR Virus Unit, ID & BG Hospital, GB-4, First Floor, 57 Dr. Suresh C. Banerjee Road, Beliaghata, Kolkata 700010, India; Tel/Fax: +913323537424-25; E-Mail: debprasadc@yahoo.co.in

Mohamed Eddouks and Debprasad Chattopadhyay (Eds)
All rights reserved-© 2012 Bentham Science Publishers

INTRODUCTION

Globally diabetes is one of the most widespread diseases in existence that increased more than ten-fold in the last 40 years. Diabetes encompasses a group of diseases, in which the body's ability to convert glucose into energy is impaired, leading to a chronic condition. This metabolic disorder arises when the pancreatic beta cells are either unable to produce enough insulin, or the body cells do not respond to the released insulin. Thus, the glucose released by the breakdown of carbohydrate food accumulates in the blood (hyperglycemia), leading to the complications in cardiovascular, nerve, retina, kidney and other systems [1, 2]. Even though diabetes itself is a big enough health problem, the side effects are equally ominous. For example, one-third of the new diabetic cases ended with diabetic nephropathy; 20% eventually die from cardiovascular diseases, and diabetes is the leading cause of amputation and blindness in elderly people [3]. There are three major types of diabetes, namely type 1, type 2 and gestational diabetes. Type 2, which occurs frequently in older people, accounts for about 90-95 percent of all diagnosed cases; while type 1 accounts for 5-10 percent of cases, usually occurs in children and young adults. Gestational diabetes, on the other hand, appears in some women during pregnancy, whereas type 2 diabetes is increasingly being diagnosed in children. The three major causes of diabetes include obesity (*obey the rule of city*), a family history of diabetes, and physical inactivity [4, 5]. Moreover, certain minority population groups and women with gestational diabetes are at greater risk of developing type 2 that usually starts as insulin resistance (a disorder in which the body cells are unable to use insulin properly). Thus, diabetes is the scourge of the modern world, after heart disease and cancer. Being a multistep process, insulin resistance (or metabolic Syndrome X) occurs before the development of full blown diabetes. The syndrome X is a cluster of factors that affect about one quarter of the world's population and among those factors insulin resistance is the precursor to diabetes and cardiovascular disorders [6].

Today diabetes mellitus (DM) occurs throughout the world, both in the developed and developing nations, particularly in Asia and Africa, where most patients will probably be found by 2030 [7]. In developing countries, rapid urbanization and lifestyle changes, particularly the "western-style" diet are the major causes of increased incidence of diabetes. Though the environmental or dietary effect is one of the major concerns, its mechanism(s) is not yet very clear [7]. Indigenous populations in first world countries showed a higher prevalence and increasing incidence than their corresponding non-indigenous populations, as found in Australia, where the age-standardized prevalence of self-reported diabetes in indigenous Australians is four times that of non-indigenous counterparts [8]. As of 2010 about 285 million (6.4%) adult (aged 20-79 years) were diabetic globally, that may increase to 7.7% (439 million) by 2030. The estimate revealed that between 2010 and 2030, there will be 69% increase in numbers of adults with diabetes in developing countries and a 20% increase in developed nations [9]. In March 2010, over 30 million people were diagnosed diabetic in India. The crude prevalence rate in urban India is about 9% while it is 3% in rural areas, and the estimated number of diabetics in India is around 40 million. In India, impaired glucose tolerance (IGT) is a mounting problem, with a prevalence around 8.7% in urban and 7.9% in rural areas, of which about 35% of IGT sufferers may develop type 2 diabetes, indicating that India is genuinely facing a healthcare crisis. Moreover, in India type 1 is rare, and one third of type 2 diabetic patients are overweight, and diabetes appears much earlier in life, which makes chronic long-term complications more and more common (http://www.diabetesindia.com/Retrieved on 22.05.2010) [10]. The top 10 countries, in numbers of sufferers are India, China, USA, Indonesia, Japan, Pakistan, Russia, Brazil, Italy and Bangladesh, where about 6 deaths occur per minute due to diabetic complications [11].

While there is no cure, the conventional treatments rely on drugs to keep blood glucose level within an acceptable range or stable, as excess glucose in the bloodstream spells trouble for the major organs leading to heart disease, kidney failure, blindness, loss of sensation in the feet and hands and may lead to an early death. Though the drugs are the first line of defence to control blood sugar, safer alternatives to control blood sugar are the change in dietary pattern from high carbohydrate, fat, sugar, sodium salt to whole grains, fresh fruit and vegetables and raw food diet with regular exercise. Thus, the basic tools for preventing and managing diabetes are healthy eating, physical activity, and blood glucose monitoring with or without prescription drugs, insulin, or both. The complementary and alternative therapies, including "nutritional medicine" along with nutraceuticals are one of the preferred areas of diabetes treatment. This review will summarize the scientific tit-bits on the effectiveness and safety of selected nutritional medicines and supplements used globally by people suffering from diabetes, particularly in type 2, along with recent information for a proper management of diabetes.

HISTORY

The term diabetes, coined by Aretaeus of Cappadocia, derives from the Greek verb *diabaínein* (διαβαίνειν). The prefix *dia-* means "across or apart", and the verb *bainein* means "to walk or stand". Thus, *diabeinein* means "to stride, walk, or stand with legs asunder", and *diabētēs* means one that "straddles", or "a compass, siphon" (disease that discharges the excessive amounts of urine). Diabetes was first recorded in 1425, while Thomas Willis in 1675 added the word *mellitus* (Latin word meaning "honey") due to the sweet taste of the urine, noticed by the ancient Greeks, Chinese, Egyptians, Indians, and Persians. In 1776, Matthew Dobson confirmed that the sweet taste was due to excess sugar in the urine and blood [12]. Diabetes mellitus was the death sentence in the ancient era, and even Hippocrates did not mention it, probably because he felt that the disease was incurable, but Aretaeus attempted to treat it as he feels that "life with diabetes is short, disgusting and painful" [13]. Renowned Indian Physician Sushruta (6th century BC) classified diabetes as *Medhumeha* (sweet urine disease) and identified it with obesity and sedentary lifestyle, and thus advised for exercises to "cure" it [14]. Later, the detailed account of diabetes mellitus was provided by Avicenna (980-1037) of medieval Persia in his book *The Canon of Medicine*. He described the abnormal appetite and the collapse of sexual functions in people having the sweet urine, and recognized primary and secondary diabetes, and diabetic gangrene. Avicenna treated diabetes with a mixture of lupine, *trigonella* (fenugreek), and zedoary seed, a treatment that reduces the urinary sugar effectively and is still prescribed today. Avicenna also described diabetes insipidus, though Johann Peter Frank (1745-1821) first differentiated between diabetes mellitus and diabetes insipidus [15]. Although diabetes has been recognized since antiquity and its treatment of various efficacy has been known since the middle Ages, its pathogenesis was understood experimentally only in 1900 [16]. However, the discovery of the role of pancreas in diabetes is attributed to Joseph von Mering and Oskar Minkowski in 1889, who showed that the dogs can develop the signs and symptoms of diabetes, when its pancreas was removed [17]. In

1910, Sir Edward Albert Sharpey-Schafer suggested that diabetic people were deficient in *insulin*, a chemical produced by the pancreas (Latin *insula* means island, in reference to islets of Langerhans). The endocrine role of the pancreas in metabolism was further clarified in 1921 by Sir Frederick Grant Banting and Charles Herbert Best who induced diabetes in dogs and reversed the condition by using an extract from the pancreatic islets of Langerhans of healthy dogs [18]. Later Banting, Best, and Collip purified insulin from bovine pancreases, which lead to an effective treatment of diabetes with insulin injections in 1922. For this, Banting and MacLeod were awarded the Nobel Prize in 1923. Insulin production and therapy rapidly spread around the world and WHO honored Banting by declaring his birthday, the 14th November as World Diabetes Day.

However, the distinction between type 1 and type 2 diabetes was first made by Sir Harold Percival Himsworth [19]. The landmark discoveries in diabetes research include the identification of the sulfonylureas in 1942 [16], the use of biguanides for type 2 diabetes in the 1950s, metformin in 1979, the determination of the amino acid sequence of insulin by Sir Frederick Sanger (for which he received Nobel Prize), and the radioimmunoassay for insulin by Rosalyn Yalow and Solomon Berson [20], for which Yalow got the 1977 Nobel Prize. In 1980 Genentech Biotech developed human insulin and in 1982 the three-dimensional structure of insulin (PDB 2INS) was discovered [21]. However, in 1988 Dr. Gerald Reaven's identified the constellation of symptoms called metabolic syndrome, and in the 1990s, thiazolidinedione was found to be an effective insulin sensitizer. The insulin is then isolated from genetically engineered bacteria (the human insulin gene was inserted in *Escherichia coli*, a bacteria that can synthesize human insulin), to produce large quantities of insulin. Later two large longitudinal studies demonstrated that intensive glycemic control in diabetes reduces chronic side effects [22].

CLASSIFICATION

Based on agreed nomenclature, the most cases of diabetes fall into the three broad categories: type 1, type 2, and gestational diabetes. Type 1 diabetes results from the body's failure to produce insulin, and thus requires insulin. Type 2 results from insulin resistance, when body cells fail to use insulin properly; while Gestational diabetes happens when a woman has a high blood glucose level during pregnancy, that later may develop into type 2 diabetes. The term type 1 diabetes has replaced the former terms like childhood-onset diabetes, juvenile diabetes, and insulin-dependent diabetes mellitus (IDDM). Likewise, type 2 diabetes has replaced its former terms like adult-onset diabetes, obesity-related diabetes, and non-insulin-dependent diabetes mellitus (NIDDM). Some sources classified gestational diabetes as type 3 [23], insulin-resistant type 1 as double diabetes, and type 2 that progresses to require insulin, and latent autoimmune diabetes of adults (LADA) or type 1.5 diabetes (Johns Hopkins Autoimmune Disease Research Center. http://autoimmune.pathology.jhmi.edu/diseases). However, another rare condition that produces a large amount of urine without taste is called diabetes insipidus.

Type 1 Diabetes: Type 1 diabetes is characterized by the loss of insulin-producing pancreatic beta cells leading to insulin deficiency and represents about 10% of diabetes cases. It can be further classified as immune-mediated or idiopathic. The majority of type 1 is of immune-mediated nature, where beta cell loss is a T-cell mediated autoimmune attack [1]. There is no known preventive measure against type 1 diabetes. In the early stage most affected people are healthy with normal weight, sensitivity and responsiveness to insulin. As it primarily affects children or young adults, and is thereby traditionally termed as juvenile diabetes.

Type 2 Diabetes: Type 2 diabetes occurs due to a defect in insulin's secretion and action, and represents about 90% of diabetes cases. It is characterized by insulin resistance or with relatively reduced insulin secretion and is a heterogeneous, multifactorial and polygenic disease. The defective responsiveness of body tissues to insulin may involve the insulin receptor. However, the specific defects are still unknown. As the disease progresses, the impairment of insulin secretion occurs, and therapeutic replacement of insulin may become necessary. In the early stage, it is characterized by reduced insulin sensitivity, when hyperglycemia can be reversed by a variety of measures and medications through improving insulin sensitivity or reducing glucose production by the liver.

Gestational Diabetes: Gestational diabetes mellitus (GDM) resembles to type 2, involving a combination of relatively inadequate insulin secretion and responsiveness. It occurs in about 2%-5% of all pregnancies and may improve or disappear after delivery. With careful medical supervision it can be fully treatable, though 20-50% of affected women develop type 2 diabetes later. However, untreated GDM can damage the health of the fetus or mother. Risks to the baby include macrosomia (high birth weight), congenital cardiac and CNS anomalies, and skeletal muscle malformations. Increased fetal insulin may inhibit fetal surfactant production leading to respiratory distress, while RBC destruction causes hyperbilirubinemia. In severe cases, perinatal death may occur due to poor placental perfusion for vascular impairment. A recent study revealed that more and more women are entering pregnancy with preexisting diabetes and the rate of diabetes in expectant mothers has doubled in the past 6 years in the USA [24]. This is particularly alarming as diabetes raises the risk of pregnancy complications, and increasing the potential of diabetic children.

Other Types: Other forms include congenital diabetes due to genetic defects of insulin secretion; cystic fibrosis-related diabetes; steroid induced diabetes due to high doses of glucocorticoids; and several forms of monogenic diabetes.

DIABETES AND ANTIDIABETIC DRUGS: A RELATIONSHIP

The recent JUPITER trial reported an increased risk for diabetes in patients using rosuvastatin [25] like the PROSPER (Prospective Study of Pravastatin in the Elderly at Risk) trial with pravastatin [26]. In a meta-analysis of 13 clinical trials with 91,140 non-diabetic participants, a small but significant relationship between statin use and risk for incident diabetes was noticed. The study showed that 4278 developed incident diabetes over a mean follow-up period of 4 years. Of the 13 trials, 6 reported incident diabetes, and 2 showed positive associations between statin therapy and incident diabetes. In the combined data, 174 more cases of incident diabetes occurred in the statin treated groups than in the placebo, representing a 9% increase in the development of diabetes during follow-up [27]. In a study with 390 type 2 diabetes patients (196 received metformin three timed daily for four years, and a placebo was prescribed to 194), revealed that 19% of the people with metformin therapy had reduction in their vitamin B_{12} levels compared with placebo. Interestingly, the reduced levels of B_{12} in the metformin group persisted and became more apparent over time [28, 29]. It is well known that Vitamin B_{12} is essential to maintain healthy nerve cells and RBC, and its deficiency leads to fatigue, mental changes, anemia and nerve damage.

SIGNS AND SYMPTOMS

The classical symptoms of DM are polyuria (frequent urination), polydipsia (increased thirst) and increased hunger or polyphagia [5]. Symptoms may develop within weeks or months in type 1, particularly in children, and cause a rapid and significant weight loss (despite normal or increased eating) and irreducible mental fatigue. However, in type 2 symptoms develop slowly and may be subtle or completely absent. Except weight loss (unexplained weight loss at the onset) other symptoms are same as type 1. Diabetic complications started when the blood glucose concentration is raised beyond its renal threshold (10 mmol/L, although altered in pregnancy), due to incomplete reabsorption of glucose in the proximal renal tubule, and thus part of the glucose remains in the urine (glycosuria). This increases the osmotic pressure of the urine and inhibits reabsorption of water by the kidney, resulting in increased urine production (polyuria) and fluid loss. The lost blood volume is thus replaced osmotically from cellular water, causing dehydration and increased thirst. The prolonged high blood glucose causes glucose absorption and thereby changes in the shape of the eye lenses, leading to a blurred vision. However, sustained sensible glucose control usually helps to return the lens to its original shape. Type 1 DM is suspected in cases of rapid vision change, whereas in type 2 vision changes are gradual. Type 1 patients initially present diabetic ketoacidosis, an extreme metabolic dysregulation characterized by the smell of acetone on the patient's breath (Kussmaul breathing), polyuria, nausea, vomiting, abdominal pain, altered states of consciousness or arousal (hostility and mania or confusion and lethargy), even coma to death. A rarer but equally severe possibility is a hyperosmolar nonketotic state in type 2, due to dehydration or loss of body water. Often, the patient is urged to drink extreme amounts of sugar-containing drinks, leading to a vicious circle of water loss. Sometimes skin rashes known as diabetic dermadromes occur in diabetic patients.

DIAGNOSIS

DM is characterized by recurrent or persistent hyperglycemia, and is diagnosed by testing any one of the following tests as presented in Table **1** [30]: Fasting plasma glucose level at or above 7.0 mmol/L (126 mg/dL); Plasma glucose at or above 11.1 mmol/L (200 mg/dL) two hours after a 75g oral glucose load (glucose tolerance test); Hyperglycemia and casual plasma glucose at or above 11.1

mmol/L (200 mg/dL); Glycated hemoglobin (hemoglobin A1$_C$) at or above 6.5, as recommended by the American Diabetes Association [31].

Table 1: Diabetes criteria (www.who.int) 1999.

Diabetes Criteria			
Condition	2 Hour Glucose	Fasting Glucose	Hb A1$_C$
	mmol/l(mg/dl)	mmol/l(mg/dl)	
Normal	<7.8 (<140)	<6.1 (<110)	3.5-5.7
Impaired fasting glycaemia	<7.8 (<140)	≥ 6.1(≥110) & <7.0(<126)	<6.5
Impaired glucose tolerance	≥7.8 (≥140)	<7.0 (<126)	>6.5
Diabetes mellitus	≥11.1 (≥190)	≥7.0 (≥126)	>7.0

About 25% of the people with type1 DM have developed some degree of diabetic ketoacidosis, *i.e.*, high concentrations of ketone bodies due to the breakdown of fatty acids and the deamination of amino acids. The diagnosis of diabetes primarily includes: health screening, hyperglycemia, and secondary symptoms like vision changes or fatigue. However, it is often detected from problems like heart attack, stroke, neuropathy, poor wound healing, foot ulcer, certain eye problems, certain fungal infections, or delivering a baby with macrosomia or hypoglycemia. A positive result, in the absence of unequivocal hyperglycemia, is confirmed by any of the above methods on a different day. Most physicians prefer to measure a fasting glucose level as it is easy, while the glucose tolerance test is time consuming (2h) and offers no prognostic advantage over the fasting test [32]. According to the current definition, two fasting glucose measurements above 126 mg/dL (7.0 mmol/L) are considered diagnostic for DM. Fasting glucose levels from 100-125 mg/dL (5.6-6.9 mmol/L) are considered as impaired fasting glucose; and when the plasma glucose is at or above 140 mg/dL (7.8 mmol/L), but not over 200 mg/dL (11.1 mmol/L) two hours after a 75 g oral glucose load, are considered as impaired glucose tolerance (IGT). Of these two pre-diabetic states, IGT in particular is a major risk factor for progression to full-blown DM and cardiovascular diseases [33].

BIOCHEMICAL PATHOPHYSIOLOGY

Insulin is the principal hormone that regulates the uptake of glucose from the blood into cells, primarily muscle and fat cells. Thus, deficiency of insulin or the insensitivity of its receptors plays a central role in diabetes. The dietary carbohydrates (starch/glycogen/sucrose), is converted to simpler glucose (main energy source) in the digestive tract within a few hours. Most disaccharides (except sucrose/lactose), and all complex polysaccharides (except starch) are processed by gut flora in the colon. In response to the rising levels of blood glucose after food, insulin is released into the bloodstream by pancreatic β-cells. Two-thirds of the body cells use insulin to absorb glucose from the blood for the production of energy and other molecules, and rest for storage. Moreover, insulin acts as the control signal for the conversion of glucose to glycogen in the liver and muscle cells. When glucose levels fall, insulin release is reduced and the reverse conversion of glycogen to glucose takes place under the control of glucagon, a hormone from pancreatic α-cells. Glucose thus forcibly produced from glycogen (liver cell stores) re-enters the bloodstream, but muscle cells lack this export mechanism. Normally liver cells do this in low insulin level (correlates with low levels of blood glucose), while higher insulin levels increase the anabolic processes like cell growth and duplication, protein synthesis, and fat storage. Insulin or its lack is the principal signal in converting many of the bidirectional processes of metabolism from a catabolic to an anabolic direction, and *vice versa*. In particular, a low insulin level is the trigger for entering or leaving ketosis (fat burning phase). If the amount of insulin available is insufficient, cells respond poorly to insulin (insulin insensitivity or resistance), or when insulin itself is defective, then glucose will not be absorbed properly by body cells nor will be stored in the liver and muscles. The net effect is persistent high levels of blood glucose, poor protein synthesis, and other metabolic derangements, such as acidosis.

Screening: Diabetes screening is recommended at various stages of life, particularly for those having one or several risk factors. According to the circumstances the screening test varies. It can be a random blood glucose test, a fasting blood glucose test, a blood glucose test 2h after taking 75 g of glucose, or a formal glucose tolerance test. A screening is usually recommended for adults at age 40-50, and then periodically. Earlier screening is recommended only for people having obesity, family history of diabetes and high-risk ethnicity, *e.g.*, Hispanic, Native American, Afro-Caribbean, Pacific Islander, or Māori [34, 35]. However, many diabetes related conditions such as: subclinical Cushing's syndrome [36], testosterone deficiency [37], high blood pressure, elevated cholesterol levels, coronary artery disease, past gestational diabetes, polycystic ovary syndrome, chronic pancreatitis, fatty liver, hemochromatosis, cystic fibrosis, mitochondrial neuropathies and myopathies, myotonic dystrophy, Friedreich's ataxia, and inherited forms of neonatal hyperinsulinism, or long term use of corticosteroids, some chemotherapeutics (L-asparaginase), antipsychotics and mood stabilizers (phenothiazines, some atypical antipsychotics) warrant screening. A diabetic patient should test routinely, like yearly urine testing for microalbuminuria and retina testing for retinopathy.

CHEMICAL PARADIGM OF DIABETES

After a meal, the digestive system convert carbohydrate into glucose, a monosaccharide or sugar, the main source of cellular fuel. The glucose enters the bloodstream *via* the small intestine and finally into the cells by the pumping action of the heart. The cell converts glucose into energy (ATP), water and other byproducts *via* glycolysis, mitochondrial Krebs cycle and electron transport chain. In diabetes, the body is unable to make enough insulin which usually helps glucose to enter the body cells, or the body cells do not respond (impaired) to insulin properly.

Usually modern diets are characterized by high carbohydrate and low fat. The foods we eat contain chemical manure/fertilizers, pesticides, herbicides, preservatives and colour, cultivated in mineral deficient soil and are refined and processed in such a way that many of the vitamins, minerals and phytofactors are destroyed. Moreover, modern food does not contain fresh fruits and vegetables that supply the major vitamins, minerals, fiber and phytonutrients. Thus, our diet is unable to fulfill our daily nutrient need and thereby creates a nutrition gap. Over the years our diet (*either eat properly or die improperly*) has taken toll. The body desires to control blood glucose, but due to less sensitivity to its own insulin beta cells forcibly produce more and more insulin to control blood sugars. With time, individuals with insulin resistance, need more and more insulin to keep the blood sugar normal. These elevated insulin level (hyperinsulinemia) may lead to serious health problem, collectively termed as syndrome X by Dr. Gerald Reavens. The symptoms include significant inflammation of the arteries, elevated blood pressure (hypertension), increased tendency to form blood clots, elevated triglycerides, increased LDL, lowered HDL, and uncontrolled weight gain usually around the middle, called as central obesity. When all the above factors are combined, the risk of developing heart disease including heart attack and stroke jumps twenty-fold. The syndrome X may last for several years (10-20 years), during which the pancreatic beta cells completely wear out and can no longer produce such high levels of insulin. At this point insulin level begins to drop and blood sugar to rise. At first, slight elevations of blood sugar takes place, which is called as glucose intolerance or preclinical diabetes. Often, both insulin production and insulin action are impaired. Therefore, instead of moving into the cells glucose builds up in the blood. Then within a year or two, if no change in lifestyle occurs, full blown diabetes mellitus will develop and the aging of the arteries accelerates faster as blood sugar begins to rise steadily. Over time, the high blood glucose levels can damage many parts of the body including the heart, blood vessels, eyes, kidneys, nerves, feet, and skin. However, these complications can be minimized or delayed by proper controlling of blood glucose, blood pressure, and cholesterol levels.

Cause of Insulin Resistance: Several theories suggest that less and less sensitivity of body to its own insulin over the years is due to several factors. However, studies revealed that the main cause of insulin insensitivity is the altered insulin secretion and utilization, and both these factors depend on dietary habits [38]. It is known that the main culprit for insulin insensitivity is the excessive use of long chain of sugars (carbohydrates) as a staple food that absorbed at various rates by the body. The white flour, rice, pasta, and potatoes release sugars into the bloodstream faster than table sugar, and thus these foods are called as high glycemic food. While most vegetables and fruits release their sugars much slowly and are thus called as low glycemic foods [39]. When we eat higher amount of high glycemic foods blood sugar rises very rapidly and thereby stimulates the release of insulin. When the blood sugar drops, the person feels hungry, and thus takes a snack or a big meal, and the whole process starts all over again. After a period of time, the release of insulin has been over stimulated so often that the body simply becomes less and less sensitive to it. In order to control the blood sugar levels, the pancreas secretes a higher amount of insulin, and that elevated level of insulin causes destructive metabolic changes leading to the insulin resistance or Syndrome X. A simple ratio of triglyceride level by the HDL cholesterol is an indication of syndrome X. If this ratio is greater than two, the person may start to develop insulin resistance. Additionally the increase of blood pressure and waistline is an indication of a serious case of Syndrome.

Pre-Diabetic Condition: When blood glucose levels are higher than normal but not high enough for a diagnosis of type 2 DM is termed as the pre-diabetic stage. Many people are destined to develop type 2 DM after spending several years in pre-diabetic stage. Thus, this pre-diabetic stage is called as healthcare epidemic [24, 40]. Some uncommon diabetes is caused when the body's tissue receptors do not respond to insulin even when insulin levels are normal. It is known that genetic mutations (autosomal or mitochondrial) can lead to defects in the beta cell function, and sometimes abnormal insulin action is genetically determined. Any disease that causes extensive damage to the pancreas may lead to diabetes (*e.g.*, chronic pancreatitis, cystic fibrosis). Moreover, diseases associated with excessive secretion of insulin-antagonistic hormones, drugs that impair insulin secretion and some toxins that damage pancreatic beta cells can cause diabetes [30] and the common complications include diabetic retinopathy, diabetic nephropathy, and cardiovascular diseases.

CAUSES OF DIABETES

Though the exact cause of this killer disease is still unknown, several factors including genetic factor, lifestyle, diet, free radical and certain medical conditions are found to be responsible. For example, type 1 DM is genetically determined while type 2 is determined primarily by lifestyle factors and partially by genetic influence [41].

Genetics: Both type 1 and type 2 diabetes are partly inherited. Type 1 may also be triggered by infections (*e.g.*, Coxsackievirus B4), and the individual susceptibility to some of these triggers is attributed to human leucocyte antigen (HLA) or HLA genotypes. However, the inherited susceptibility requires an environmental trigger. In type 2 there is a stronger inheritance pattern, as the people whose first-degree relatives are diabetic have a much higher risk of developing type 2. Concordance among monozygotic twins is close to 100%, and about 25% of victims have a family history of DM. Genes significantly associated with type 2 include *TCF7L2, PPARG, FTO,*

KCNJ11, *NOTCH2*, *WFS1*, *CDKAL1*, *IGF2BP2*, *SLC30A8*, *JAZF1* and *HHEX* [42]. The gene *KCNJ11* (potassium rectifying channel, subfamily J, member 11), encodes the islet ATP-sensitive potassium channel Kir6.2, and TCF7L2 (transcription factor 7-like 2) regulates proglucagon gene expression and the production of glucagon-like peptide-1 [1]. Moreover, obesity (*obey the rule of city*) is an independent risk factor for type 2 and is strongly inherited [43]. Monogenic forms (MODY) constitute about 1-5 % of all cases [44]. Moreover, various hereditary conditions may feature diabetes *e.g.*, myotonic dystrophy and Friedreich's ataxia. Wolfram's syndrome, an autosomal recessive neuro-degenerative disorder in childhood consists of diabetes insipidus, diabetes mellitus, optic atrophy and deafness (DIDMOAD) [45]. Gene expression promoted by a diet of high fat and glucose plus high levels of inflammatory cytokines in the obese person, results in cells that "produce fewer and smaller mitochondria than normal," and are thus prone to insulin resistance (http://www.economist.com/sciencetechnology/displayStory.cfm?story_id =1435057).

Lifestyle: Several lifestyle factors are important for the development of type 2 DM. Study revealed that high levels of physical activity, a healthy diet, non smokers and non-alcoholics have an 82% lower rate of diabetes; when the weight is normal, the rate is 89% lower. A healthy diet includes a lot of fiber, high polyunsaturated to saturated fat ratio and a lower mean glycemic index [4]. Obesity alone is found to contribute about 55% in type 2 [46], while a decreasing consumption of saturated fats and trans fatty acids or replacing them with unsaturated fats may reduce the risk [41, 47]. Interestingly, the increased rate of childhood obesity is believed to increase the type 2 DM in children and adolescents [48]. Moreover, environmental toxins may contribute to the recent increases in type 2 DM, as positive correlation is evident between the concentration of bisphenol A, a constituent of some plastics, in the urine and the incidence of type 2 DM [49].

Free Radical Theory: Reactive oxygen species (ROS); a by-product of normal metabolism, are produced during the transfer of electrons along the respiratory chain to generate ATP in aerobic respiration. In a perfect system, oxygen accepts the electron to yield water. However, as the system is not perfect, ROS are produced due to inappropriate electron donation (at least in 2% time), involving ubiquinone at Complex III [50]. In order to prevent oxidative damage to cellular components, a number of protective enzymes, *e.g.*, superoxide dismutase's (SODs) have been evolved to remove superoxide anions (O_2^-) by catalysing their conversion into hydrogen peroxide (H_2O_2), which in turn converted into oxygen and water by catalase. Other antioxidant enzymes involved in maintaining the redox status of glutathione is glutathione peroxidase that removes H_2O_2 by using it to oxidize GSH to GSSG; while glutathione reductase regenerates GSH from GSSG, with NADPH as a source of reducing power. Observations in a number of species show that oxidative damage accumulates with age in a wide variety of tissues [51], and the efficiency of cellular antioxidant defences decline with age [52, 53], lending strong support to the free radical theory of aging and diseases [54] like artherosclerosis, diabetes, arthritis, macular degeneration, neurodegenerative diseases, cancer *etc.*

Certain *medical conditions* like the subclinical Cushing's syndrome (cortisol excess) may be associated with type 2 DM [36], as found in about 9% of the diabetic population [55]. Diabetic patients with a pituitary microadenoma are found to improve insulin sensitivity after the removal of microadenomas [56]. Moreover, hypogonadism is often associated with cortisol excess, and testosterone deficiency is associated with type 2 DM [37], though the exact mechanism by which testosterone improves insulin sensitivity is still not known.

NUTRITION AND NUTRITIONAL MEDICINE

About 2500 years ago, Hippocrates, the *Father of Medicine*, said "*Let thy food be thy medicine and thy medicine be thy food*". The great 12th century physician Moses Maimonides repeated the Hippocratic statement as "*No illness which can be treated by diet should be treated by any other means*". Actually, Hippocrates and Maimonides insisted that their students should practise nutrient therapy. This type of therapy is being used by very few doctors today, but at large by nutritionists. One of the major causes is the very little training in nutrition at medical schools and unless a doctor pursued the study of nutrition out of choice, he/she is unlikely to be sufficiently informed to give advice about optimum nutrition. Secondly, the practitioners of modern medicine are largely unaware of nutritional medicine; as continuing medical education is conducted by drug companies seeking to promote particular drugs, and not nutrition. In 1968 one of the great minds, twice Nobel prize winner Linus Pauling advocated Orthomolecular (the right molecule) Nutrition, *i.e.*, by giving the body the right molecules (optimum nutrition) most diseases can be eradicated.

Nutritional medicine involves the use of essential nutritional components like low glycemic carbohydrates, essential amino acids, essential fatty acids, dietary fiber, vitamin, minerals and phytofactors (like bioflavonoids) from natural source, either through food or as supplements. In order to function adequately, the living organism needs a whole series of complex carbohydrates, essential amino acids (Isoleucine, Leucine, Lysine, Methionine, Phenylalanine, Threonine, Tryptophan, Valine and Histidine), essential fatty acid (omega 3 and omega 6), vitamins (A to E), and trace elements such as zinc, magnesium, chromium, selenium *etc.* In 1753, a naval physician James Lind first observed that the sailors on long voyages who did not eat fresh fruit and vegetables may develop scurvy, and the addition of lime juice to their diet could prevent the disease. From the 1920s to the 30s a series of specific nutritional deficiency diseases, such as pellagra and beriberi (deficiency diseases of Vitamin B group) were carefully documented. As a consequence, the dietary recommendations tend to be more focused on the specific intakes of vitamins and minerals that avoid deficiency rather than promote optimal health. Though scientists are almost certain about the nutritional requirements to avoid illness, there is often little information, and much argument about the doses of nutritional supplements required to sustain optimal health, particularly during a disease process or competitive sport or unusual mental demands. This can be illustrated by the differences in Reference Nutrient Intakes (RNI) between the US and the UK, as the average UK population falls below the recommended intakes. Generally the industrialized world eat enough to suffer from increasing obesity, while a significant minority are suffering from nutritional deficiencies, probably associated with the high fat, high carbohydrate, and low nutrient junk food. Due to the industrialisation of farming, modern food is cultivated with fertilizers, pesticides, herbicides, and stored with preservatives and colour, that yield relatively lower levels of trace elements and vitamins. The medical community scoff at vitamins and food supplements as a way of producing "expensive urine". But this view is now changing due to the better understanding of the molecular basis of disease, and the role of free radicals in heart disease, diabetes, arthritis and autoimmune diseases, such as scleroderma, systemic lupus erythematosus, rheumatoid arthritis *etc.* In these diseases, food supplements in anti-oxidant doses act as nutritional medicine [57, 58]. Basically, to counter a disease, doctors have two options: either to go the "*anti*" way with drugs like antibiotics, anti-allergics, anti-inflammatories, anti-depressants, immune suppressants *etc.* or to build positive organ and body health with nutritional foods, exercises, proper sleep, the positive mental attitude and nutritional supplements when required. Though the ideal way is to emphasise the latter and use the former only if absolutely indicated. Modern medicine believed largely in the "*anti*" approach based on the discoveries of *anti-agents* in the 20th Century. However, in this new millennium, the latter is gaining more importance due to clinical experience of clinicians round the globe.

Historically, nutritional medicine began in Asia when Dr. Carl Rehnborg, a nutritional scientist, started work on plant based food supplements in China. He felt that plant components (phytofactors) and other cofactors extracted from organically farmed plants, would synergistically work with cellular proteins, vitamins and minerals to potentiate their effect. To test out his hypothesis, half a century ago, Rehnborg used an ingenious method, by offering the organically grown health foods to consumers directly, and asking them if-you-find-it-useful-you-can-recommend it-to-your-friends. As a scientist, Rehnborg wanted to know the honest truth and therefore he avoided the conventional marketing system. Rehnborg's successors have further ensured best digestibility and absorption indices, which makes them a natural choice to use not only in the elderly and the ailing whose digestion and absorption power are impaired but for all people. Dr. Ray Dr. Strand, a South Dakota-based family practitioner and author of two bestseller books is a pioneer in the field of nutritional medicine. His own conversion came as an eyewitness when his wife turned to nutritional medicine in desperation, because a string of specialists and the best drugs, even steroids did not help her fibromyalgia, asthma, allergy and propensity to recurrent infections. Nutritional supplements finally brought about profound improvement over three months! Some 'weird vitamins and minerals' had restored his wife's health when all the medical expertise and medication could not help. Dr. Strand found that the patients who used these recovered steadily from degenerative and auto-immune diseases [58]. In a similar manner, continents away, Dr. Hiramalini Seshadri, a Bombay based rheumatologist had the same experience. A sixth sense and desperation had prompted Dr. Seshadri to try nutritional supplements for a host of chronic disorders; for the side effects and cost with high powered drugs. He had tried anti-oxidant doses of vitamin E, folic acid, *Acerola cherry* derived vitamin C, grape seed extract, and flavonoids on patients having chronic rheumatological disorders and the results were most gratifying. Dr. Seshadri feels that people who need fitness could benefit from food supplementation, not out of choice but out of necessity. Indeed, good nutrition is the best medicine!

NUTRITIONAL MEDICINE: CONVENTIONAL OR COMPLEMENTARY?

The discoveries of the physiological functions of various vitamins and minerals represent a very important part of the development of conventional medicine. However, it is interesting that conventional physicians assume that the average diet is nutritionally adequate, and that they investigate the nutritional status only in specific illnesses such as eating disorders or anaemia. A point frequently raised within the context of complementary medicine is that of individuality. One of the underlying principles of nutritional medicine is that each person is unique and has unique nutritional requirements due to *nutritional polymorphism*, so that what might be an adequate nutritional intake for one person may be inappropriate for another [59]. A natural question is: why aren't we getting these nutrition and phytofactors from our daily diet? The readymade food concentrates are only for the ill or elderly people, who need proper nourishment and anti-oxidant till recovery and then put on dietary sources gradually. But here again, it is necessary to take organically grown vegetables and fruits as elderly or ill people have compromised liver and renal function; and the fertilisers, pesticides, weedicides, preservatives and colours in marketed fruits and vegetables could tip the balance unfavourably. However, the aim of Nutritional medicine is to understand (i) the molecular functions of nutrients present in the diet; (ii) the regulatory mechanisms that control metabolism in normal and disease states; (iii) how metabolism and regulation of nutrients are integrated; (iv) how nutrients affect pathogenesis and health, and (v) critical analysis of nutrient claims and fads. Thus, nutritional medicine is both conventional and complementary. The word diet and nutrition are thought to be synonymous to many people. Actually the Dietetics or the study of diet (die-eat; die improperly if not eat properly), its composition, interpretation and communication about its nutritional role help in informed and practical choices of food and lifestyle, while nutrition is the study of nutrients in food, how the body uses it, and the relationship between diet, health and disease. It is the science of consuming and utilizing foods. Actually nutritional science investigates the metabolic and physiological responses of the body to diet. Due to the tremendous advancement of molecular biology, biochemistry and genetics, nutrition is more focused on the biochemical sequences of metabolic pathways. It also focuses on how diseases or health problems can be prevented or lessened with a healthy diet, and how certain diseases or conditions are caused by dietary factors (like poor diet, food allergies, metabolic diseases) *etc.* Thus, nutrition focuses on food, and its effect on health; while dietetics looks at the human, and then the role of food on human's health. Nutrition is required in all processes of life, right from the very moment the sperm fertilizes an egg, through fetal development in the uterus, to the birth, growth, maturity, old age, and eventual death. Even after death the living body serves as nutrition for other organisms. Anything that involves life and chemical or biochemical movement has nutrition at its core, and a living organism depends on energy, that comes from the combustion of food. Thus, food is such a fuel that not only gives us energy to work, but also gives us energy to grow, to develop, to repair damage, to fight diseases, to motivate, to socialize and to sustain creativity.

THE NUTRITIONAL NEEDS OF THE HUMAN BODY

Classically the food is classified into seven categories *e.g.* carbohydrate, protein, fat, vitamin, mineral, fiber and water. Some nutrients are required in relatively large quantities (Macronutrients), while others in small amounts (Micronutrients). The macronutrient like carbohydrate, fat and protein provide energy, while micronutrients like vitamins and minerals help in growth and development. Carbohydrates are made up of carbon, hydrogen and oxygen, and further classified as monosaccharides (glucose, fructose, glactose), disaccharides (sucrose, lactose), oligo-saccharide (few monosaccharide units, *eg.* Inulin) and polysaccharides (starch, glycogen, chitin). Nutritionally, polysaccharides are favored as they are complex sugar chains, take longer time to break down and are absorbed into the bloodstream, and usually do not spike blood sugar levels. Proteins are usually made up of nitrogen, carbon, hydrogen, and oxygen and are either simple (monomers) or complex (polymers) that build and repair tissue, and when used as a fuel, they break down to release nitrogen. Fats are also made up of carbon, hydrogen, and oxygen.

Basically fats are triglycerides (polymers) having three molecules of fatty acid (monomers) combined with one molecule of the alcohol (glycerol). Complete breakdown of one gram of carbohydrate or protein yields 4.1 kcal energy, while each gram of fat yields 9.2 kcal of energy. Another crucial and essential macronutrient that does not provide energy is fiber, which is a carbohydrate with limited absorption. About 70% of the non-fat mass of the human body is water. Though the exact amount of water needed by a human being is unknown, but estimates vary between 1-7 liters per day, as water requirements are linked to size, age, environmental temperatures, physical activity, health status, and dietary habits. The variables that influence water requirements are so vast that accurate advice on water intake needs individual evaluation.

We are not all alike due to DNA polymorphism, and hence, our dietary needs for a particular lifestyle must be adequately covered, through eating more of the appropriate kinds of foods. Nutritional supplements may be helpful when silent nutritional deficiencies cause health problems in the long run. For example in smokers, alcoholics, pregnant women, pollution and high stress occupation, emotional stress, allergies, diseases and degenerative illness or inherited weakness, the nutritional needs may be increased [60]. The poor nutritional quality of many foods is another factor. Depleted soils, lengthy storage, toxicity from pesticides, herbicides, fertilizers, preservatives, additives, antibiotics and so on can make an apparently healthy food of little value. Tests have shown that most people do not obtain adequate selenium, zinc, folic acid or essential fatty acids in their diet, and thus suffer from physical and mental problems [61]. Deficiency of any of the essential nutrients (below the RDA amount) will, over a period of time, result in illness. Recent studies showed that most of the population in industrialized countries is deficient in one or more nutrients, like zinc, selenium, vitamin B complex, vitamin C, and is literally on the edge of illness [62]. Moreover, individual nutritional needs are frequently higher than the RDA amounts, and to reverse the effects of decades of poor diet and the dietary toxicity and to attain optimum health, larger amounts are required through improved diet and or supplements. The well being and good health depend on nutritional status and social life style patterns also. Thus nutrition equals life, and there is a saying "*you are what you eat*". All foods contain nutrients but not all nutrients are present in one food. Thus our body needs a variety of nutrients like protein, carbohydrate, fats, vitamins, minerals and phytonutrients, dietary fiber and water. The food we take/get on regular basis is not only lacking vitamins, minerals and fiber, but also contains high amounts of trans fat and cholesterol with empty calories. As a whole today's life style and food create more physical and psychological stress to produce more and more free radicals, which can damage heart, lungs, skin, brain and tissues.

Over the last decades, the prevalence of obesity and diabetes related diseases have increased rapidly. Obesity is a disorder of energy imbalance and is associated with hyper-insulinemia, insulin resistance, and abnormalities in lipid metabolism, and is the most important risk factor for Type 2 diabetes, cardiovascular disease, atherosclerosis, and certain cancers. The lower frequency of these diseases in Asian countries is thought to be due to its diet containing soy and soy-based products, and the health benefits associated with soy consumption are linked to the soy isoflavones, a class of phytoestrogen. Due to their structural similarities to endogenous estrogens, isoflavones elicit weak estrogenic effects by competing with 17β-estradiol (E2) for binding to the intranuclear estrogen receptors (ERs) and exert estrogenic or anti-estrogenic effects in various tissues. The estrogenic activities of soy isoflavones seem to play an important role in their health- enhancing properties. Additionally, the isoflavones exert non-ER-mediated effects through many pathways. Genistein, daidzein, and glycitein are the principal and most active isoflavones in soy that have higher binding affinity for the ER. Epidemiologic and laboratory data suggest that these compounds could have health benefits in obesity [63]. A recent study showed that soy isolates can reduce the risk of type 2 diabetes in overweight women [64]. Several studies also indicate that isoflavones of soy isolates with essential amino acids, can improve several cellular functions, although a few reports suggest that a soy-based diet impaired infants' immune functions [65]. However, the prospective longitudinal study of Arkansas Children's Nutrition Center shows no adverse effects in the soy-fed children, and their results suggest that soy supports normal growth and may have advantages in promoting bone development [66]. The major illness causes by improper nutrition are presented in Table **2**:

Table 2: Illnesses Caused by Improper Nutrient Consumption.

Nutrients	Deficiency	Excess
Calories	Starvation, Marasmus	Obesity, diabetes mellitus, Cardiovascular disease

Table 2: cont….

Simple carbohydrates	None	Diabetes mellitus, Obesity, Cardiovascular disease
Complex carbohydrates	None	Obesity, Cardiovascular disease (high glycemic index foods)
Protein	Kwashiorkor	Starvation, Ketoacidosis (in diabetics)
Saturated fat	Possible essential fatty acid (EFA) deficiency	Obesity, Cardiovascular Disease
Trans fat	None	Obesity, Cardiovascular Disease
Unsaturated fat	Fat-soluble vitamin deficiency, EFA deficiency	Obesity, Cardiovascular disease

DIET OF DIABETICS

Diet has a profound role to control the insulin resistant syndrome [67-69]. It was found that rural diet is diabetogenic, and the large amount of proteins in the diet causes a reduction of abdominal fat [68, 69]. Ornish (1996) [70] had advocated that a low fat diet is beneficial to health but reduces the HDL level in the blood. Hence, a diet with adequate fat having a good ratio of omega-3 and omega-6 fatty acids is best for health, and vegetarian diet has a role in reducing the incidence of insulin resistance [71, 72].

Diets prescribed for diabetics show dramatic changes after the discovery of insulin. In insulin-dependent diabetics, the carbohydrate content is reduced to 10-20 gm/day, with increased fat and protein content. Diabetic diets in the post-insulin era derived 40%, 20% and 40% of their calories from carbohydrates, proteins and fats respectively. Currently prescribed diabetic diets are high carbohydrate (low glycemic), high fiber and low fat diets, to derive 50-60% of calories from carbohydrates, 15-20% from fats and the rest from proteins [73]. Sweetener should be both nutritive and non-nutritive, while Sodium should be restricted to 1000 mg/10000 kcal, not to exceed 3000 mg/day to minimize symptoms of Hypertension, and vitamins/minerals should meet recommended levels. Supplements are helpful if caloric intake is low or the variety of foods consumed is limited. Low carbohydrate diet cannot reduce hyperglycaemia in type 2 diabetics because low carbohydrate decreases pro-insulin synthesis and insulin secretion and results in diminished peripheral responsiveness to insulin. Thus, a more effective approach is to provide good quantities of complex carbohydrates that are digested and absorbed slowly so that the rate of glucose delivery into the extra-cellular space is modest and sustained, thereby giving endogenous insulin a diminished task and a longer time to effect glucose disposal [74]. High fiber diets and guar gum have been used in diabetics to decrease and delay the carbohydrate digestion and absorption [75]. The human body contains mostly water thus, the body adopts various strategies to emulsify the fatty food using cholesterol, lecithin, and bile. Then the body forms complexes with the lipids, initially with very-low density lipoproteins (VLDL), then to LDL and finally to HDL. The relative quantity of the latter in the blood is thus, a fair measure of the efficiency of transfer of fat, and is a positive indicator for the prevention of fat deposition in the blood vessels [70]. Researchers examined the long-term relationship between different types of dietary fat and the risk of Type 2 diabetes and found that trans-fatty acids are responsible for the increased prevalence of type 2 diabetes [76]. This leads to a reduced intake of vanaspati and a replacement of traditional mustard oil, coconut oil and *ghee* with olive oil that can be helpful for prevention of diabetes [77, 78].

Effects of Low-Fat, High-Carbohydrate Diet: A person on a low-fat, high-carbohydrate diet utilizes the fatty acid synthetic pathway extensively. This requires citrate to leave the mitochondria and generate malonyl-CoA. The high concentration of malonyl-CoA inhibits the activity of the enzyme responsible for the fatty acid oxidation. That's why extreme low-fat diets do not result in fast weight loss. The burning of excess fat is inhibited by the high carbohydrate intake. In persons with low body fat and good lean mass high carbohydrate intake spares the use of fatty acids that are otherwise quickly used for energy, and may accumulate in the membrane [79].

Apart from carbon, hydrogen, oxygen and nitrogen, the human body needs certain amount of dietary vitamins and minerals, more specifically "dietary ions" on daily basis, which the body cannot make and must be obtained from a well balanced diet. However, an excess the vitamins and minerals may cause toxic effects. The requirement, functions, deficiency and toxicity along with the daily intakes recommended by health experts and agencies are presented here to provide an overview of recommended daily allowances of all vitamins and minerals [80].

Minerals: Minerals are often artificially added to some foods to make up for dietary shortages and prevent subsequent health problems, *e.g.*, iodine is added in 'iodized salt' to prevent iodine deficiency, that affects about two billion people with mental retardation and thyroid gland problems, a serious public health concern globally [81]. Several experts opine that 16 key minerals are essential for structural, functional and biochemical processes as well as electrolytes. The requirements, deficiency and role of some essential mineral ions in nutrition are depicted in Table **3**.

Table 3: Role and Daily Requirements of Minerals or Mineral Ions as Nutritional Medicine.

Name & Source	Requirements	Function	Deficiency	Excess
Boron *Source:* Pears, pulses, tomatoes, apples, banana, beans, broccoli, carrot, cashew, dates, grape, honey, potato.	Men and women < 20 mg	Helps to maintain mineral and hormone level, bone health; prevent loss of calcium (osteoporosis) raises testosterone levels in to builds muscles.	Osteomalacia, osteoarthritis, depression, Reduce metabolism of calcium, Mg, P; And increase stress.	Above 100 mg can cause red rash, vomiting, diarrhea, less circulation, shock and coma.
Calcium *Natural Sources*: Dairy products, soybeans, sunflower seeds, legumes, sardines.	Men 1000 mg Women 1200 mg	Restore muscle, heart, nerve and digestive health; builds bone & teeth; help in iron utilization, blood coagulation, synthesis and function of blood cells; relieves pain and cramps; eases insomnia.	Hypocalcaemia leading to muscle cramps, spasms, hyperactive tendon reflexes.	Above 1500 mg cause stomach problem; hypercalcaemia (weekend muscle, constipation, low impulses in heart, stones in urinary tract, impaired kidney function, and iron absorption.
Chloride	700-3400 mg	HCl production in stomach, and for cellular pump functions	Hyperchloremia	Hyperchloremia
Chromium *Sources*: Brewer's yeast, Wheat germ, Rye bread, Oysters, Peas, Potatoes.	0.12- 0.35 mg	Regulates glucose use and hunger; control storage of fats, cholesterol, protein, and carbohydrates; reduces cravings; protect DNA and RNA; help in heart function.	Cold sweats, dizziness, irritability, frequent hunger, excessive sleep, drowsiness, addiction to sweet, excess thirst, Frequent urination.	Above 200 µg may cause concentration problems and Fainting.
Copper *Natural Sources*: Shrimp, beef liver, whole wheat, prunes, nuts, raw oysters.	2 mg	Component of redox enzymes; facilitates iron absorption; synthesizes enzymes, skin pigments; promotes protein metabolism; produces RNA, haemoglobin, RBC, hair color.	Anemia or pancytopenia (reduction of RBC, WBC, platelets number) and neuro-degeneration.	About 10 mg is toxic, interfere with formation of blood cells; convulsions, palsy, insensibility and eventually death.

Table 3: cont….

Fluorine *Sources:* Tea, fish, drinking water, toothpaste, mouthwash with fluoride, sea food.	Men 1.5 mg Women 4.0 mg	*Calcium or sodium* fluoride develop strong teeth and bones, prevent dental caries by increasing tooth enamel to resist acid; promotes re-mineralization and inhibits the cariogenic microbial process.	Increased cavities and unstable bones	Chronic dental fluorosis; Over 2.5 ppm cause dark brown stains on teeth. Over 20-80 mg/day for many years cause skeletal Fluorosis.
Iodine *Natural Sources:* Kelp, seafood, green leafy vegetables.	Child 90 µg Adult 150 µg	Help in synthesis of thyroxine, prevents goitre; helps burn fat; converts carotene to Vitamin A; carbohydrate absorption; promotes growth; regulates energy production; maintains hair, nails skin and teeth.	Delayed development	Affect functioning of thyroid gland.
Iron *Natural Sources:* Liver, meat, raw clams, oysters, oatmeal, nuts, beans, wheat germ	Men 10 mg; Women 15 mg	Need for proteins, enzymes, and hemoglobin formation.	Anemia.	Above 20 mg cause stomach upset, constipation, blackened stools, and iron deposits in organs.
Magnesium *Natural Sources:* Nuts, figs, seeds, dark-green vegetables, wheat bran, avocados, bananas.	1-3 y 80 mg, 4-8 y 130 mg; 9-13 y 240 mg; 14-18 y 360- 410 mg; Adult female 310-320 mg; Breastfeed and pregnancy 350-400 mg; Adult males 400-420mg.	Processes ATP, maintain bones; reduce cholesterol; form tooth enamel, fight tooth decay; convert sugar into ATP; help nerve function, utilize B, C, E; regulate body temperature; help mineral absorption; prevents calcium deposits in bladder, heart attacks, depression, polio.	Hypo-magnesemia (irritability of nervous system with spasms in hands and feet, muscular twitching and cramps, and larynx spasms).	Above 400 mg cause stomach problems, diarrhoea; Hypermagnesemia (nausea, vomiting, impaired breathing, low blood pressure.
Manganese	5.0 mg	Act as a cofactor with many enzymes.	Wobbliness, fainting, hearing loss, weak ligament and tendons; may cause diabetes.	Excess amount may hinder dietary iron adsorption.
Molybdenum	75 µg	Need for Xanthine oxidase, aldehyde & sulfite oxidases; uric acid formation, iron utilization, carbohydrate metabolism, and sulfite detoxification.	Affect metabolism and blood counts.	Above 200 µg cause kidney problems and copper deficiencies.

Table 3: cont….

Nickel *Sources*: lentils, oats and nuts.	<1 mg	Iron absorption, RBC formation	Hamper iron absorption and RBC production.	May cause skin rash, allergies.
Phosphorus	Men 800 mg, Women 1200 mg	Component of bones, help in energy processing.	Hypo-phosphatemia like rickets.	Above 250 mg cause stomach problems; Hyperphosphatemia, kidney failure.
Potassium	2000-3500 mg	As electrolyte, essential in co-regulating ATP with sodium.	Hypokalemia; affect nervous system and heart.	Stomach upsets, heart rhythm disorder Hyperkalemia.
Selenium	Men 0.07mg Women 0.05mg.	Essential cofactor of antioxidant enzymes.	Keshan disease (myocardial necrosis/weak heart), Kashing-Beck disease (degeneration & necrosis of cartilage)	Garlic-smelling breath, hair loss, gastrointestinal disorders, sloughing of nails, fatigue, irritability, neural damage. Above 200 µg is toxic.
Sodium	Men 1100 mg Women 3300 mg	A systemic electrolyte, regulate ATP with potassium.	Hyponatremia causing cellular malfunctioning.	Hypernatremia cause cellular malfunctioning.
Vanadium *Sources*: Cereals, Corn, Meat, Soy, Mushroom, Olive, Radish, Seafood, Vegetable oils, Whole grains.	< 1.8 mg	Help in formation of RBC, bone, teeth, fat metabolism; prevents dental caries, heart attacks, high sugar (mimicking insulin); slow down cholesterol formation. Vanadyl sulfate improve glucose control in type 2 DM [82].	Not known.	Vanadium is very toxic and cause manic depression, cramping, diarrhea and a green tongue.
Zinc *Natural Sources:* Eggs, cheese, beef, pork, wheat germ, brewer's yeast, pumpkin seeds, popcorn.	Men 15 mg Women 12 mg	Made enzymes and insulin; eliminate cholesterol deposits; absorb B complex, metabolize carbohydrates; help in healing, prostate function; prevents prostate cancer and sterility; keeps hair glossy and smooth.	Short stature, anemia, increased skin pigmentation, enlarged liver and spleen, impaired gonadal function, wound healing, and immune deficiency.	Above 25 mg cause anemia and copper deficiency, suppresses copper and iron absorption.

Revised in 1989 by the Food and Nutrition Board, National Academy of Sciences, National Research Council, Washington DC, USA.

Vitamins: Vitamins are organic compounds required in small amounts. They cannot be synthesized by the body, and thus have to be obtained from food on a daily basis [83]. Vitamins are classified on the basis of their bioactivity as water soluble or fat soluble. There are altogether 13 vitamins, of which fat-soluble are A, D, E and K while water-soluble vitamins are seven B vitamins (some are manufactured by bacteria in gut) and vitamin C [84]. Water soluble vitamins need to be consumed more regularly as they are eliminated faster through urine and are not stored, thus, urinary output is a good predictor of water soluble vitamin consumption. Fat soluble vitamins on the other hand, are absorbed through the intestines with the help of fats (lipids), and can accumulate in the body as they are harder to eliminate quickly. Excess levels of fat soluble vitamins thus create hypervitaminosis, and cystic fibrosis. Thus, patients of these diseases need to monitor their fat-soluble vitamins level closely. It is known that most vitamins have many different reactions, or functions [85]. Table **4** represents the known vitamins, their source, functions and deficiency symptoms.

Table 4: Important Vitamins, their Daily Requirement and Role as Nutritional Medicine

Name	Chemical Name	Function	Deficiency & Source	Excess
Vitamin A *Requirement*: 600 μg	Retinol, Retinoids, Carotenoids. Beta carotene is a precursor to A and acts as an antioxidant to protect from free radical damage.	Eye health, supports immune system. Help in bone growth, normal tooth, healthy mucous membranes, skin, and hair; essential for night vision.	Lack of vitamin A causes Night-blindness, and intestinal infections. *Sources*: Fish oils, liver, carrots, green and yellow vegetables, dairy products.	At 9000 mg cause dry, scaly skin; fatigue, nausea, loss of appetite; bone & joint pains, headaches; and Keratomalacia (cornea degeneration), blurred vision, growth retardation.
B Complex: **Vitamin B₁** *Requirement*: 1.4 mg	Thiamine	Convert sugar into energy; promotes appetite, digestion; strong heart muscle, nerves, growth; prevents fatigue, fat deposit in arteries.	Beriberi, Wernicke-Korsakoff syndrome (mental confusion, muscle weakness). *Sources*: Wheat, yeast, oatmeal, peanuts, pork, bran, sunflower seeds, soybean sprouts.	Rarely hypersensitive reactions (anaphylactic shock and drowsiness).
Vitamin B₂ *Requirement*: 1.6 mg/day.	Riboflavin.	Help in releasing energy; utilization of fats, proteins, sugars; and healthy vision.	Mouth lesions, seborrhea, corneal vascularization; insufficient intake result dermatitis. *Sources*: Dairy products, liver, kidney, yeast, leafy vegetables, fish, eggs.	No complications; higher than 200 mg may cause urine colour alteration.
Vitamin B₃ *Requirement*: 18 mg/day.	Niacin	Help in healthy skin, nerves, GI tract; converting carbohydrates into energy.	Pellagra; mental confusion, muscle weakness. *Sources*: Liver, lean meat, wheat, brewer's yeast, fish, eggs, poultry, nuts, sesame seed.	Above 150 mg cause facial flushing, liver damage, skin, gastrointestinal and other problems.
Vitamin B₅ *Requirement*:	Pantothenic acid	Crucial in energy and hormone	Paresthesia; insufficient intake cause fatigue, nausea, abdominal cramping.	None reported, however, 1200 mg cause nausea and

Table 4: cont….

			Sources: Eggs, fish, dairy products, whole-grain cereals, legumes, yeast, broccoli, cabbage, potatoes	heartburn.
6 mg/day.		production.		
Vitamin B$_6$ *Requirement*: 2 mg	Pyridoxamine, Pyridoxal	Metabolism of protein, fat, carbohydrate; RBC formation, control cholesterol; prevents water retention; builds hemoglobin.	Anemia, peripheral neuropathy; Insufficient intake result dermatitis. Sources: Brewer's yeast, wheat germ, meats, milk, eggs, avocados, bananas.	Above 100 mg cause numbness and tingling in hands and feet, nerve damage, impaired ability to sense stimuli
Vitamin B$_7$ *Requirement*: 30 μg	Biotin	Release energy from carbohydrates, and to synthesize fat.	Dermatitis, enteritis; anemia; insufficient intake cause fatigue, nausea, abdominal cramping. Sources: Eggs, Fish, Whole-cereals, Legumes, vegetables of cabbage family.	None reported.
Vitamin B$_9$ *Requirement*: 400 μg	Folic acid	Essential for A, D, E, K functions; RBC and nucleic acid formation; protein digestion. Prevent neural tube defects. Reduces homocystein level.	Neural tube defect; cause anemia. Natural Sources: Dark-green leafy vegetables, carrots, liver, eggs, soybeans, oranges, beans, whole wheat.	Seizure threshold diminished; Above 400 μg cause anemia, mask vitamin B$_{12}$ deficiency.
Vitamin B$_{12}$ *Requirement*: 6 μg.	Cyanocobalamin, hydroxy or methyl cobalamin	Use of protein, fats, carbohydrates; RBC formation; healthy nerves, nucleic acid; prevent pernicious anemia	Megaloblastic anemia . Sources: Liver, beef, pork, eggs, dairy products, shellfish, fortified cereals.	Above 3000 μg cause eye problems.
Vitamin C *Requirement*: 75 mg	Ascorbic acid	For collagen, neuro-transmitters; iron, protein & folic acid absorption; prevents vitamin oxidation, cold, infections, fatigue & stress; help in calcium & amino acid metabolism; promotes stamina; reduces allergies; heals wounds.	Lack of C cause infection, reduced wound healing, and scurvy. Natural Sources: Citrus fruits, berries, green and leafy vegetables, tomatoes cauliflower, potatoes	Diarrhea, nausea, skin irritation, burning urination, copper depletion, risk of kidney stones, abdominal cramping and bloating in mega doses.
Vitamin D *Requirement*: 5 μg	Ergo or Chole-calciferol	Bone and tooth development; Ca & P absorption and use; maintains nerve and heart action; prevents rickets.	Deficiency cause rickets in children, osteomalacia in adults, risk of some cancers. Sources: Cheese, Butter, Margarine Cream, Fish, Cereals.	Above 50 μg cause hyper-vitaminosis (headache, weakness, blood pressure, indigestion, tissue calcification; nausea, weight loss, kidney damage, coma and death.

Table 4: cont....

Vitamin E *Requirement*: 10 mg.	Tocopherol. As antioxidant protect healthy cells.	Protects body's Vitamin A storage, tissues and fat oxidation, breakdown of RBC; strengthens capillary walls; regulates protein and calcium metabolism, menstrual cycle; prevents vitamin loss; lowers cholesterol	Very rare, sometimes hemolytic anemia in newborn babies. *Natural Sources*: Soybeans, vegetable oils, broccoli, brussels sprouts, leafy greens, whole grain cereals, eggs.	Toxicity uncommon. Above 1000 mg may cause blood clotting, haemorrhage, risk of congestive heart failure, nausea and digestive tract disorder.
Vitamin K *Requirement*: 80 μg.	Phylloquinone, Menaquinones (K_3).	blood clotting.	Tendencies to bleed. *Sources*: Cabbage, cauliflower, spinach, soybeans, cereals.	Large doses damage liver, cause anemia.

These are reference values (not for diagnosis), based on a 2000 calorie intake, on daily basis, obtained from The Recommended Daily Intake of the old RDA proposed by FDA, WHO, European Union Directive. Values from WHO are lower than those of the FDA (*e.g.*, Mg 60 mg, B_6 0,5 mg, B_{12} 4 μg, C 15 mg, K 35 mg, folate 220 μg). Elements that have a recommended daily intake within μg range are referred as trace elements (*e.g.* chromium, copper, selenium).

Most foods contain a combination of some or all of the seven nutrient classes. The human body requires some nutrients regularly and others less frequently. Poor health may be the result of an imbalance, either not enough or too much of one or more nutrient [86]. The function of vitamins in the human body is extensive and complex as they serve multiple roles and work together, from reducing infection to aiding metabolism. Generally, vitamins and minerals work hand in hand to help in the prevention of diseases. *Many vitamins and minerals interact with each other in groups e.g.* a good balance of vitamin D, calcium, phosphorus, magnesium, zinc, fluoride, chloride, manganese, copper and sulphur is required for healthy bones. The combined action of beta carotene, vitamin E and C protects cells from free radical damage and reduces the risk of cancer. Usually E and C work hand in hand, and once E serves its purpose as an antioxidant it becomes inactive, but vitamin C then regenerate vitamin E. Vitamin D's role in bone health is to prevent osteoporosis; while Folate's can lower homocystein levels to reduce the risk of cardiovascular diseases. Many of them enhance or impair another vitamin or mineral's absorption and function (*e.g.*, an excessive amount of iron can cause zinc deficiency). Thus, taking insufficient amounts of vitamins may result in deficiencies, while an excess may cause toxicities. Deficiency is rare in fat-soluble vitamins due to their storage, but mild deficiencies can occur due to the lack of a balanced diet. However, deficiencies in water soluble vitamins are common and toxicity due to high doses is rare in water-soluble vitamins. A well-rounded diet with a variety of foods is ideal for an appropriate amount of vitamins to function to the best of its ability.

TODAY'S NUTRITION

Detectable levels of pesticides are present in almost all fruits and vegetables sold in most countries. Studies suggest that children exposed to higher levels of pesticides from commercially grown fruit and vegetables are more likely to develop attention deficit hyperactivity disorder (ADHD). A study with 1,139 children across the US revealed that children with above-average levels of pesticide by-products in the urine have the double chance of getting ADHD [87]. Studies on Farm workers revealed that exposure to the organophosphate pesticides is linked to behavioural and cognitive problems in children [88]. Organophosphates are designed for toxic effects on the nervous system of pests; however in humans these compounds act on some neurotransmitters [87]. Though the Environmental Protection Agency regulations have eliminated most residential uses of pesticides (www.ams.usda.gov/AMSv1.0/getfile?dDocName_STELPRDC5081750), but it become the largest sources of exposure for children through the commercially grown foods, in which children are more sensitive than adults.

NUTRITIONAL GOAL IN DIABETES

All forms of diabetes can be managed with insulin. However, type 2 can be controlled with drugs, while a chronic condition cannot be cured. In type 1 DM pancreas transplants have been tried with limited success; while gastric bypass surgery has been successful in morbid obesity and type 2 diabetes. Diabetes without proper treatments can cause many serious complications like hypoglycemia, ketoacidosis or nonketotic hyperosmolar coma, as well as long term complications like cardiovascular disease, chronic renal failure, retinal damage which require treatment as well as the control of blood pressure and lifestyle factors including smoking. Diet (*die if you not eat properly*) is the one of the most important behavioural aspect of diabetes treatment. However, basic principles of nutritional management are often poorly understood, both by clinicians and patients. Dietary compliance is a major factor in achieving glycemic control in type 2, as glycemic control can reduce nephropathy and retinopathy [89]. Moreover, weight reduction can improve or even reverse glucose intolerance in type 2 DM [90, 91]. Several studies indicated that the diabetic patients commonly fail to adhere to the recommended diet and exercise schedule. A study showed that less than 40 percent of diabetic patients follow 20 percent of their prescribed diet [92]; while another study showed that the noncompliance rates among diabetics were 62 percent for diet and 85 percent for exercise [93]. As soon as a person begins developing insulin resistance, it is advisable to go for lifestyle changes, because cardiovascular damages really begin during this time. Therefore, physicians need to be aware of the early signs of insulin resistance like the triglyceride/HDL cholesterol ratio, as insulin resistance is totally reversible at this point. Treatment for insulin resistance by lifestyle changes not only prevents accelerated damage of the arteries but can avoid full blown diabetes itself. Most physicians are aware that diet and exercise can help diabetic patients, but do not invest enough time in helping the patients to understand the necessity of changing life style habits to prevent diabetic complications without overdependence on medications. This is due to the fact that it is easier to write a prescription than to educate and motivate a patient for regular exercise and good nutrition.

PRINCIPLES OF NUTRITIONAL MEDICINE

We all know that the primitive people do not consume processed foods and probably do not have degenerative diseases [94]. In contrast, typical modern diets are insufficient for good health, necessitating the use of supplements of vitamins, dietary minerals, proteins (mainly essential amino acids), antioxidants, omega 3 (ω-3) fatty acids, dietary fiber, some medium chain triglycerides, lipotropes, systemic and digestive enzymes, other digestive factors, and prohormones to ward off hypothetical metabolic anomalies at an early stage [95]. Nutritionists opine that it is better to provide prescriptions for optimal amounts of micronutrients after the diagnoses of diabetes, based on blood tests and personal history [96, 97]. As the changes in lifestyle and diet can prevent and reduce diabetes and hypertension [98], primarily by avoiding high carbohydrate and high fat diet [99], weight management and meal planning [100] even for obese [101].

NUTRITIONAL SUPPLEMENTATION IN DIABETES

It is true that diet and exercise are important not only in diabetes but also in the prevention of many other diseases. However, the need to take supplements is seldom discussed. Yet they are needed as today's food lacks the essential amount of nutrients needed to stay healthy, like most of the modern school students who need special tuition. Whatever food we are taking are depleted of nutrients as it comes from farms whose soils contain little minerals and organic nutrients. For diabetes management six essential nutritional medicines have been shown to control blood sugar and were used long before Frederick Banting discovered insulin. Many people with diabetes use acupuncture or biofeedback to get relief from painful symptoms, dietary supplements to improve blood glucose control, and manage other symptoms, as well as to lessen the risk of developing serious complications [102, 103]. The following nutritional medicine is especially helpful in diabetes, some of which has passed in clinical trials (placebo control), such as alpha-lipoic acid, omega-3 fatty acids, chromium, and polyphenols, mostly available in fresh fruits and vegetables.

Alpha-Lipoic Acid (ALA or lipoic acid or thioctic acid) is an antioxidant that protects against cellular damage by free radicals. It also improves blood flow and increases cell sensitivity to insulin for a better glucose absorption. ALA is found in spinach, broccoli, potatoes, and liver. Many people with type 2 diabetes use ALA to lower blood glucose levels by improving the body's ability to use insulin; and to prevent or treat diabetic neuropathy. ALA has been found to help in better insulin sensitivity, glucose metabolism, and reduce diabetic neuropathy in some studies [103]. Intravenous use of ALA can lower blood sugar too much, so people with diabetes must monitor their blood sugar levels carefully [102]. However, to use ALA in diabetes much research is needed.

Omega-3 Fatty Acids: Since its discovery in 1970s, the role of omega 3 fatty acids has been studied against several diseases. Omega 3 fatty acid is a family of essential (as the human body cannot produce it) polyunsaturated (more than one double bond) fatty acids (PUFA). Unsaturated means extra hydrogen can be inserted chemically, has lower melting points and thus liquid in nature. PUFA are divided into two sub-groups: omega 6 (first double bond between 6th and 7th carbon atoms) and omega 3 (first double bond between 3rd and 4th carbon atom), and both are essential for normal growth and good health. Both omega 6 and omega 3 are essential in a ratio of 2:1, which is absent in today's diet. Currently the average ratio of omega 6: omega 3 in UK is around 8:1; in the US 10:1, in

Australia 12:1 and in India 20:1 [104]. Because of their wide-ranging roles, virtually the entire human body and every stage of life is susceptible to several diseases, particularly inflammatory diseases, if the balance of the two PUFAs becomes out of kilter. The role of Omega 3 fatty acid in diabetes, hypertension and related conditions are presented in Table **5**.

Table 5: How Omega 3 Fatty Acids Help in Diabetes, Hypertension and Related Complications.

Uses of Omega 3 Fatty Acid Based on Scientific Evidence	Evidence For Use
High blood pressure: Multiple human trials report small reductions in blood pressure with intake of omega-3 fatty acid, and DHA have greater benefits than EPA. However, high intakes of omega-3 fatty acids daily may be necessary to get clinically relevant effects, which may increase the risk of bleeding.	Strong
Hypertriglyceridemia: Strong scientific evidence from human trials that omega-3 fatty acids from fish or supplements significantly reduce triglyceride levels dose-dependently. Fish oil supplements can improve HDL along with increased LDL. However, due to conflicting evidence it is unclear whether plant based omega 3 alpha-linolenic acid can affects triglyceride levels, or not. There is growing evidence that omega 3 fatty acid can reduce C-Reactive Protein, but additional research is needed, as the data are mixed.	Fair
Hypercholesterolemia: Beneficial effects on blood cholesterol levels have not been demonstrated. Fish oil supplements cause small improvements in HDL, but increases in LDL, and do not appear to affect CRP levels.	Fair
Primary cardiovascular disease prevention: Several epidemiological studies showed that significantly lower rate of death from heart disease for regular fish eaters. Whether the benefits only occur in people at risk of developing heart disease is unclear. However, evidence suggests overall benefits of regular consumption of fish oil.	Good
Primary cardiovascular disease prevention (α-linolenic acid, ALA) Added research is necessary to conclude.	Unclear
Secondary cardiovascular disease prevention: Several randomized controlled trials in people with a history of heart attack, report that regular consumption of oily fish/fish oil/omega-3 supplements reduces the risk of heart attack, sudden death, and all-cause mortality. Most patients in these studies were also in conventional treatments, suggesting that the benefits of fish oils may add to the effects of other therapies.	Strong
Secondary cardiovascular disease prevention: Several randomized controlled trials showed that alpha-linolenic acid in people with a history of heart attack proved mixed results; some studies suggest benefits, others do not. Thus more research is necessary for a conclusion.	Unclear
Cardiac arrhythmias: Promising evidence that omega-3 fatty acids decrease the risk of cardiac arrhythmias, in people who regularly ingest fish oil or EPA+DHA. But more research can help for a firm conclusion.	Unclear
Atherosclerosis: Some studies report regular intake of fish/fish oil supplements reduces the risk of developing arterial plaques, while other is not. Thus, additional evidence is required before a firm conclusion.	Unclear
Angina pectoris: Preliminary studies report reductions in angina associated with fish oil intake. Further research is necessary for a definite conclusion.	Unclear

Table 5: cont….

Stroke prevention: Some epidemiologic studies showed benefits, while others do not. Effects are found on ischemic or thrombotic stroke risk, while large intakes of omega-3 may increase the risk of hemorrhagic stroke. Thus, it is unclear whether benefits in people with or without a history of stroke, or due to the effects of fish oil.	Unclear
Nephrotic syndrome: Insufficient reliable evidence for a clear conclusion.	Unclear
Prevention of restenosis after coronary angioplasty: Several randomized controlled trials on omega-3 fatty acid intake showed reduce blockage of arteries following balloon angioplasty but the evidence remains inconclusive.	Unclear

The parent alpha linolenic acid (ALA) is essential and must come from foods such as vegetable oil (canola, flaxseed and soybean oils), walnuts, and wheat germ. The dietary ALA has 18 carbon atoms and 3 double bonds (18:3), and needs to be converted by the human body into eicosapentaenoic (EPA, 20:5) and docosahexaenoic acid (DHA, 22:6) by a twenty-stepped process, but this conversion process is found to be inefficient in the majority of adults [105,106]. Thus, EPA and DHA should be obtained from fish or fish oil. Omega-3 fatty acids are believed to have a multi-factorial mode of action including a structural and functional component of membrane lipids, nerve tissues, brain and retina. Omega 3 is the precursors of eicosanoids (highly reactive prostaglandins and leukotrienes, responsible for anti-inflammatory functions), and help in the movement of calcium and other substances in and out of cells, as well as in the relaxation and contraction of muscles, blood clotting, digestion, fertility, cell division, and growth (www.fda.gov, 2008). Moreover, it can have antiarrhythmic, antithrombotic, anti-inflammatory, and antiatherosclerotic effects, along with improvement in endothelial function, lowering of blood pressure and triglyceride [107-113]. The triglyceride-lowering effects of omega 3 fatty acids are due to decreased hepatic lipogenesis [108]; while anti-thrombogenic effects are for the reduction of collagen-induced platelet aggregation that affects homeostasis [111], and by changing cell membrane properties. Omega 3 also interacts with cell signalling systems, promote anti-inflammatory actions and cause endothelial relaxation, mediated by nitric oxide [107]. It also has blood pressure lowering effect [113], but the strongest evidence is related to antiarrhythmic effects [112]. Omega-3 can decrease ventricular arrhythmias through the electrical stabilisation of myocytes [110], and reduce the risk of sudden cardiac death *via* increased heart rate variability [109]. Further studies revealed that Omega 3 can protect heart disease, reduce inflammation, and lower triglyceride levels [114, 115], but does not affect blood glucose control, total cholesterol, or HDL cholesterol in diabetes [116]. The accumulated findings suggest that omega 3 can reduce hypertension and diabetes related cardiovascular diseases by reducing platelet aggregation (clumping of RBC in coronary arteries), triglyceride, blood pressure, blood viscosity, heartbeat abnormalities (ventricular tachycardia), arterial inflammation caused by free radical damage and its plaque formation, and can increase arterial elasticity [108, 117]. Even in some studies omega-3 fatty acids are shown to raise LDL cholesterol. However, long-term studies on heart disease in people with diabetes are needed. Omega-3 appears to be safe for most adults at low-to-moderate doses [115]. Though sea fish is the best source for omega 3, but some species of fish are found to be contaminated by mercury, pesticides, PCBs (www.fda.gov/Food/FoodSafety/ProductSpecificInformation/Seafood/FoodbornePath ogensContaminants/Methylmercury/ucm115662.htm, January 21, 2008), and in high doses fish oil can interact with blood thinners and drugs used for high blood pressure [115].

Chromium: is an essential trace mineral for a proper enzymatic function. It is found in foods like meat, fish, cheese, whole grains, legumes, whole wheat, brewer's yeast, some fruits, vegetables, and spices. In a supplement it is available as chromium picolinate, chromium chloride, and chromium nicotinate. Chromium with insulin helps the cell membranes to absorb glucose and remove the excess glucose from the bloodstream, and thereby improves glucose tolerance [118], decreases cholesterol and triglycerides, and increases HDL. A placebo controlled trial using 100 and 500 µg chromium picolinate twice a day on 180 non-insulin dependent diabetics showed that chromium improves blood sugar (glycated haemoglobin test) level significantly [119, 120]. Studies with chromium supplementation on glucose control in diabetics (www.ods.od.nih.gov/factsheets/chromium.asp, 2008) showed mixed results. Some researchers have found benefits, but many of the studies are not well designed [120], and thus high-quality research is needed. At low doses, short-term use of chromium appears to be safe for most adults [121]. However, people with diabetes should be aware that chromium might cause blood sugar levels to go too low, and high doses can cause serious side effects including kidney problems [120, 121].

What we are Missing in Our Diet: Even if we eat a diet rich in fresh whole natural foods, we are not getting everything our body needs. Because in order to get all the bodily needed vitamins and minerals, we have to take a mountain of food every day. Moreover, due to less consumption of fresh vegetables and fruits we are missing a whole series of dietary phytonutrients.

PHYTONUTRIENTS OR PHYTOCHEMICALS

A growing area of interest is the effect of plant nutrients, collectively called phytonutrients or phytochemicals. These nutrients are found in colored fruits and vegetables, seafood, algae, and fungi. One of the principal classes of phytochemicals is polyphenols that provide health benefits to the cardiovascular and immune system, by down-regulating the formation of ROS, key chemicals in many diseases. Polyphenols are antioxidants found in tea and dark chocolate. They are studied for possible effects on vascular health (including blood pressure) and on the body's ability to use insulin [122, 123]. Laboratory studies suggest that epigallocatechin gallet (EGCG), a polyphenol of green tea, may protect against cardiovascular disease and have a beneficial effect on insulin activity and glucose control [124, 125]. However, a few trials with EGCG and green tea in diabetes have not shown such effects [126]. Green tea is safe for most adults in moderate amounts [127] though caffeine of green teas can cause insomnia, anxiety, or irritability in some people. Green tea also contains small amounts of vitamin K that can make anticoagulant drugs, such as warfarin, less effective [127]. The most rigorously tested phytochemical is zeaxanthin, a yellow-pigmented carotenoid of yellow and orange fruits and vegetables. Repeated studies have shown a strong correlation between the use of zeaxanthin and the prevention of age-related macular degeneration [128], and cataracts [129]. Another carotenoid lutein has also been shown to lower the risk of contracting macular degeneration. Both these compounds are found to concentrate in the retina when ingested orally, and serve to protect the rods and cones against the destructive effects of light. Similarly beta-cryptoxanthin appears to protect against chronic joint inflammatory diseases arthritis [130]. Substantial evidence suggests that another red phytochemical lycopene has negative association with the development of prostate cancer. As indicated above, some of the correlations between the ingestion of certain phytochemicals and the prevention of disease are, in some cases, enormous in magnitude. Yet, even when the evidence is obtained, translating it to practical dietary advice can be difficult and counter-intuitive. Lutein, for example, occurs in many yellow and orange fruits and vegetables that protect the eyes against various diseases. However, it does not protect the eye nearly as well as zeaxanthin, and the presence of lutein in the retina will prevent zeaxanthin uptake. Additionally, it was found that the lutein present in egg yolk is more readily absorbed than from vegetable sources, possibly because of fat solubility [131]. Moreover, it is difficult to answer whether we eat eggs that contain cholesterol and saturated fat. Lycopene is prevalent in tomatoes but more highly concentrated in tomato sauce, or soup yet, such sauces tend to have high amounts of salt, sugar, and preservatives. Role of major phytochemicals and their health benefits are presented in Table **6**.

Table 6: Common Benefits of Some Major Phytochemicals.

Group	Sources	Possible Benefits
Flavonoids	Berries, herbs, vegetables, wine, grapes, tea.	Prevent oxidation of LDLs, arteriosclerosis and heart disease.
Isoflavones	Soy, red clover, kudzu root.	Prevent arteriosclerosis, heart disease, cancer and easing symptoms of menopause .
Isothiocyanates	Cruciferous vegetables.	Cancer prevention.
Monoterpenes	Citrus peels, essential oils, herbs, spices, green plants [29].	Cancer prevention, treating gallstones.
Organosulfur	Chives, garlic, onions.	Cancer prevention, lowered LDLs, assist immune system.
Saponins	Beans, cereals, herbs.	Hypercholesterolemia, Hyperglycemia, cancer prevention, Anti-inflammatory.
Capsaicinoids	Chile peppers.	Topical pain relief, cancer prevention, apoptosis.

Flavonoids are a family of about 5000 phytochemicals with common chemical structures called polyphenols, and are divided into chemically-related subclasses like isoflavones (soy), flavanones (naringenin of citrus), flavanols (catechins of tea, cocoa), flavonols (quercetin from fruits and vegetables) and anthocyanidins (berries, grapes). Following ingestion, flavonoids undergo a chemical change by stomach acids and enzymes. Flavonoids are poorly absorbed into the blood and rapidly eliminated from the body. Thus, they have low 'bioavailability', as evident from studies that the bioavailability of soy isoflavones and citrus flavonones is only 10% of total intake, while it is about 2% for most of the other flavonoids like anthocyanidins, catechins, quercetin [132, 133]. Many *in vitro* experiments reported strong antioxidant activity of parent flavonoids in high, unphysiological concentrations rather than the metabolites of flavonoids. Thus, misunderstanding about the actual biological significance of flavonoids may lead to believe incorrectly that flavonoids have a strong antioxidant value. As per FDA the nutrient with recognized antioxidant activity *i.e.*, after ingestion and absorbed from the gastrointestinal tract it can participate in cellular processes to inactivate free radicals or prevent free radical-initiated reactions and is included as an antioxidant (21 CFR 101.54(g)(2)). Thus, the regulatory document excludes polyphenols as physiological antioxidants because: polyphenols are unable to survive the gastric acid-enzymes in its parental chemical form in the natural fruit; they do not have a biochemically confirmed mechanism of action or participation in any biological processes *in vivo*; and have not been proven to inactivate free radicals or block radical-initiated events in physiological studies [133, 134].

POSSIBLE ACTIONS OF DIETARY FLAVONOIDS OR BIOFLAVONOIDS IN HUMANS

Minimal or No Direct Antioxidant Activity: Flavonoids showed antioxidant activity *in vitro* by scavenging free radicals. However, in the human body, flavonoids are not so effective antioxidants because, even with high levels of dietary intake, cellular flavonoid concentrations are 100-1000 times lower than concentrations of other cellular antioxidants like vitamins C, E, and glutathione [134]. Moreover, flavonoid metabolites often have a lower antioxidant activity than their parent flavonoids. Thus, the antioxidant function of dietary flavonoids in the body is very small and physiologically negligible [132-134].

Potential Estrogenic and Anti-Estrogenic Activities: Soy isoflavones are called "phytoestrogens" (plant- compounds having estrogen-like effects). Estrogen is a hormone that binds to its receptors located in the bones, liver, heart, brain and reproductive tissue. Soy isoflavones can either mimic the effects of estrogen or block its effects in others. Estrogenic effects in various tissues could help to maintain bone density and improve cholesterol levels, while anti-estrogenic effects in the reproductive tissue could potentially decrease the risk of hormone-associated cancers (*e.g.*, breast, uterine and prostate cancers).

Potential Effects on Cell-Signaling Pathways: Cells can respond to a variety of stresses or signals by increasing or decreasing the activity of cell-signaling pathways or signal transduction pathways that regulate cell growth, proliferation and removal of damaged cells (programmed cell death or "apoptosis"). It is now clear that flavonoids antioxidant effects may be due to their ability to modulate cell-signaling pathways [133]. Inside cells, the concentration of flavonoids needed to affect cell-signalling mechanisms is much lower than that needed for its cellular antioxidant capacity. The results of laboratory experiments suggest that flavonoids may selectively inhibit a group of cell-signaling enzymes called kinases, required to maintain normal cell function. Increased activity of these kinases is responsible for the initiation of various chronic diseases generated due to silent inflammation. As flavonoids may selectively inhibit kinases and thereby lower the risk of chronic diseases [133].

In most experiments flavonoids in their native chemical form, if applied directly into the experimental set in relatively high concentrations, can change and regulate the cell signalling process. The regulation of cell signaling can help (i) to prevent diseases like cancer by increasing the levels of detoxification enzymes that help to excrete potentially toxic or carcinogenic compounds; (ii) to maintain and preserve normal cell cycle that leads to growth, replication and division of a cell (when DNA is damaged the cycle can be transiently arrested, and allow the DNA to be repaired. If the damage is irreparable, removal of damaged cell takes place, and if DNA mutations are propagated, cancer may develop as found in defective cell cycle regulation; (iii) to inhibit proliferation and induce Apoptosis (unlike normal cells, cancer cells proliferate rapidly and cannot respond to cell signals that initiate apoptosis). Flavonoids stimulate apoptosis in isolated cancer cells, and thus, treated as important dietary agents to combat cancer); (iv) to inhibit tumor invasion and angiogenesis (the development of new blood vessels or angiogenesis is necessary for the growth and invasiveness of cancerous tumors by matrix-metalloproteinases, and flavonoids can oppose both the invasion process and angiogenesis); (v) to decrease inflammation that leads to inhibit apoptosis, production of free radicals, release of inflammatory mediators responsible for cell proliferation and angiogenesis. Thus modulation of cell-signaling pathways by flavonoids can prevent many diseases like cardiovascular diseases by (i) decreasing inflammation. Atherosclerosis is an inflammatory disease of the arterial wall and several markers of inflammation like C-reactive protein (CRP) are found to be associated with increased risk of heart attacks and strokes. *In vitro* and *in vivo* studies with animals and humans showed that dietary flavonoids may lower CRP, and inhibit atherosclerosis resulting from inflammation of the arterial wall [135]; (ii) Decreasing vascular endothelial cell adhesion. Early in the development of atherosclerosis, inflammatory WBC is recruited from the blood to the arterial wall. This event is dependent on adhesion molecules produced by vascular endothelial cells that line the inner walls of blood vessels which is found to be inhibited by flavonoids [136]; (iii) Decreasing platelet aggregation, an initial step in the formation of a blood clot, which can occlude a coronary or cerebral artery leading to a heart attack or stroke. Thus, inhibiting platelet aggregation by flavonoids is important in the prevention of cardiovascular diseases; (iv) Increasing endothelial nitric oxide (NO) production. The endothelial nitric oxide synthetase (eNOS) produces NO to maintain normal blood vessel relaxation (vasodilation), while impaired NO-dependent vasodilation is linked to an increased risk of cardiovascular diseases. Nitric oxide also reduces inflammation and inhibits smooth muscle proliferation, an important factor in atherosclerosis. Dietary flavonoids (from tea, cocoa) may increase eNOS activity by binding to estrogen receptors and stimulating cell-signalling pathways that activate eNOS [137]. Thus, dietary flavonoids are not significant antioxidants in humans, but may affect a variety of cell-signaling pathways, thereby possibly influencing the onset and progression of cancer or cardiovascular diseases [138]. Plant derived phytofactors, vitamins and minerals are presented with their food equivalence in Table **7**.

Table 7: Phytonutrient and its Food equivalence of one daily serving

Requirements of some major Phytofactors, Vitamins and Minerals			
Lycopene (1.25 tomato) 150-250 mg	Vitamin E (33 spoons peanut butter)	Vitamin C (7cups Cantaloupe pieces)	Vitamin B12 (3.78 kg beef)
Lutein (1.3 cups spinach) 6-10 mg	Folate (6 cups of baked beans)	Niacin (1.5 whole chicken breast)	Thiamine (3 kg of Pork loin)
Quercetin (5 whole apple) 150-200 mg	Riboflavin (7.7 quarts of milk)	Vitamin B6 (22 medium Bananas)	Magnesium of 4.2 cups Peas)
Ellagic acid (1.5 cups Rasp berries); 40-60 mg	Hesperidin (3 whole Orange); 60-75 mg	EGCG (2 cup green teas); 90-100 mg	Omega 3 (1.5 oz sea fish)

Other supplements studied for diabetes and its complications include magnesium, CoQ10, vanadium, isoflavones, garlic, ginseng *etc.* with mixed results. Magnesium is an important mineral, lacking in the average diet, which helps to improve insulin response and enhances the fluidity of RBC membranes for a better absorption of glucose. It is available in seeds, nuts, legumes and green leafy vegetables. The recommended dose is 25 mg and vitamin B-6 should be needed to assimilate magnesium. Some studies on the effects of magnesium supplementation on blood glucose control showed mixed results (Office of Dietary Supplements *Magnesium* ods.od.nih.gov/factsheets/magnesium. asp, 2008), although several studies revealed that diet high in magnesium may lower the risk of diabetes [139-141].

Coenzyme Q10 triggers pancreatic beta cell function as antioxidant, and thus, produces the required insulin to get glucose into the cells. It can decrease heart damage in an adequate dose (50-100 mg per day); and the patients taking statins should take a CoQ10 supplement as statins markedly reduce CoQ10 levels [142]. However, its ability to control glucose is not consistent. Similarly the use of garlic is found to be beneficial for diabetes in epidemiological studies, however few preliminary studies with garlic for lowering blood glucose levels did not yield consistent results [143, 144]. It was noted that ginseng and vanadium can help to control blood glucose levels, and vanadium was used to help diabetics long before insulin was discovered, as vanadyl sulfate is reported to help to control the rise of glucose after every meal [145]. The source of Vanadium is mushrooms, shellfish, dill, parsley and black pepper. Some people with diabetes may also use botanicals such as prickly pear cactus, gurmar, *Coccinia indica*, *Aloe vera*, fenugreek, and bitter melon to control glucose levels [103]. A study with Indian herb *Gymnema sylvestre* showed enhanced insulin action, when 200 mg of gymnema extract was given to 22 diabetic (type 2) patients twice daily along with their oral medications. All patients experienced improved blood glucose control and five of them even able to discontinue their drug. In another study with the soluble fiber of Fenugreek seed revealed that soluble fibre (15-50 grams twice daily after meal) can effectively control blood sugar, probably due to its alkaloid trigonelline [102]. In diabetes the maintainance of blood sugar is important, but it may be of little help unless the lifestyle that causes diabetes is addressed. Thus, eliminating fast foods, plenty of exercise, cutting out habits of smoking, drinking and enough sleep are all important along with supplementation.

GOALS OF NUTRITIONAL THERAPY

Nutrition therapy for type 2 DM can optimally manage the "ABCs" of diabetes control. A is hemoglobin $A1_C$, B is blood pressure, and C is LDL-cholesterol. Thus, the prescription must be tailored for the individual patient, to address existing or at-risk complications of diabetes.

Healthy Diet is Not Only Important But a Must to Prevent Metabolic Disorders

Foods that should be avoided completely include bread, white flour, white rice, sugar, white potatoes, as these simple carbohydrates are digested so fast that they cause a spike in blood sugar levels. It is absolutely critical to avoid ALL trans-fatty acid, hydrogenated oils, canola oil, margarine and "bad fats" of omega 6, because they are the PLAGUE on humanity!! Fruits, vegetables, whole grains (oatmeal, wild rice), beans, legumes, fish and seafood, soy, Asian mushrooms, herbs, spices, cinnamon and unsweetened teas can be the dietary staples. Even if a person regularly takes fish and seafood, a fish oil supplement is recommended for all of the health benefits of omega-3 fatty acids. A list of nutritional medicines recommended for some major health problems are presented in Table **8**.

Table 8: Symptoms and Solutions for Some Health Problems with Nutritional Medicine

Health Problems	Nutritional Medicine Recommendations
Impaired Glucose metabolism and preclinical Diabetes	Essential amino acid, Omega 3 Fatty acid, B complex, Vitamin C, Grape seed extract, Co-Q10, Calcium, Magnesium, Chromium, Selenium, Vanadium, Soluble Fiber, *Garcinia cambogia*, *Gymnema sylvestre*
High Cholesterol	Green tea leaf extract, Omega 3 Fatty acid.
High Blood Pressure	Omega 3 Fatty acid, Garlic, Calcium, Magnesium.
Overall Heart Health	Omega 3 Fatty acid, Co-Q10, Garlic, Green Tea leaf extract, B complex, Calcium, Magnesium.
Liver Function	Fruit and vegetable concentrates, Milk Thistle, Dandelion.
Overweight/Obesity	Essential amino acid, Omega 3 Fatty acid, Co-Q-10, Calcium, Magnesium, Fiber, *Garcinia, Gymnema*

MANAGEMENT AND PREVENTION OF DIABETES: MODERN PERSPECTIVE

Management: Diabetes mellitus is a chronic disease which is difficult to cure. Thus, its management concentrates on keeping blood sugar levels as close to normal (euglycemia) without undue patient danger, and by dietary management, exercise, and appropriate medications (insulin in type 1, and oral medications with insulin in type 2). To keep blood glucose levels within acceptable range, patients should be educated on the complications of the diseases as well as the role of dietetic support and sensible exercise. Additionally, to reduce associated risks of cardiovascular disease lifestyle modifications are the only answer to control blood pressure (for hypertensive patients), and cholesterol for dyslipidemia with regular exercise, and prohibited smoking [146]. Patients with foot problems are recommended to wear diabetic socks, and diabetic shoes. The treatment of type 1 DM needs the support of insulin, and/or insulin analogs; while for type 2 oral medications and or insulin will be helpful. Another vital part of diabetes management is support or diabetic care. Such care is usually available from general practitioners outside hospitals or from hospital-based specialists for complicated cases or together as a team, like Optometrists, podiatrists/chiropodists, dietitians, physiotherapists, nursing specialists or Certified Diabetes Educators may jointly provide multidisciplinary expertise. Peer support also links diabetics through government or non-government organizations. However, in many countries of Asia and Africa, such network is still very poor.

Prevention: The risk of Type 1 diabetes depends upon a genetic predisposition based on HLA types (DR3, DR4), unknown environmental trigger (*e.g.*, infection), and an uncontrolled autoimmune response that attacks insulin producing beta cells [147]. Some studies have suggested that breastfeeding decreases the risk of type 1 diabetes in later life [148, 149]. However, no firm evidence has been found in studies with various other nutritional risk factors [150]. It is reported that children who received 2000 IU of Vitamin D during their first year of life have reduced risk of type 1 diabetes, but the causal relationship is obscure [151]. A 7 years study on children with antibodies to beta cell proteins (*i.e.* at early stages of an immune reaction) but no overt diabetes, when treated with vitamin B_3 (niacin), showed less than half the diabetes onset incidence compared to the general population, and those who received no vitamin B3 [152]. Several studies revealed that the risk of type 2 diabetes can be reduced by making changes in diet, increasing physical activity [153-155], meal planning [156], and diet with exercise [157]. The American Diabetes Association recommends at least 2½ h of exercise per week or brisk sustained walks for maintaining a healthy weight, a modest fat intake, and eating sufficient fiber from whole grains. Interestingly, moderate alcohol intake is thought to be helpful to reduce the risk but not recommended. The relationship between a low dose alcohol consumption and heart disease is called the *French Paradox*. Despite recommendations of dietary interventions, there is inadequate evidence that only eating foods of low glycemic index are clinically helpful [158-162]. It is found that diets that are very low in saturated fats can reduce the risk of becoming insulin resistant and diabetic [163-165]. Study showed that people whose dietary, smoking, and alcohol habits are in the low-risk group and whose physical activity level is high have an 82% lower incidence of diabetes [4]. Another study of dietary practice showed a direct relationship with the incidence of diabetes [41]. Numerous studies suggest connections between some aspects of type 2 diabetes with certain foods, like high protein low carbohydrate diets, lifestyle intervention with or without drugs [71, 166-170], and even breastfeeding can help to prevent type 2 diabetes [171]. Interestingly, some studies have reported the delayed progression of diabetes in predisposed patients through prophylactic use of metformin [154], rosiglitazone [172], or valsartan [173]. It is also reported that the use of hydroxychloroquine for rheumatoid arthritis can reduce the incidence of diabetes by 77% though an unknown mechanism [174]. However, lifestyle interventions are more effective than metformin at preventing diabetes regardless of weight loss [175].

Prognosis: Patient education, understanding, and participation are vital as the complications of diabetes are less common and less severe in people having well-managed blood sugar levels through dietary interventions [176, 177]. Except in type 1, which always requires insulin replacement, the type 2 diabetes management may change with age. Insulin production decreases because of age-related impairment of pancreatic beta cells. Additionally, increased insulin resistance and decreased tissue sensitivity to insulin are due to the loss of lean tissue and the accumulation of fat, particularly intra-abdominal fat. Glucose tolerance progressively declines with age, leading to a high prevalence of type 2 DM and post challenge hyperglycemia in the older population [178]. Age-related glucose intolerance is often accompanied by insulin resistance, but circulating insulin levels are similar to those of younger people [179]. Treatment goals for older patients with diabetes vary with the individual, considering the health status, as well as life expectancy, the level of dependence, and the willingness to adhere to the treatment regimen [180].

CONCLUSIONS

In 1990 international efforts to improve the quality and life expectancy of people with diabetes led to the "*St Vincent Declaration*" [181, 182]. Today several countries have successful national diabetes control programs [183], however, the rehabilitation of diabetic people in many countries is very poor. A recent study shows that diabetic patients with neuropathic symptoms (numbness or tingling in feet or hands) are twice as likely to be unemployed as those without the symptoms [184].

The management of diabetes with drugs of zero side effects is still a great challenge for the biomedical scientists. The toxicity, side effects, long term therapy, regular glucose monitoring have led to increase in the demand for dietary intervention along with nutraceuticals, and natural fruits and vegetables that have antihyperglycemic activity. The metabolic imbalance that causes diabetes mellitus is a characteristic of the materialistic world. However, differences in social structure, psychic stress, obesity, sedentary lifestyle, hormonal imbalance and heredity are optimizing the growth of diabetic pandemic. Increasing population with diabetes has a huge requirement of effective remediation. The vast variety of plants, both as food and medicine, are used traditionally for diabetic prevention or anti-diabetic property in many countries. However, careful assessment, including sustainability of such plant based nutraceuticals or pharmaceuticals, the ecological and seasonal variation in activity of phyto-constituents, metal contents of crude anti-diabetic phytocompounds, thorough toxicity study and cost effectiveness are required for their popularity. The use of food supplements comes only when the regular food does not serve the nutrients required by the body, particularly in persons having high demand. Supplementation is not only a way to increase intake of the nutrients without increasing caloric intake, but also the way to get measured content of nutrients. That's important because 70-90% of type II diabetes sufferers are overweight. To cope with the modern lifestyle, modern diet is insufficient to fulfill all the required essential nutrients, particularly high quality essential amino acid, essential fatty acid like omega 3, several vitamins and minerals, dietary fibers and especially the fresh phytonutrients or color wheel, that help the liver to release P450 II cytochrome enzymes to detoxify the body. Moreover, we need supplements as they promote well being, fill the nutrition gap and determine how we live tomorrow. These efforts may provide treatment for all and justify the role of novel traditional plants based therapy having anti-diabetic potentials. Thus, the medicine of the future will no longer be remedial, but preventive; not based on drugs alone but on the optimum nutrition for health.

The exact cause of the increasing prevalence of diabetes throughout the globe, particularly in the Asian subcontinent, is unknown. However, probably both nature and nurture may have a role. While we have a little to do, at present with 'nature', we can definitely modulate 'nurture' for desirable results. Dietary control in insulin resistance, intake of culturally acceptable diabetic preventive food and discouraging sedentary habits help to reduce the prevalence of diabetes and are most beneficial in the present context, since they do not cost much.

ACKNOWLEDGEMENTS

The authors extend their thanks to Bentham Science Publishers.

DECLARATION OF CONFLICT OF INTEREST

No conflict of interest was declared by the authors.

REFERENCES

[1] Rother KI. Diabetes treatment-bridging the divide. New England J Medicine 2007; 356(15): 1499–1501.

[2] Tierney LM, McPhee SJ, Papadakis MA. Current medical Diagnosis & Treatment. International edition. New York: Lange Medical Books/McGraw-Hill. 2002. pp. 1203-1215. ISBN 0-07-137688-7.Deshpande AD, Harris-Hayes M, Schootman M. Epidemiology of Diabetes and Diabetes-Related Complications. Phytotherapy 2008; 88(11): 1254-1264.

[4] Mozaffarian D, Kamineni A, Carnethon M, Djoussé L, Mukamal KJ, Siscovick D. Lifestyle risk factors and new-onset diabetes mellitus in older adults: the cardiovascular health study. Archives of Internal Medicine 2009; 169(8): 798-807.

[5] Cooke DW, Plotnick L. Type 1 diabetes mellitus in pediatrics. Pediatr Rev 2008; 29(11): 374-384.

[6] Belletti DA, Zacker C, Wogen J. Effect of cardiometabolic risk factors on hypertension management: a cross-sectional study among 28 physician practices in the United States. Cardiovascular Diabetology 2010; 9:7. Doi:10.1186/1475-2840-9-7.

[7]   Wild S, Roglic G, Greent A, Sicree R, King H. Global prevalence of Diabetes: Estimates for the year 2000 and projections for 2030. Diabetes Care 2004; 27(5):1047-1053.

[8]   Australian Institute for Health and Welfare. Diabetes, an overview. http://www.aihw.gov.au/ indigenous/health/diabetes.cfm. Retrieved 2008-06-23.

[9]   Shaw JE, Sicree RA, Zimmet PZ. Global estimates of the prevalence of diabetes for 2010 and 2030. Diabetes Res Clin Pract 2010; 87(1): 4-14.

[10]   Gupta R, Mishra A. Type 2 Diabetes in India: Regional disparities. British J Diabetes vascular disease 2007; 7 (1): 12-16.

[11]   Yang W, Lu J, Weng J, Jia W, Ji L, Xiao J, Shan Z, Liu J, Tian H, Ji Q, Zhu D, Ge J, Lin L, Chen L, Guo X, Zhao Z, Lie Q, Zhou Z, Shan G, He J. For the China National Diabetes and Metabolic Disorder study group. Prevalance of Diabetes among Men and Women in China. New England J Medicine 2010; 362 (12): 1090-1101.

[12]   Dobson M. Nature of the urine in diabetes. Medical Observations and Inquiries 1776; 5: 298-310.

[13]   Cornelius MV. The history of clinical endocrinology. Carnforth, Lancs, U.K: Parthenon Pub. Group. 1993; pp. 23-34. ISBN 1-85070-427-9.

[14]   Dwivedi G, Dwivedi S. History of Medicine: Sushruta -the Clinician- Teacher par Excellence. National Informatics Centre (Government of India) 2007.

[15]   Nabipour, I. Clinical Endocrinology in the Islamic Civilization in Iran. International Journal of Endocrinology and Metabolism 2003; 1: 43-45.

[16]   Patlak M. New weapons to combat an ancient disease: treating diabetes. The FASEB Journal 2002; 16(14): 1853.

[17]   Von Mehring J, Minkowski O. Diabetes mellitus nach pankreasexstirpation. Arch Exp Pathol Pharmakol 1990; 26: 371-387.

[18]   Banting FG, Best CH, Collip JB, Campbell WR, Fletcher AA. Pancreatic extracts in the treatment of diabetes mellitus: preliminary report. CMAJ 1991; 145(10): 1281-1286.

[19]   Himsworth H. Diabetes mellitus: its differentiation into insulin-sensitive and insulin-insensitive types. Lancet 1936; i: 127-130.

[20]   Yalow RS, Berson SA. Immunoassay of endogenous plasma insulin in man. The Journal of Clinical Investigation 1960; 39: 1157-1175.

[21]   Smith GD, Duax WL, Dodson EJ, Dodson GG, Degraaf RAG, Reynolds CD. The Structure of Des-Phe B1 Bovine Insulin. Acta Crystallogr Sect B 1982; 38: 3028.

[22]   The Diabetes Control and Complications Trial Research Group. The effect of intensive treatment of diabetes on the development and progression of long-term complications in insulin-dependent diabetes mellitus. The Diabetes Control and Complications Trial Research Group. New England J Medicine 1993; 329(14): 977-986. American Diabetes Association (2005). Total Prevalence of Diabetes and Pre-diabetes. http://www. diabetes.org/diabetes-statistics/ prevalence. jsp. Retrieved 2006-03-17.

[23]   Lawrence JM, Contreras R, Chen W, Sacks DA. Trends in the prevalence of preexisting diabetes and gestational diabetes mellitus among a racially/ethnically diverse population of pregnant women, 1999-2005. Diabetes Care 2008; 31(5): 899-904.

[24]   Ridker PM, Danielson E, Fonseca FA. JUPITER Study Group. Rosuvastatin to prevent vascular events in men and women with elevated C-reactive protein. N Engl J Med 2008; 359: 2195-2207.

[25]   Shepherd J, Blauw GJ, Murphy MB. PROSPER Study Group, Prospective Study of Pravastatin in the Elderly at Risk. Pravastatin in elderly individuals at risk of vascular disease: a randomised controlled trial. Lancet 2002; 360:1623-1630.

[26] Sattar N, Preiss D, Murray HM. Statins and risk of incident diabetes: A collaborative meta-analysis of randomised Statin trials. *Lancet* 2010; 375:735-742.

[27] Liu KW, Dai LK, Jean W. Metformin-related vitamin B12 deficiency. Age and Ageing 2006; 35(2): 200-201.

[28] De Jager J, Kooy A, Lehert P, Wulffele M, van der Kolk J, Bets D, Verburg J, Donker A, Stehouwer C (2010). Long term treatment with metformin in patients with type 2 diabetes and risk of vitamin B-12 deficiency: randomised placebo controlled trial. British Medical J 340: c2181. DOI: 10.1136/bmj.c2181.

[29] WHO Department of Noncommunicable Disease Surveillance (1999). Definition, Diagnosis and Classification of Diabetes Mellitus and its Complications. http://whqlibdoc.who.int/hq/1999/WHO_NCD_NCS_99.2.pdf.

[30] Diabetes Care January 2010. http://care.diabetesjournals.org/content/33/Supplement_1/S3.full. Retrieved 2010-01-29.

[31] Saydah SH, Miret M, Sung J, Varas C, Gause D, Brancati FL. Post challenge hyperglycemia and mortality in a national sample of U.S. adults. Diabetes Care 2001; 24(8): 1397-402. Santaguida PL, Balion C, Hunt D, Morrison K, Gerstein H, Raina P, Booker L, Yazdi H. Diagnosis, Prognosis, and Treatment of Impaired Glucose Tolerance and Impaired Fasting Glucose. Summary of Evidence Report/Technology Assessment, No. 128. Agency for Healthcare Research and Quality. http://www.ahrq.gov/clinic/epcsums/ impglusum.htm. Retrieved 2008-07-20.

[32] Lee CM, Huxley RR, Lam TH. Prevalence of diabetes mellitus and population attributable fractions for coronary heart disease and stroke mortality in the WHO South-East Asia and Western Pacific regions. Asia Pacific Journal of Clinical Nutrition 2007; 16(1): 187-192.

[33] Seidell JC. Obesity, insulin resistance and diabetes-a worldwide epidemic. The British Journal of Nutrition 2000; 83 Suppl 1: S5-8.

[34] Iwasaki Y, Takayasu S, Nishiyama M. Is the metabolic syndrome an intracellular Cushing state? Effects of multiple humoral factors on the transcriptional activity of the hepatic glucocorticoid-activating enzyme (11β-hydroxysteroid dehydrogenase type 1) gene. Molecular and Cellular Endocrinology 2008; 285(1-2): 10-18.

[35] Saad F, Gooren L. The role of testosterone in the metabolic syndrome: a review. J Ster Biochem M Biol 2009; 114(1-2): 40-43.

[36] Mitra A, Basu B, Mukherjee S. Significance of Different Dietary Habits in Sections of Indian Diabetics. J Hum Ecol 2009; 26(2): 89-98.

[37] Thomas D, Elliott EJ. Low glycaemic index, or low glycaemic load, diets for diabetes mellitus. Cochrane Database Syst Rev 2009; CD006296.

[38] Yehuda Handelsman. A Doctor's Diagnosis: Prediabetes. Power of Prevention, 2009; Vol 1, Issue 2.

[39] Risérus U, Willett WC, Hu FB. Dietary fats and prevention of type 2 diabetes. Progress in Lipid Research 2009; 48(1): 44-51.

[40] Lyssenko V, Jonsson A, Almgren P. Clinical risk factors, DNA variants, and the development of type 2 diabetes. New England J Medicine 2008; 359(21): 2220-2232. Walley AJ, Blakemore AI, Froguel P. Genetics of obesity and the prediction of risk for health. Human Molecular Genetics 2006; 2: R124-30.

[41] Monogenic Forms of Diabetes: Neonatal Diabetes Mellitus and Maturity-onset Diabetes of the Young. National Diabetes Information Clearinghouse (NDIC), National Institute of Diabetes &

Digestive and Kidney Diseases, NIH. http://www.diabetes. niddk.nih.gov/dm/pubs/mody. Retrieved 2008-08-04.

[42]   Barrett TG. Mitochondrial diabetes, DIDMOAD and other inherited diabetes syndromes. Best Practice and Research. Clinical Endocrinology & Metabolism 2001; 15(3): 325-343.

[43]   Centers for Disease Control and Prevention. Prevalence of overweight and obesity among adults with diagnosed diabetes-United States, 1988–1994 and 1999–2002. MMWR. Morbidity and Mortality Weekly Report 2004; 53(45): 1066-1068.

[44]   Pastors JG, Waslaski J, Gunderson H. Diabetes meal-planning strategies. In: Diabetes Medical Nutrition Therapy and Education, Ross, RA, Boucher, JL, O'Connell, BS (Eds), American Dietetic Association, Chicago, IL 2005.

[45]   Rosenbloom A, Silverstein JH (2003). Type 2 Diabetes in Children and Adolescents: A Clinician's Guide to Diagnosis, Epidemiology, Pathogenesis, Prevention, and Treatment. American Diabetes Association, U.S. pp. 1. ISBN 978-1580401555.

[46]   Lang IA, Galloway TS, Scarlett A. Association of urinary bisphenol A concentration with medical disorders and laboratory abnormalities in adults. JAMA 2008; 300(11): 1303-1310.

[47]   Finkel T, Holbrook NJ. Oxidants, oxidative stress and the biology of ageing. Nature 2000; 408: 239-247.

[48]   Sohal RS, Weindruch R. Oxidative stress, caloric restriction, and aging. Science 1996; 273(5271): 59-63.

[49]   Beckman KB, Ames BN (1997). In: Oxidative Stress and the Molecular Biology of antioxidant Defences (Scandalios JG ed.), pp. 201-246, CSHL Press, New York. Wei YH, Lee HC. Oxidative stress, mitochondrial DNA mutation and impairment of antioxidant enzymes in aging. Exp Biol Med 2002; 227: 671-682.

[50]   Parke DV. Nutritional antioxidants and disease prevention: Mechanism of action. In: Antioxidants in Human health (TK Basu, NJ Temple, ML Garg Eds.), CAB International., London, 1999; pp. 1-13.

[51]   Chiodini I, Torlontano M, Scillitani A. Association of subclinical hypercortisolism with type 2 diabetes mellitus: a case-control study in hospitalized patients. European Journal of Endocrinology 2005; 153(6): 837-844.

[52]   Taniguchi T, Hamasaki A, Okamoto M. Subclinical hypercortisolism in hospitalized patients with type 2 diabetes mellitus. Endocrine Journal 2008; 55(2): 429-432.

[53]   Farrell JB, Deshmukh A, Baghaie AA. Low testosterone and the association with type 2 diabetes. The Diabetes Educator 2008; 34(5): 799-806.

[54]   Strand RD. What your Doctor does not know about Nutritional Medicine may be killing you. Magna Publishing Co Ltd, Mumbai, India. ISBN 81-7809-170-4, 2003; pp. 2-9; 147-181.

[55]   Lewith GT, Breen A, Filshie J, Fisher P, McIntyre M, Mathie RT, Peters D. Complementary Medicine: Evidence base, competence to practice and regulation. Clin Med 2003; 3:235-240.

[56]   Marlow HJ, Hayes WK, Soret S, Carter RL, Schwab ER, Sabaté J. Diet and the environment: does what you eat matter? American J Clin Nutr 2009; 89: 1699S-1703S.

[57]   Lakhan SE, Vieira KF. Nutritional therapies for mental disorders. Nutrition J 2008; 7: 2. Doi:10.1186/1475-2891-7-2.

[58]   Newby PK. Plant foods and plant based diets: protective against childhood obesity? American J Clin Nutr 2009; 89(suppl):1572S-1587S.

[59]   Ørgaard A, Jensen1 L. The effects of soy isoflavones on obesity. Exp Biol Med 2008; 233:1066-1080. Nanri A, Mizoue T, Takahashi Y, Kirii K, Inoue M, Noda M, Tsugane S. Soy

product and isoflavones intakes are associated with a lower risk of Type 2 diabetes in overweight Japanese Women. J Nutr 2010; 140(3): 580-586.

[60] Yellayi S, Naaz A, Szewczykowski MA, Sato T, Woods JA, Chang J, Segre M, Allred CD, Helferich WG, Cooke PS. The phytoestrogen genistein induces thymic and immune changes: A human health concern? Proceedings National Academy of Sciences USA 2002; 99:7616-7621.

[61] Badger TM, Gilchrist JM, Pivik RT, Andres A, Shankar K, Chen J-R, Ronis MJ. The health implications of soy infant formula. American J Clin Nutr 2009; 89: 1668S-1672S.

[62] Sanders TAB, Oakley FR, Miller GJ, Mitropoulous KA. Influence of N-6 *Versus* N-3 Polyunsaturated Fatty Acids in Diet Low in Saturated Fatty Acid Decreases During Long Term Compliance with a Lipid Lowering Diet. J Internal Medicine 1985; 59: 249-258.

[63] Luscombe ND, Clifton PM, Noakes M, Parker B, Wittert G. Effects of Energy-Restricted Diets Containing Increased Protein on Weight Loss, Resting Energy Expenditure, and The Thermic Effect of Feeding in type 2 Diabetes. Diabetes Care 2002; 25: 652-657.

[64] Mitra A, Bhattacharya D. Effects of Overall Consumption, Dietary Patterns, Cooking, on Patients Suffering From Non Insulin Dependent Diabetes Mellitus. J Interacademicia 2005; 9(4): 635-642.

[65] Ornish D (1996). Program for Reversing Heart Disease. New York: Ivy Books.

[66] Franz MJ, Bantle JP, Beebe CA. Evidence-based nutrition principles and recommendations for the treatment and prevention of diabetes and related complications. Diabetes Care 2002; 25: 148.

[67] Fisher M, Levine PH, Weiner B. The Effect of Vegetarian Diets on Plasma Lipid and Platelet Levels. Archives of Internal Medicine 1986; 146:1193-1197.

[68] Macrae R, Robinson RK, Sadler MJ. Encyclopedia of Food Science, Food Technology and Nutrition. 2nd Volume. London: Academic Press. 1993.

[69] Kahn CR, Weir GC. Joslin's Diabetes Mellitus. New Delhi: B. I. Waverly Pvt. Ltd. 1996. Per-Henrik Group, Antti A, Svante S, Lief G. Long-Term Effects of Guar Gum in Subjects with Non-Insulin-Dependent Diabetes Mellitus. American J Clinical Nutrition 1993; 58: 513-518.

[70] Salmeron J, Hu FB, Manson J. Dietary Fat Intake and Risk of Type 2 Diabetes in Women. American J Clinical Nutrition 2001; 73: 1019-1026.

[71] Singh RB, Niaz MA, Ghosh S, Beegom R, Rastogi V, Sharma JP, Dube GK. Association of Trans Fatty acids (vegetable ghee) and clarified butter (Indian ghee) intake with higher risk of Coronary Artery Disease in Rural and Urban populations with low fat consumption. International J Cardiology 1996; 56: 289-298.

[72] Enig MG (2006). Coconut Oil- Health and Nutritional Benefits. Retrieved from http: //www.shirleys-wellnesscafe.com/coconut.htm on 16.01.2006.

[73] Chaudhuri SK. Concise Medical Physiology. 1st Edition. Calcutta: New Central Book Agency. 1988.

[74] Sullivan K (2002). *Vitamins and Minerals: A Practical Approach to a Health Diet and Safe Supplementation*. Harper Collins.

[75] World Health Organization/International Council for the Control of the Iodine Deficiency Disorders/United Nations Childrens Fund (2007). Assessment of iodine deficiency disorders and monitoring their elimination. Geneva: World Health Organization, 3rd Ed. ISBN 978 92 4 159582 7.

[76] Goldfine AB, Patti ME, Zuberi L, Goldstein BJ, Leblanc R, Landaker EJ, Jiang ZY, Willsky GR. Metabolic effects of vanadyl sulfate in humans with non-insulin-dependent diabetes mellitus: *in vivo* and *in vitro* studies. Metabolism 2000; 49(3): 400-410.

[77]   Mason JB (2007). Vitamins, trace minerals, and other micronutrients. In: Goldman L, Ausiello D, eds. Cecil Medicine. 23rd ed. Philadelphia, Pa: Saunders Elsevier, Chap 237.

[78]   Anderson RA (2007). Prescribing antioxidants. In: Rakel D, ed. Integrative Medicine. Chap 103, 2nd ed. Philadelphia, Pa: Saunders Elsevier. Hamrick I, Counts SH. Vitamin and mineral supplements. Wellness and Prevention 2008; 35(4): 729-747.

[79]   Jacobs Dr. Jr, Gross MD, Tapsell LC. Food synergy: an operational concept for understanding nutrition. American J Clin Nutr 2009; 89(suppl): 1543S-1548S.

[80]   Bouchard MF, Bellinger DC, Wright RO, Weisskopf MG. Attention-deficit/Hyperactivity Disorder and urinary metabolites of organophosphate pesticides. Pediatrics 2010; E1270-E1277. DOI: 10.1542/peds.2009-3058.

[81]   Furlong CE, Holland N, Richter RJ, Bradman A, Ho A, Eskenazi B. PON1 status of farmworker mothers and children as a predictor of organophosphate sensitivity. Pharmacogenet Genomics 2006; 16(3): 183-190.

[82]   UK Prospective Diabetes Study (UKPDS) Group. Intensive blood-glucose control with sulphonylureas or insulin compared with conventional treatment and risk of complications in patients with type 2 diabetes (UKPDS 33). Lancet 1998; 352: 837.

[83]   Long, SD, O'Brien, KO, MacDonald, KD. Weight loss in severely obese subjects prevents the progression of impaired glucose tolerance to type II diabetes. A longitudinal interventional study. Diabetes Care 1994; 17: 372.

[84]   Wing, RR, Blair, EH, Bononi, P. Caloric restriction *per se* is a significant factor in improvements in glycemic control and insulin sensitivity during weight loss in obese NIDDM patients. Diabetes Care 1994; 17: 30.

[85]   Close, EJ, Wiles, PG, Lockton, JA. The degree of day-to-day variation in food intake in diabetic patients. Diabet Med 1993; 10:514.

[86]   Hernandez-Ronquillo L, Tellez-Zenteno JF, Garduno-Espinosa J, Gonzalez-Acevez E. Factors associated with therapy noncompliance in type-2 diabetes patients. Salud Publica Mex 2003; 45: 191.

[87]   Price W. Nutrition and Physical Degeneration (8th Ed.), Price-Pottenger Nutrition Foundation. 2008. ISBN 0916764206. Huemer RP. A theory of diagnosis for orthomolecular medicine. J Theor Biol 1977; 67(4): 625-635.

[88]   Hoffer A, Walker M. Smart nutrients. Avery 2000. ISBN 0895295628.

[89]   Syd Baumel. Dealing with depression naturally: complementary and alternative therapies for restoring emotional health (2nd ed). Los Angeles: McGraw-Hill 2000. ISBN 0658002910. OCLC 43641423.

[90]   Dasgupta K, Grover SA, Da Costa D. Impact of modified glucose target and exercise interventions on vascular risk factors. Diabetes Res Clin Pract 2006; 72: 53.

[91]   Shah M, Adams-Huet B, Bantle JP. Effect of a high-carbohydrate *versus* a high--cis-monounsaturated fat diet on blood pressure in patients with type 2 diabetes. Diabetes Care 2005; 28: 2607.

[92]   Quinn RD. Five-year self-management of weight using meal replacements: comparison with matched controls in rural Wisconsin. Nutrition 2000; 16: 344.

[93]   Metz JA, Stern JS, Kris-Etherton P, Reusser ME, Morris CD, Hatton DC, Oparil S, Haynes B, Resnick LM, Pi-Sunyer FX, Clark S, Chester L, McMahon M, Snyder GW and McCarron DA. A randomized trial of improved weight loss with a prepared meal plan in overweight and obese patients. Arch Intern Med 2000; 160: 2150.

[94]   Yeh GY, Eisenberg DM, Kaptchuk TJ. Systematic review of herbs and dietary supplements for glycemic control in diabetes. Diabetes Care 2003; 26(4):1277-1294.

[95]   Halat KM, Dennehy CE. Botanicals and dietary supplements in diabetic peripheral neuropathy. Journal of the American Board of Family Practice 2003; 16(1): 47-57.

[96]   MacLean CH, Issa AM, Newberry SJ, Mojica WA, Morton SC, Garland RH, Hilton LG, Traina SB, Shekelle PG (2005). Effects of Omega-3 Fatty Acids on Cognitive Function with Aging, Dementia, and Neurological Diseases. Evidence Report/Technology Assessment No. 114, Prepared by the Southern California Evidence-based Practice Center, under Contract No. 290-02-0003. AHRQ Publication No. 05-E011-2. Rockville, MD. Brenna JT. Efficiency of conversion of alpha-linolenic acid to long chain n-3 fatty acids in man. Curr Opin Clin Nutr Metab Care 2002; 5(2): 127-132.

[97]   Burdge GC, Calder PC. Conversion of alpha-linolenic acid to longer-chain polyunsaturated fatty acids in human adults. Reprod Nutr Dev 2005; 45(5): 581–597.

[98]   Harris WS. Omega-3 fatty acids and cardiovascular disease: a case for omega-3 index as a new risk factor. Pharmacol Res 2007; 55:217-23.

[99]   Harris WS, Bulchandani D. Why do omega-3 fatty acids lower serum triglycerides? Curr Opin Lipidol 2006; 17: 387-393.

[100]   Albert CM, Campos H, Stampfer MJ. Blood levels of long-chain n-3 fatty acids and the risk of sudden death. New Engl J Med 2002; 346: 1113-18.

[101]   Kang JX, Leaf A. Prevention of fatal cardiac arrhythmias by polyunsaturated fatty acids. American J Clin Nutr 2000; 71: 202S-207S.

[102]   Knapp HR. Dietary fatty acids in human thrombosis and hemostasis. American J Clin Nutr 1997; 65: 1687S-1698S.

[103]   Nair SS, Leitch JW, Falconer J, Garg ML. Prevention of cardiac arrhythmia by dietary (n-3) polyunsaturated fatty acids and their mechanism of action. J Nutr 1997; 127: 383-93.

[104]   Morris MC, Sacks F, Rosner B. Does fish oil lower blood pressure? A meta-analysis of controlled trials. Circulation 1993; 88: 523-33.

[105]   Agency for Healthcare Research and Quality (2004). Effects of Omega-3 fatty acids on lipids and glycemic control in Type II Diabetes and the Metabolic Syndrome and on Inflammatory Bowel Disease, Rheumatoid Arthritis, Renal Disease, Systemic Lupus Erythematosus, and Osteoporosis. Evidence Report/Technology Assessment no. 89. Rockville, MD: Agency for Healthcare Research and Quality; AHRQ Publication No. 04-E012-2.

[106]   Hartweg J, Perera R, Montori V. Omega-3 polyunsaturated fatty acids for type 2 diabetes mellitus: review. The Cochrane Database of Systematic Reviews 2008; (1): CD003205. Hartweg J, Farmer AJ, Perera R. Meta-analysis of the effects of n-3 polyunsaturated fatty acids on lipoproteins and other emerging lipid cardiovascular risk markers in patients with type 2 diabetes. Diabetologia 2007; 50(8): 1593-1602.

[107]   von Schacky C. The role of omega-3 fatty acids in cardiovascular disease. Curr. Atheroscler Rep 2003; 5(2): 139-145.

[108]   Unsitup MI. Effect of inorganic chromium supplementation on glucose tolerance, insulin response and serum lipids in non-insulin dependent diabetics. American J Clinical Nutrition 1983; 38(3): 404-410.

[109]   Anderson, RA. Elevated intakes of supplemental chromium improve glucose insulin variables in individuals with type 2 diabetes. Diabetes 1997; 46(11): 1786-1791.

[110]   Althuis MD, Jordan NE, Ludington EA. Glucose and insulin responses to dietary chromium supplements: a meta-analysis. American Journal of Clinical Nutrition 2002; 76(1): 148-155.

[111]   Balk EM, Tatsioni A, Lichtenstein AH. Effect of chromium supplementation on glucose metabolism and lipids: A systematic review of randomized controlled trials. Diabetes Care 2007; 30(8): 2154-2163.

[112] Collins QF, Liu HY, Pi J. Epigallocatechin-3-gallate (EGCG), a green tea polyphenol, suppresses hepatic gluconeogenesis through 5'-AMP activated protein kinase. Journal of Biological Chemistry 2007; 282(41): 30143-30149.

[113] Kim J, Formoso G, Li Y. Epigallocatechin gallate, a green tea polyphenol, mediates NO-dependent vasodilation using signaling pathways in vascular endothelium requiring reactive oxygen species and Fyn. Journal of Biological Chemistry 2007; 282(18): 13736-13745.

[114] Fukino Y, Shimbo M, Aoki N. Randomized controlled trial for an effect of green tea consumption on insulin resistance and inflammation markers. Journal of Nutritional Science and Vitaminology 2005; 51(5): 335-342. Ryu OH, Lee J, Lee KW. Effects of green tea consumption on inflammation, insulin resistance and pulse wave velocity in type 2 diabetes patients. Diabetes Research and Clinical Practice 2006; 71(3): 356-358.

[115] Mackenzie T, Leary L, Brooks WB. The effect of an extract of green and black tea on glucose control in adults with type 2 diabetes mellitus: double-blind randomized study. Metabolism 2007; 56(10): 1340-1344.

[116] Potenza MA, Marasciulo FL, Tarquinio M. EGCG, a green tea polyphenol, improves endothelial function and insulin sensitivity, reduces blood pressure, and protects against myocardial I/R injury in SHR. American Journal of Physiology, Endocrinology, and Metabolism 2007; 292(5): E1378-E1387.

[117] Seddon JM, Ajani UA, Sperduto RD. Dietary carotenoids, vitamins A, C, and E, and advanced age-related macular degeneration. Eye Disease Case-Control Study Group. JAMA 1994; 272(18): 1413-1420.

[118] Lyle BJ, Mares-Perlman JA, Klein BE, Klein R, Greger JL. Antioxidant intake and risk of incident age-related nuclear cataracts in the Beaver Dam Eye Study. Am J Epidemiol 1999; 149(9): 801-809.

[119] Pattison DJ, Symmons DP, Lunt M. Dietary beta-cryptoxanthin and inflammatory polyarthritis: results from a population-based prospective study. Am J Clin Nutr 2005; 82(2): 451-455.

[120] Handelman GJ, Nightingale ZD, Lichtenstein AH, Schaefer EJ, Blumberg JB. Lutein and zeaxanthin concentrations in plasma after dietary supplementation with egg yolk. Am. J. Clin Nutr 1999; 70(2): 247-251.

[121] Lotito SB, Frei B. Consumption of flavonoid-rich foods and increased plasma antioxidant capacity in humans: cause, consequence, or epiphenomenon? Free Radic Biol Med 2006a; 41: 1727-1746. Williams RJ, Spencer JP, Rice-Evans C. Flavonoids: antioxidants or signalling molecules? Free Radic Biol Med 2004; 36: 838-849.

[122] Frei B, Higdon JV. Antioxidant activity of tea polyphenols *in vivo*: evidence from animal studies. J Nutr 2003; 133: 3275S-3284S.

[123] Gross P (2009). New roles for polyphenols. A 3-Part report on Current Regulations & the State of Science; http://www.nutraceuticalsworld.com/contents/ view/14064

[124] Lotito SB, Frei B. Dietary flavonoids attenuate tumour necrosis factor alpha-induced adhesion molecule expression in human aortic endothelial cells. Structure-function relationships and activity after first pass metabolism. J Biol Chem 2006b; 281: 37102-37110.

[125] Anter E, Chen K, Shapira OM, Karas RH, Keaney JF Jr. p38 Mitogen-activated protein kinase activates eNOS in endothelial cells by an estrogen receptor alpha-dependent pathway in response to black tea polyphenols. Circ Res 005; 96:1072-1078.

[126] Frei B. Antioxidant Expertise of the Linus Pauling Institute. Nutraceuticals World, March 2009.

[127] Song Y, He K, Levitan EB, *et al.* Effects of oral magnesium supplementation on glycaemic control in type 2 diabetes: a meta-analysis of randomized double-blind controlled trials. Diabetic Medicine 2006; 23(10): 1050-1056.

[128] Larsson SC, Wolk A. Magnesium intake and risk of type 2 diabetes: a meta analysis. Journal of Internal Medicine 2007; 262(2): 208-214.

[129] Schulze MB, Schulz M, Heidemann C. Fiber and magnesium intake and incidence of type 2 diabetes: a prospective study and meta-analysis. Archives Internal Medicine 2007; 167(9): 956-965.

[130] Bonadkdar RA, Guarneri E. Coenzyme Q10. American Family Physician 2005; 72(6): 1065-1069. Agency for Healthcare Research and Quality (2000). Garlic: Effects on cardiovascular risks and disease, protective effects against Cancer, and clinical adverse effects. Evidence Report/Technology Assessment no. 20. Rockville, MD, AHRQ publication no. 01-E023.

[131] Banerjee SK, Maulik SK. Effect of garlic on cardiovascular disorders: a review. Nutrition Journal 2002; 1(1): 4.

[132] Bhanot S, McNeill JH, Bryer-Ash MV. Vanadyl sulfate prevents fructose-induced hyperinsulinemia and hypertension in rats. Hypertension 1994; 23(3): 308-312.

[133] Adler AI, Stratton IM, Neil HA. Association of systolic blood pressure with macrovascular and microvascular complications of type 2 diabetes (UKPDS 36): prospective observational study. BMJ 2000; 321 (7258): 412-419.

[134] Daneman D. Type 1 diabetes. Lancet 2006; 367(9513): 847-858.

[135] Borch-Johnsen K, Joner G, Mandrup-Poulsen T. Relation between breast-feeding and incidence rates of insulin-dependent diabetes mellitus. A hypothesis. Lancet 1984; 2 (8411): 1083-1086.

[136] Shehadeh N, Shamir R, Berant M, Etzioni A. Insulin in human milk and the prevention of type 1 diabetes. Pediatric Diabetes 2001; 2(4): 175-177.

[137] Virtanen SM, Knip M. Nutritional risk predictors of beta cell autoimmunity and type 1 diabetes at a young age. American J Clinical Nutrition 2003; 78(6): 1053-1067.

[138] Hyppönen E, Läärä E, Reunanen A, Järvelin MR, Virtanen SM. Intake of vitamin D and risk of type 1 diabetes: a birth-cohort study. Lancet 2001; 358(9292): 1500-1503.

[139] Elliott RB, Pilcher CC, Fergusson DM, Stewart AW. A population based strategy to prevent insulin-dependent diabetes using nicotinamide. Journal of Pediatric Endocrinology & Metabolism 1996; 9(5): 501-509.

[140] Lindström J, Ilanne-Parikka P, Peltonen M. Sustained reduction in the incidence of type 2 diabetes by lifestyle intervention: follow-up of the Finnish Diabetes Prevention Study. Lancet 2006; 368(9548): 1673-1679. Knowler WC, Barrett-Connor E, Fowler SE. Reduction in the incidence of type 2 diabetes with lifestyle intervention or metformin. The New England Journal of Medicine 2002; 346(6): 393-403.

[141] Diabetes Prevention Program Research Group. 10-year follow-up of diabetes incidence and weight loss in the Diabetes Prevention Program Outcomes Study. Lancet 2009; 374(9702): 1677-1686.

[142] Pi-Sunyer FX, Maggio CA, McCarron DA. Multicenter randomized trial of a comprehensive prepared meal program in type 2 diabetes. Diabetes Care 1999; 22: 191.

[143] Brooks GA, Butte NF, Rand WM, *et al.* Chronicle of the Institute of Medicine physical activity recommendation: how a physical activity recommendation came to be among dietary recommendations. American J Clin Nutr 2004; 79: 921S.

[144] Bantle JP, Wylie-Rosett J, Albright AL. Nutrition recommendations and interventions for diabetes-2006: a position statement of the American Diabetes Association. Diabetes Care 2006; 29(9): 2140-2157.

[145] Bantle JP, Wylie-Rosett J, Albright AL. Nutrition recommendations and interventions for diabetes: a position statement of the American Diabetes Association. Diabetes Care 2008; 31(Suppl 1): S61.

[146] Jenkins DJ, Kendall CW, McKeown-Eyssen G. Effect of a low-glycemic index or a high-cereal fiber diet on type 2 diabetes: a randomized trial. JAMA 2008; 300: 2742.

[147] Boden G, Sargrad K, Homko C. Effect of a low-carbohydrate diet on appetite, blood glucose levels, and insulin resistance in obese patients with type 2 diabetes. Ann Intern Med 2005; 142: 403.

[148] Sheard NF, Clark NG, Brand-Miller JC *et al.* Dietary carbohydrate (amount and type) in the prevention and management of diabetes: a statement by the American Diabetes Association. Diabetes Care 2004; 27:2266. Barnard ND, Katcher HI, Jenkins DJ, Cohen J, Turner-McGrievy G. Vegetarian and vegan diets in type 2 diabetes management. Nutrition Reviews 2009; 67(5): 255-263.

[149] Neal Barnard. "13". Dr. Neal Barnard's Program for Reversing Diabetes: The Scientifically Proven System for Reversing Diabetes without Drugs. New York, NY: Rodale/Holtzbrinck Publishers 2007. ISBN 978-1-59486-528-2.

[150] Lovejoy JC, Smith SR, Champagne CM *et al.* Effects of Diets Enriched in Saturated (Palmitic), Monounsaturated (Oleic), or trans (Elaidic) Fatty Acids on Insulin Sensitivity and Substrate Oxidation in Healthy Adults. Diabetes Care 2002; 25: 1283.

[151] Esposito K, Maiorino MI, Ciotola M. Effects of a Mediterranean-style diet on the need for antihyperglycemic drug therapy in patients with newly diagnosed type 2 diabetes: a randomized trial. Ann Intern Med 2009; 151:306.

[152] Nuttall FQ, Gannon MC. The metabolic response to a high-protein, low-carbohydrate diet in men with type 2 diabetes mellitus. Metabolism 2006; 55: 243.

[153] Gannon MC, Nuttall FQ. Effect of a high-protein, low-carbohydrate diet on blood glucose control in people with type 2 diabetes. Diabetes 2004; 53: 2375.

[154] The Diabetes Prevention Program: description of lifestyle intervention. Diabetes Care 2002; 25: 2165.

[155] Franz MJ, Monk A, Barry B *et al.* Effectiveness of medical nutrition therapy provided by dieticians in the management of non-insulin-dependent diabetes mellitus: a randomized, controlled clinical trial. J Am Diet Assoc 1995; 95: 1009.

[156] Stuebe AM, Rich-Edwards JW, Willett WC, Manson JE, Michels KB. Duration of lactation and incidence of type 2 diabetes. JAMA 2005; 294(20): 2601-2610.

[157] Gerstein HC, Yusuf S, Bosch J. Effect of rosiglitazone on the frequency of diabetes in patients with impaired glucose tolerance or impaired fasting glucose: a randomised controlled trial. Lancet 2006; 368(9541): 1096-1105. Kjeldsen SE, Julius S, Mancia G. Effects of valsartan compared to amlodipine on preventing type 2 diabetes in high-risk hypertensive patients: the VALUE trial. J Hypertension 2006; 24(7): 1405-1412.

[158] Wasko MC, Hubert HB, Lingala VB. Hydroxychloroquine and risk of diabetes in patients with rheumatoid arthritis. JAMA 2007; 298(2): 187-193.

[159] Knowler WC, Fowler SE, Hamman RF. 10-year follow-up of diabetes incidence and weight loss in the Diabetes Prevention Program Outcomes Study. Lancet 2009; 374(9702): 1677-1686.

[160] Nathan DM, Cleary PA, Backlund JY. Intensive diabetes treatment and cardiovascular disease in patients with type 1 diabetes. The New England Journal of Medicine 2005: 353(25): 2643-2653.

[161] The Diabetes Control and Complications Trial Research Group. The effect of intensive diabetes therapy on the development and progression of neuropathy. The Diabetes Control and Complications Trial Research Group. Annals of Internal Medicine 1995; 122(8): 561-568.

[162] Harris MI, Flegal KM, Cowie CC. Prevalence of diabetes, impaired fasting glucose, and impaired glucose tolerance in U.S. adults. The Third National Health and Nutrition Examination Survey, 1988–1994. Diabetes Care 1998; 21(4): 518-524.

[163] Chang AM, Halter JB. Aging and insulin secretion. American Journal of Physiology. Endocrinology and Metabolism 2003; 284(1): E7-12.

[164] Diabetes and Aging. Diabetes Dateline. National Institute of Diabetes and Digestive and Kidney Diseases. 2002. http://diabetes.niddk.nih.gov/ about/dateline/spri02/8.htm. Retrieved 2007-05-14.

[165] Theodore H. Tulchinsky, Elena A. Varavikova (2008). The New Public Health, Second Ed. New York: Academic Press. p. 200. ISBN 0-12-370890-7.

[166] Piwernetz K, Home PD, Snorgaard O, Antsiferov M, Staehr-Johansen K, Krans M. Monitoring the targets of the St Vincent Declaration and the implementation of quality management in diabetes care: the DIABCARE initiative. The DIABCARE Monitoring Group of the St Vincent Declaration Steering Committee. Diabetic Medicine 1993; 10(4): 371-377.

[167] Dubois, HFW and Bankauskaite, V. Type 2 diabetes programmes in Europe. Euro Observer 2005; 7(2): 5-6.

[168] Stewart WF, Ricci JA, Chee E, Hirsch AG, Brandenburg NA. Lost productive time and costs due to diabetes and diabetic neuropathic pain in the US workforce. J Occup Environ Med 2007; 49(6): 672-679.Steffen LM. Eat your fruit and vegetables. Lancet 2006; 367: 278-279. The Diabetes Prevention Program: description of lifestyle intervention. Diabetes Care 2002; 25: 2165.

[170] Franz MJ, Monk A, Barry B *et al.* Effectiveness of medical nutrition therapy provided by dieticians in the management of non-insulin-dependent diabetes mellitus: a randomized, controlled clinical trial. J Am Diet Assoc 1995; 95: 1009.

[171] Stuebe AM, Rich-Edwards JW, Willett WC, Manson JE, Michels KB. Duration of lactation and incidence of type 2 diabetes. JAMA 2005; 294(20): 2601-2610.

[172] Gerstein HC, Yusuf S, Bosch J. Effect of rosiglitazone on the frequency of diabetes in patients with impaired glucose tolerance or impaired fasting glucose: a randomized controlled trial. Lancet 2006; 368(9541): 1096-1105.

[173] Kjeldsen SE, Julius S, Mancia G. Effects of valsartan compared to amlodipine on preventing type 2 diabetes in high-risk hypertensive patients: the VALUE trial. J Hypertension 2006; 24(7): 1405-1412.

[174] Wasko MC, Hubert HB, Lingala VB. Hydroxychloroquine and risk of diabetes in patients with rheumatoid arthritis. JAMA 2007; 298(2): 187-193.

[175] Knowler WC, Fowler SE, Hamman RF. 10-year follow-up of diabetes incidence and weight loss in the Diabetes Prevention Program Outcomes Study. Lancet 2009; 374(9702): 1677-1686.

[176] Nathan DM, Cleary PA, Backlund JY. Intensive diabetes treatment and cardiovascular disease in patients with type 1 diabetes. The New England Journal of Medicine 2005: 353(25): 2643-2653.

[177] The Diabetes Control and Complications Trial Research Group. The effect of intensive diabetes therapy on the development and progression of neuropathy. The Diabetes Control and Complications Trial Research Group. Annals of Internal Medicine 1995; 122(8): 561-568.

[178] Harris MI, Flegal KM, Cowie CC. Prevalence of diabetes, impaired fasting glucose, and impaired glucose tolerance in U.S. adults. The Third National Health and Nutrition Examination Survey, 1988–1994. Diabetes Care 1998; 21(4): 518-524.

[179] Chang AM, Halter JB. Aging and insulin secretion. American Journal of Physiology Endocrinology and Metabolism 2003; 284(1): E7-12.

[180] Theodore H. Tulchinsky, Elena A. Varavikova (2008). The New Public Health, Second Ed. New York: Academic Press. p. 200. ISBN 0-12-370890-7.

[181] Piwernetz K, Home PD, Snorgaard O, Antsiferov M, Staehr-Johansen K, Krans M. Monitoring the targets of the St Vincent Declaration and the implementation of quality management in diabetes care: the DIABCARE initiative. The DIABCARE Monitoring Group of the St Vincent Declaration Steering Committee. Diabetic Medicine 1993; 10(4): 371-377.

[182] Dubois, HFW and Bankauskaite, V. Type 2 diabetes programmes in Europe. Euro Observer 2005; 7(2): 5-6.

[183] Stewart WF, Ricci JA, Chee E, Hirsch AG, Brandenburg NA. Lost productive time and costs due to diabetes and diabetic neuropathic pain in the US workforce. J Occup Environ Med 2007; 49(6): 672-679.

[184] Steffen LM. Eat your fruit and vegetables. Lancet 2006; 367: 278-279.

CHAPTER 2

Diabetes and Hypertension: A Cause and Effect Synergy?

Debprasad Chattopadhyay[1,*], Hemanta Mukherjee[1], Paromita Bag[1], Chitralekha Saha[2] and Tapan Chatterjee[2]

[1]ICMR Virus Unit, ID & BG Hospital, General Block 4, 57 Dr. Suresh C. Banerjee Road, Kolkata 700010; [2]Diabetic Clinic, Salt lake City, Kolkata 700 064 and [3]Pharmaceutical Technology Department, Jadavpur University, Kolkata 700 032, India

Abstract: Diabetes is a disease that affects millions of people worldwide and is characterized by elevated levels of glucose in the blood due to its overproduction mainly by liver, and underutilization by insulin requiring organs such as liver, adipose and muscle tissues. There is, however, glucose over utilization in tissues not dependent on insulin for glucose transport like kidney, nerve and brain. Due to the excess tissue glucose there are serious complications and its reversal is important for a good metabolic control and normalization of body. Diabetes adversely affects the arteries, predisposing them to atherosclerosis, which in turn cause high blood pressure and other cardiovascular problems. If not treated, it can lead to blood vessel damage, stroke, heart failure, heart attack, or kidney failure. Diabetes comes in a variety of types with the most common being type 1 and type 2. Type 1 is an auto-immune disease resulting from an insulin deficiency; while type 2 is characterized by an insulin resistance resulting from genetic factors, poor diet, excess weight and inactivity. Compared to people with normal blood pressure, hypertensive people have an increased risk of coronary artery disease, strokes, peripheral vascular disease (hardening of the arteries in the legs and feet) and heart failure. This paper will discuss the biochemical events of these metabolic disorders and the relationship between diabetes and hypertension to understand how the intervention process for its management can be initiated in personal level.

Keywords: Diabetes, hypertension, complications, blood pressure, insulin, heart, vascular, management.

INTRODUCTION

Diabetes is a disorder or imbalance of glucose utilization and insulin availability that affects the way body uses food for energy. Normally, the carbohydrate food is

*Address correspondence to Debprasad Chattopadhyay: ICMR Virus Unit, ID & BG Hospital, GB-4, First Floor, 57 Dr. Suresh C. Banerjee Road, Beliaghata, Kolkata 700010, India; Tel/Fax: +913323537424-25; E-mail: debprasadc@yahoo.co.in

Mohamed Eddouks and Debprasad Chattopadhyay (Eds)
All rights reserved-© 2012 Bentham Science Publishers

digested and broken down into glucose in the digestive tract and the glucose then enters cells to be used as fuel *via* blood. Insulin, a storage hormone produced by the β (beta) cells of the Islets of Langerhans of pancreas, helps move the glucose into cells. A healthy pancreas adjusts the amount of insulin based on the level of glucose. But, if this process is broken down, the blood sugar levels become too high, leading to a condition called "*diabetes*". Hence, it is a heterogeneous metabolic disorder characterized by hyperglycaemia resulting from defective insulin secretion, or resistance to insulin action or both [1]. There are two main types of full-blown diabetes, called as *diabetes mellitus* (DM) Type 1 and Type 2. People with Type 1 diabetes are completely unable to produce insulin, while Type 2 people can produce insulin, but their cells don't respond to it. In either case, the glucose can't move into the cells and blood glucose levels become high. Over time, these high glucose levels can cause serious complications [2, 3]. A metabolic disorder is caused by biochemical abnormality due to the malfunctioning or non-functioning of enzymes or hormones. When the metabolism or any of its biochemical steps is blocked or defective, it can cause a build-up of toxic substances or a deficiency of substances within the cell, that lead to serious symptoms. Some metabolic diseases are inherited and those inborn errors can lead to serious complications or even death. The type 1 diabetes mellitus occurs when the pancreas doesn't produce and secrete enough insulin; however, when the body can't respond normally to its own insulin it causes type 2. For the most part, the causes of diabetes remain a mystery. However, certain habits, environments, and predispositions are thought to increase the chances of diabetes. Often the onset of diabetes is related to hypertension, high blood sugar and high blood cholesterol. Genetic factors, poor diet, less physical activity or inactivity, and environment are believed to be catalysts for this metabolic disorder.

Diabetes affects the arteries and predisposing them to atherosclerosis (hardening of the arteries), which in turn causes high blood pressure (hypertension) and other cardiovascular problems. If untreated, it can lead to blood vessel damage, stroke, heart failure, heart attack, or kidney failure [4]. On the other hand, high blood pressure (BP) is an important risk factor for the development and worsening of many complications of diabetes, including diabetic retinopathy [5] and or nephropathy [6], that affects up to 60% of people with diabetes [7]. Compared to people with normal BP, men and women with hypertension have an increased risk of coronary artery disease, strokes, peripheral vascular disease (hardening of the arteries in the legs and feet) and heart failure [8]. Studies with pre-hypertensive (BP 120-139/80-89 is even high yet normal) people over a 10 year period of follow up time, revealed two to three fold increased risk of heart disease [9].

TYPES OF DIABETES

Type 1 Diabetes: Type 1 diabetes (T1D), also called as *insulin dependent diabetes mellitus* (IDDM), or *juvenile diabetes*, caused when pancreas can't make any insulin. Most often it occurs before age of 30, but may strike at any age. The origins of Type 1 diabetes are not fully understood, but there are several theories. However, the recent evidence indicated that when pancreas undergoes an attack by its own immune cells (autoimmune attack), the immune system mistakenly manufactures antibodies and inflammatory cells that rendered β-cells incapable of making insulin. Abnormal antibodies against β-cells, found in the majority of type 1 diabetes cases, are responsible for pancreatic tissue damage. It is reported that this tendency to develop abnormal antibodies is partly genetically inherited [10, 11], though certain viral infections (congenital rubella, coxsackie virus B, cytomegalovirus, adenovirus, and mumps) or some environmental toxins may trigger such abnormal antibody responses. Some of these antibodies are: anti-islet antibodies, anti-insulin antibodies and anti-glutamic acid decarboxylase antibodies, which help to determine the risk of developing type 1 diabetes [10]. Moreover, the genetic predisposition based on human leucocyte antigen (HLA) types (particularly DR3 and DR4), environmental trigger (*e.g.*, certain viral infection and environmental toxins), and uncontrolled autoimmune response attacks the insulin producing β-cells [12]. Interestingly some studies have suggested that breastfeeding decreased the risk of diabetes in later life [13], however no firm evidence with other nutritional factors has been found [14]. Although the use of Vitamin D (2000 IU) during first year of life seems to be associated with reduced risk of type 1 diabetes, but this causal relationship is obscure [15]. Children with antibodies to beta cell proteins (*i.e.* at early stages of immune reaction) but no overt diabetes when treated with vitamin B-3 (niacin), showed less onset of diabetes in a 7-year time, but is not supported in other studies [16].

Symptoms of T1D Include: excessive thirst and urination, hunger, and weight loss. Over the time the disease can cause kidney problems, pain due to nerve damage, blindness, and heart and blood vessel disease. Kids and teens with type 1 need regular insulin injections for control of blood sugar levels and to reduce the risk of developing these problems. At present, the American Diabetes Association does not recommend general screening of the population for type 1 diabetes, but high risk individuals, those with a first degree relative (sibling or parent) with type 1 diabetes, should be screened. Type 1 diabetes tends to occur in young, lean individuals, usually before 30 years of age, but occasionally in older people. This subgroup called as *latent autoimmune diabetes* in adults (LADA) is slow progressive form. Usually about 10% of the patients have type 1 and the remaining 90% have type 2 diabetes. Thus, T1D is an autoimmune metabolic disorder, characterized by T-cell-mediated destruction of pancreatic β cells, resulting in insulin deficiency and hyperglycaemia. It was reported that 4,37,500 children were affected by T1D worldwide [17], and about 70,000 children under 14 years are affected each year [17], with an annual global increase of about 3%, particularly in younger children [18]. Though the exact etiology of T1D is largely unknown, its genetic predisposition, environmental and metabolic changes are responsible for the initiation, development and progression of this disease. Insulin deficiency in T1D leads to increased gluconeogenesis and lipolysis, elevated metabolism of free fatty acids, and the generation of ketone bodies, resulting in ketoacidosis. The primary clinical signs of ketoacidosis can lead to chronic hyperglycaemia, coma and death. Chronic hyperglycaemia is the primary cause of several macrovascular and microvascular complications, including cardiovascular disease, renal disease, diabetic retinopathy and peripheral neuropathy [19].

Type 2 Diabetes: People with Type 2 diabetes (T2D) or *non-insulin dependent diabetes mellitus* (NIDDM), or *adult onset diabetes mellitus* (AODM) has adequate insulin, but the cells become resistant to it. It usually occurs in adults over 35 years, but can affect anyone, including children. T2D is determined primarily by lifestyle factors and genes [20]. According to the National Institutes of Health, USA 95 percent of all diabetes is Type 2. Being a lifestyle disease, it triggered by obesity, lack of exercise, increased age, and to some degree genetic predisposition [11, 21, 22]. In T2D, pancreas produces relatively inadequate (in insulin resistance) or more than normal amount of insulin, but the cells (particularly fat and muscle cells) lack the sensitivity to insulin. In addition to the problems with increased insulin resistance, the release of insulin by the pancreas may also be defective and suboptimal. In fact, there is a steady decline in β-cells that contribute to worsening glucose control. Hence, many patients require insulin therapy. Moreover, despite elevated glucose levels, the liver continues to produce glucose through gluconeogenesis as its control becomes compromised.

The symptoms of T2D are similar to type 1. As overweight plays a role in decreased responsiveness to insulin the kids who develop type 2 are overweight. Some can be successfully treated with dietary changes, exercise, and oral medication, or with insulin injections, particularly to reduce the risk of long-term health problems. Usually it occurs in individuals over 30 years of age and increases with age, but an alarming number of patients are now affected in their teen years. In fact, T2D is now more common than T1D in childhood [23], mostly due to poor eating habits, higher body weight, and lack of exercise. Moreover, a strong genetic component and obesity are other risk factors, and there is a direct relationship between the degree of obesity and the risk of developing type 2 diabetes.

It is estimated that the chance of developing T2D doubles for every 20% increase over desirable body weight. Data shows that for each decade after 40 years of age, regardless of weight, there is an increase in incidence of diabetes [24]. The prevalence of diabetes in 65 to 74 years of age is nearly 20%, and is more common in certain ethnic groups like 6% in Caucasians, 10% in African and Asian Americans, 15% in Hispanics and 20-50% in certain Native American communities [1, 24]. It has been reported that diabetes affects about 23.6 million (7.8%) people in US, and is a leading cause of death and disability, that costs $174 billion per year [25]. Though it is a disease of any age, but family history of diabetes, age, overweight and sedentary life style, African Americans, Alaska Natives, American Indians, Asian Americans, Native Hawaiians, Pacific Islander Americans, and Hispanics/Latinos are more vulnerable [26].

Gestational Diabetes: The third type of diabetes is minor one, called *gestational diabetes* (GD). During pregnancy it can occur temporarily, as significant hormonal changes during pregnancy can lead to blood sugar elevation in genetically predisposed individuals. The GD affects about 4% of all pregnant women globally [27], usually during the second trimester and resolves once the baby is born. However, 25%-50% of women with GD will eventually develop T2D later in life, especially those who require insulin during pregnancy, and who remain overweight after their delivery. If GD is not controlled, complications can affect both mother and baby. Therefore, a diet and exercise plan, along with medication is necessary. Patients with GD are advised to undergo an oral glucose tolerance test about six weeks after giving birth to determine if their diabetes has persisted beyond the pregnancy, or if any evidence, such as impaired glucose tolerance, is present that may be a clue to the patient's future risk for developing diabetes.

Other Types of Diabetes: A number of other types of diabetes exist and a person may exhibit more than one type. For example, in LADA (or type 1.5 diabetes or double diabetes) people show signs of both type 1 and type 2. The types of diabetes caused by genetic defects of beta cell are *maturity-onset diabetes of the young* (MODY) or *neonatal diabetes mellitus* (NDM). The genetic defects in insulin action, resulting inability to control blood glucose levels is seen in *leprechaunism* and the *Rabson-Mendenhall syndrome*. The diseased or damaged pancreas (like pancreatitis and cystic fibrosis) may lead to diabetes. Even the excess amounts of hormone like cortisol in *Cushing's syndrome* work against the action of insulin. Medications, such as glucocorticoids, or chemicals that destroy beta cells, infections (like congenital rubella, cytomegalovirus), rare immune-mediated disorders (such as *stiff-man syndrome*, an autoimmune disease of the central nervous system found in one third of people), genetic syndromes (such as *Down syndrome*, *Klinefelter's syndrome*, *Huntington's chorea*, *porphyria* and *Prader-Willi syndrome*) and *diabetes insipidus* also reduce insulin action. In other autoimmune diseases like systemic lupus erythematosus, patients may have anti-insulin receptor antibodies that cause diabetes by interfering with the binding of insulin to body tissues [4].

Thus, the development of this heterogeneous, polygenic disease is a multifactorial, multi step process characterized by a defect in insulin's secretion and action. Long before the development of full blown diabetes the body cells undergoes a pre-diabetic condition when the cells becoming resistant to insulin or pancreas is unable to produce as much insulin as required. Thus, the blood glucose levels are higher than normal, but not high enough to be called diabetes; and this is known as "pre diabetic" or *impaired fasting glucose* or *impaired glucose tolerance.* Thus, diagnosis of pre-diabetes is a warning sign of future diabetes. The good news is anyone can prevent the development of Type 2 diabetes by losing weight, making changes in diet, using food supplements if required and exercising.

Genetic defects in beta cells and Insulin action cause several forms of diabetes. The inheritable monogenic forms of diabetes result from mutations, or changes, in a single gene. Most mutations in monogenic diabetes (NDM and MODY) reduce the body's ability to produce insulin. Genetic testing can diagnose most forms of monogenic diabetes. NDM occurs in the first 6 months of life and infants cannot produce enough insulin, leading to increased blood glucose level. MODY usually occurs during adolescence or early adulthood, but sometimes remains undiagnosed until later in life. A number of different gene mutations have been shown to cause MODY, all of which limit the pancreas' ability to produce insulin and ultimately high blood glucose levels. While the genetic defects in insulin action, changes in insulin receptor leads to mild hyperglycaemia, high blood glucose or severe diabetes. Symptoms include *acanthosis nigricans*, characterized by darkened skin patches, enlarged and cystic ovaries plus virilization and the development of excess facial hair. In children, *leprechaunism* and the *Rabson-Mendenhall syndrome* cause extreme insulin resistance.

The injuries to the pancreas from trauma or disease (pancreatitis, infection, pancreatic cancer, cystic fibrosis and hemochromatosis) or surgical removal may cause "secondary" diabetes. A number of *medications* and *chemicals* (pentamidine, nicotinic acid, glucocorticoids, thyroid hormone, phenytoin, anti HIV/AIDS drugs *etc.*) can interfere with insulin secretion, leading to diabetes in people with insulin resistance. Diabetes can also result from the disturbances of certain hormones, such as excessive growth hormone production (*acromegaly*), excess cortisol from adrenal glands (*Cushing's syndrome*), glucagon in glucagonoma, and epinephrine in pheochromocytoma. In acromegaly, a pituitary gland tumor at the base of the brain causes excessive production of growth hormone, leading to hyperglycaemia.

Metabolic Changes in Carbohydrate Metabolism: Although human diets are variable, carbohydrate accounts for the bulk proportion of daily intake. Depending on food habit (meal eater or feeder) some of the dietary carbohydrate is converted and metabolized as fat (lipogenesis). In human the frequency of taking meals and extent of carbohydrates converting to fat has a direct relationship with artherosclerosis, obesity and diabetes mellitus. The carbohydrate is metabolized to glucose, fructose (from sucrose) and galactose (from lactose). Both fructose and galactose are readily converted to glucose by the liver. The metabolism of carbohydrate takes place by glycolysis (oxidation of starch/glycogen to pyruvate and lactate by Embden-Meyerhof pathway), glycogenesis (synthesis of glycogen from glucose), glycogenolysis (the breakdown of glycogen to glucose in liver, and pyruvate and lactate in muscle), and oxidation of pyruvate to acetyl coenzyme A by hexose monophosphate shunt or pentose phosphate pathway and gluconeogenesis.

Source of Blood Glucose: Glucose in blood is mainly derived from the dietary carbohydrate, other glucogenic compounds (by gluconeogenesis), and from liver glycogen (by glycogenolysis). Dietary carbohydrate (starch from plant/glycogen from animal food), and disaccharides (sucrose from refined sugar, lactose in milk) undergoes digestion in the gut to monosaccharide's (glucose/fructose/galactose), that are transported to the liver and converted to glucose. The liver has a central role in the storage and distribution of all fuels. Then the glucose is either: (i) catabolised to ATP in peripheral tissues like brain, muscle and kidney; (ii) stored as glycogen in liver and muscle; or (iii) converted to fatty acids. The fatty acids are stored in adipose tissue as triglycerides. The conversion of glucose from other glucogenic compounds by gluconeogenesis includes some amino acids, propionate and the products of some partial metabolites of glucose in liver and kidney (glucose), and skeletal muscle and RBC (lactate), which goes to blood *via Cori cycle*. On the other hand, the acylglycerol of adipose tissue is hydrolysed to glycerol and then diffuse to blood for its transport and finally converted to glucose by gluconeogenesis in liver and kidney.

Glucose Catabolism: Glucose is oxidised by tissues to synthesise ATP. During the complete oxidation of glucose by *glycolysis* six carbon glucose molecule ($C_6H_{12}O_6$) cleaves into two molecules of the three carbon pyruvate ($C_3H_3O_3^-$), with the net production of two molecules of ATP per glucose. In the later part of this path one oxidation occurs, using NAD (a co-factor) as the electron acceptor.

The NAD is limited in cell and once reduced (NADH), must be re-oxidised for recycling. This re-oxidation occurs by *anaerobic glycolysis* where pyruvate is reduced to lactate (by oxidation of NADH to NAD) in absence of oxygen (in exercising muscle where oxygen supplies are often insufficient for aerobic metabolism). However, when molecular oxygen is available the pyruvate is transported inside mitochondria for *aerobic* oxidation into acetyl coenzyme A, using NAD as electron acceptor. By a further series of reactions (*citric acid cycle*) acetyl CoA is oxidised to CO_2. These reactions are coupled to *electron transport chain* which harness chemical bond energy from a series of oxido-reduction reactions to the synthesis of ATP and re-oxidising NADH to NAD. Fast twitch muscle fibres utilise the first mechanisms; while heavily exercising muscle can use this pathway as the sole source of ATP synthesis for a short period of time. This probably evolved as a defence mechanism in humans. The formation of lactate as an end product from glucose extracts small amount of the bond energy of glucose and accumulation of lactate reduce intracellular pH. Thus, lactate is either (i) converted back to pyruvate, and then further oxidised by the second mechanism described above, to produce a large amount of ATP; or (ii) converted back to glucose in the liver by *gluconeogenesis*. It uses some of the reactions of glycolysis in the reverse direction along with some unique reactions to re-synthesise glucose, using ATP. Thereby maintaining a circulating glucose concentration in the bloodstream (even in the absence of dietary supply) and also maintaining glucose supply to fast twitch muscle fibres. The partially oxidising glucose as lactate (in muscle), is transported to the liver for conversion back to glucose and then re-supplying it to muscle, with a much higher energy yield than the 2 ATP/glucose produced by glycolysis alone. This co-operative cycle utilising both the muscle and liver tissue is called the **Cori cycle** (Fig. **1**). Both of these mechanisms illustrate the interdependence of tissues on each other and the co-operative activities between organs responsible for total metabolic activities.

Interconversion of Glycogen and Glucose: Glycogen, a highly branched polymer of glucose is a compact polar molecule efficiently stored in the limited space in liver and muscle tissue with associated water, and as aggregates of glycogen molecules within cells (as glycogen granules) of which up to 70% is water. The glycogen store of liver and muscle tissues are presented in Table **1**:

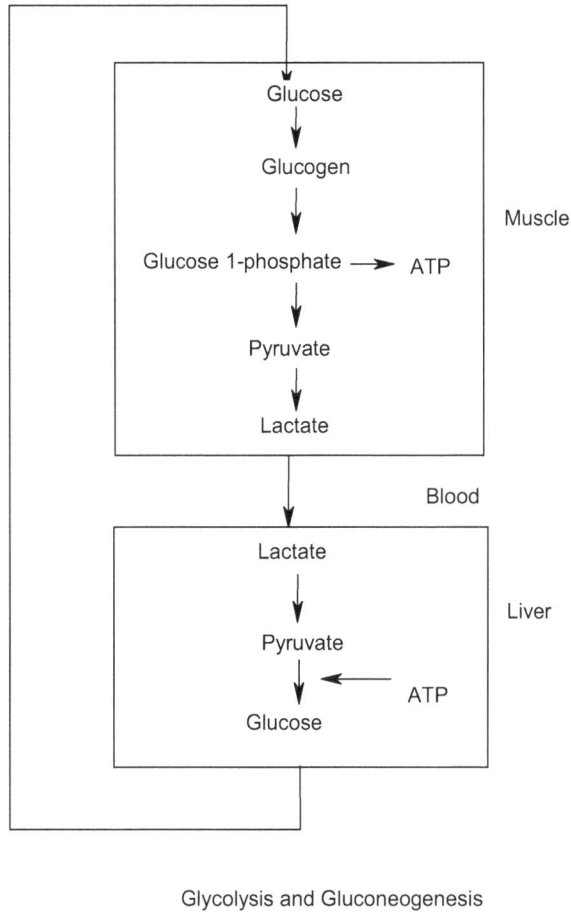

Glycolysis and Gluconeogenesis

Figure 1: Cori Cycle

Table 1: Glycogen Store of Liver and Muscle Tissues.

Organ/tissue	Mass (Kg)	Glycogen (gm/kg tissue)	Total Glucose (gm)
Liver	1.6	56	~ 100
Muscle	28	14	~ 400

The amount of glycogen in muscle changes substantially between the fed state and following heavy exercise, while its store in the liver is more constant and falls substantially after prolonged starvation. In both muscle and liver there is interconversion between the monomer glucose and the polymer glycogen. This has the potential to be a futile cycle wasting energy if the interconversion occurred continuously to meet the body's glucose requirements at a particular time.

ACTION OF INSULIN

Hormonal Control of Glycogen Metabolism: The control operates through different enzymes catalysing the synthesis and breakdown of glycogen, only one is active at any one time and thus the pathway can proceed in only one direction, either towards glycogen synthesis or towards glycogen breakdown and mobilisation of free glucose. The control is exerted by hormones on the activity of the key enzymes, though there are some differences in the hormone action in liver and muscle (Table **2**).

Table 2: Hormones of Sugar Metabolism, their Source and Action on Target Tissue

Hormone	Source	Target Tissue	Action
Glucagon	Pancreas	Liver	Stimulates glycogen breakdown
Adrenaline	Adrenals	Muscle	Stimulates glycogen breakdown
Insulin	Pancreas	Liver and Muscle	Stimulates glycogen synthesis

The storage hormone insulin acts as an off and on switches on several enzymatically controlled pathways as shown in Fig. **2**.

In normal subjects, fasting blood glucose is maintained constant by hepatic glucose output, while after an overnight fast nearly 75% of hepatic glucose output is by glycogenolysis and the rest by gluconeogenesis from lactate, alanine, glycerol and pyruvate in order of preference. Hepatic output is controlled by basal levels of insulin and glucagon (as their concentration in peripheral circulation is lower than portal vein). At least 70% of extra hepatic glucose utilization occurs in insulin-insensitive tissues like brain, RBC, renal medulla. In T2D fasting blood glucose is raised proportionately to hepatic glucose output [28] as fasting plasma insulin are normal and elevated hepatic glucose output is likely to reflect a degree of hepatic insulin insensitivity [29]. The fast pass hepatic glucose extraction in normal subjects is low and over 90% of an oral glucose load reaches the peripheral circulation [30]. Over subsequent few hours about one third of glucose is cleared by the liver. The post meal hyperinsulinemia inhibits lypolysis and stimulates storage of fatty acids and glycogen as glycogen in muscle and liver and as triacylglycerol in adipose tissue.

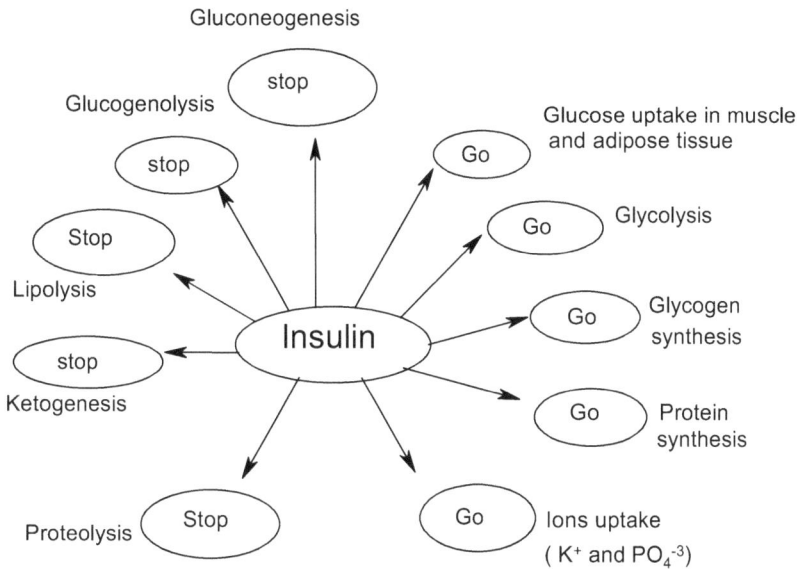

Figure 2: Schematic representation of insulin action.

GLUCOSE METABOLISM IN ABSENCE OF INSULIN

Diabetes type 1 is a fatal disease when insulin secretion totally fails following an autoimmune attack on the pancreatic beta-cells. This is in sharp contrast to starvation where insulin secretion, while reduced, is sufficient to regulate fat and carbohydrate metabolism. The total lack of insulin or lack of its response (insulin resistance) leads to two metabolic crises; a marked increase in lipolysis in adipose tissue and activation of hepatic gluconeogenesis in spite of high plasma glucose levels. The dramatically increased rate of lipolysis in adipose tissue follows the lack of insulin-inhibition of hormone-sensitive lipase. The increase in fatty acids results to a massive synthesis of ketone bodies in the liver. These ketone bodies then exceed the buffer capacity of the blood, leading to ketoacidosis. As excess acid (ketoacidosis) is a poison for the brain, leading to coma and death. In spite of this many-fold increase in blood glucose levels hepatic gluconeogenesis (using amino acids as a substrate) becomes activated in diabetes. This is because insulin is an important inhibitor of glucagon secretion and hepatic gluconeogenesis (Fig. **2**). Hyperglycemia causes loss of glucose to urine and, as urine is isoosmotic with blood, loss of water and electrolytes follows. Thus, untreated type 1 diabetics can lose carbohydrate equivalent to two loafs of bread per day!

The high levels of glucose in diabetes 1 and 2 are toxic, that lead to the formation of sorbitol in the lens of the eye, increasing osmotic pressure and disturbing protein synthesis. This is one explanation of the development of gray star in diabetics. The major toxic effect of glucose is probably glycation of proteins. It is believed that much of the neurological and circulatory defects in diabetes are due to glycation. Thus, glycated haemoglobin HbA_{1c} levels are used as indicators of long-term blood sugar levels.

REGULATION OF HEPATIC GLUCOGENESIS AND POSTPRANDIAL BLOOD GLUCOSE BY HYPOTHALAMIC K_{ATP} CHANNELS

Blood sugar levels dependent upon glucose uptake after meals and hepatic release of glucose between meals. The sugar released from the liver comes either from stored glycogen or production of glucose from lactate and amino acids, which largely responsible for stabilization of postprandial blood sugar levels. The hyperglycemia in type 2 diabetes partially results from lack of control over hepatic glucose formation due to resistance to insulin. Recently it is known that part of insulin effect occurs indirectly through insulin-sensitive receptors in the hypothalamus. Pocai *et al.*, (2005) [31] demonstrated that insulin stimulates the hypothalamic K_{ATP} channels with neural control of hepatic gluconeogenesis. Insulin stimulation of hypothalamic K_{ATP} channels results in vagus nerve signalling to the liver and inhibition of gluconeogenesis. This is part of the normal response to meals and following insulin release from the pancreatic β-cells. Thus, signalling from the brain is one of the important controls which establish correct level "between-meal". Thus hypothalamic insulin resistance and loss of control over hepatic gluconeogenesis is one of the important factors for the development of type 2 diabetes.

The overall metabolism in diabetes, both type 1 and type 2 is summarized in Fig **3**.

BIOCHEMISTRY OF DIABETES

The hallmark of diabetes mellitus (DM) is body's inability to control blood glucose, which is manifested by two major chemical syndromes: one characterized by insulin dependence (IDDM) at early age with weight loss and ketonuria, while the second characterized by relatively later onset, with insulin

Insulin Deficiency and Glucose Excess

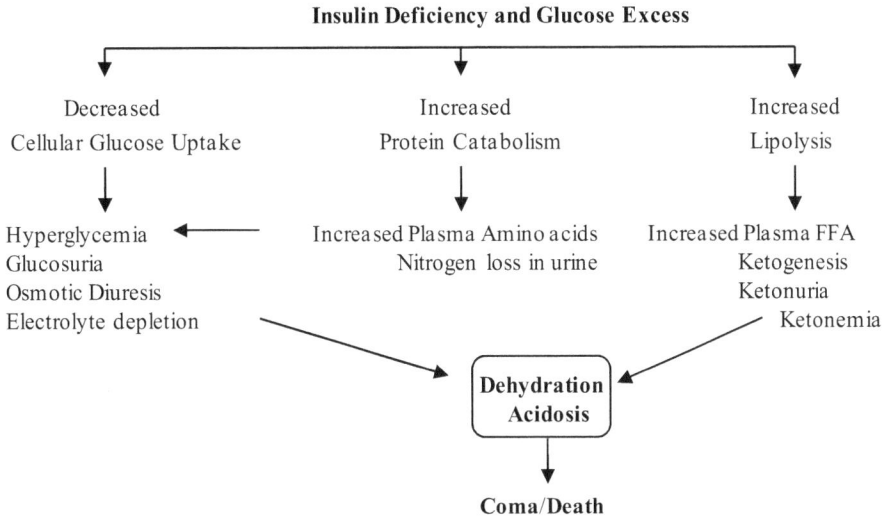

Figure 3: A summary of metabolism in uncontrolled (type I) and severe uncontrolled (type 2) diabetes (Redrawn from *Harper review of Biochemistry*).

insensitivity and partial insulin deficiency (NIDDM). First one is the consequence of an autoimmune-mediated destruction of pancreatic β-cells, leading to insulin deficiency, while second one is due to insulin resistance and relative insulin deficiency. It usually occurs in obese individuals and is associated with hypertension and dyslipidaemia. The capacity of nutrients to stimulate insulin release from the β-cell can augment oxidative fluxes in the islet cells [32]. Moreover, oxidative stress associated with insulin resistance and NIDDM [33] contributes to poor insulin action [34]. Thus, the treatment aims to reduce insulin resistance (diet, exercise and drug therapy) and to stimulate insulin secretion. In DM, oxidative stress appears to be due to an increased production of free radicals and or a sharp reduction of antioxidant defences [35-38]. Oxygen-derived free radicals have been implicated in the pathophysiology of various diseases, including diabetes mellitus [39]. It is well known that superoxide anion (the primary radical) formed by the reduction of molecular oxygen may lead to secondary radicals or reactive oxygen species (ROS) such as hydrogen peroxide and hydroxyl radical [40, 41]. It was reported that increased oxidative stress is involved in the pathogenesis and progression of diabetic tissue damage [42] and diabetes induces changes in antioxidant enzymes in various tissues [35]. Diabetes mellitus is characterized by (i) increased glycoxidation associated with the advanced oxidative stress [43]; (ii) presence of higher glucose or glycated protein that enhances lipid peroxidation and lipid peroxides that may increase the glycation end-products [44, 45]; (iii) oxidative stress results from autoxidation of glucose [46] and increased level of ROS that contribute hypercoagulable state, and the accumulation of oxidation products [47]. As hyperglycemia and hyperinsulinemia are the causes of enhanced free radical production, so, important biochemical defects caused by ROS need to be explained.

MECHANISMS OF OXYGEN FREE RADICALS (ROS) PRODUCTION

Hyperglycemia is a widely known cause of enhanced plasma free radical concentrations, where free radical production occurs through four different routes: (i) increased glycolysis; (ii) intercellular activation of sorbitol (polyol) pathway; (iii) auto-oxidation of glucose and (iv) non-enzymatic protein glycation.

Increased Glycolysis: Hyperglycemia seems to enhance non-oxidative metabolism of glucose to lactate through increasing glucose-6-phosphate, and $NADH/NAD^+$ ratio. In accelerated glycolysis, oxidation of glyceraldehydes 3-phosphate (GAP) to 1,3-biphosphoglycerate (1,3-DPG) by GAP dehydrogenase becomes rate limiting, by reduction of NAD^+ to NADH. In the cytosol NADH is oxidized to NAD^+ by lactate dehydrogenase, coupled to the reduction of pyruvate to lactate. Thus, the increase in the ratio of $NADH/NAD^+$ will reflect increased lactate/pyruvate ratio. The increased rate of glycolysis increases free cytosolic $NADH/NAD^+$ ratio (redox imbalance) resulting from a disequilibrium between the rate of oxidation of GAP to 1,3-DPG and the rate of reduction of pyruvate. This indicates that, the increased glycolysis, a consequence of diabetes, is related to an increase in $NADH/NAD^+$ ratio due to impaired oxidation of NADH to NAD^+. *Increased sorbital pathway*: One of the consequences of hyperglycemia in diabetes is increased metabolism of glucose by the sorbitol pathway (Fig. **4**), an insignificant pathway in normal glycemic condition. It leads to the accumulation of both sorbitol (not permeable to cell membrane) and fructose is one of the main metabolic disturbances in diabetic hyperglycemia [48]. Here, glucose is reduced to sorbitol by aldose reductase, coupled with oxidation of $NADH/NAD^+$. Sorbitol is then oxidized to fructose by the reduction of NAD^+ to NADH using sorbitol dehydrogenase. NADH is required for the conversion of

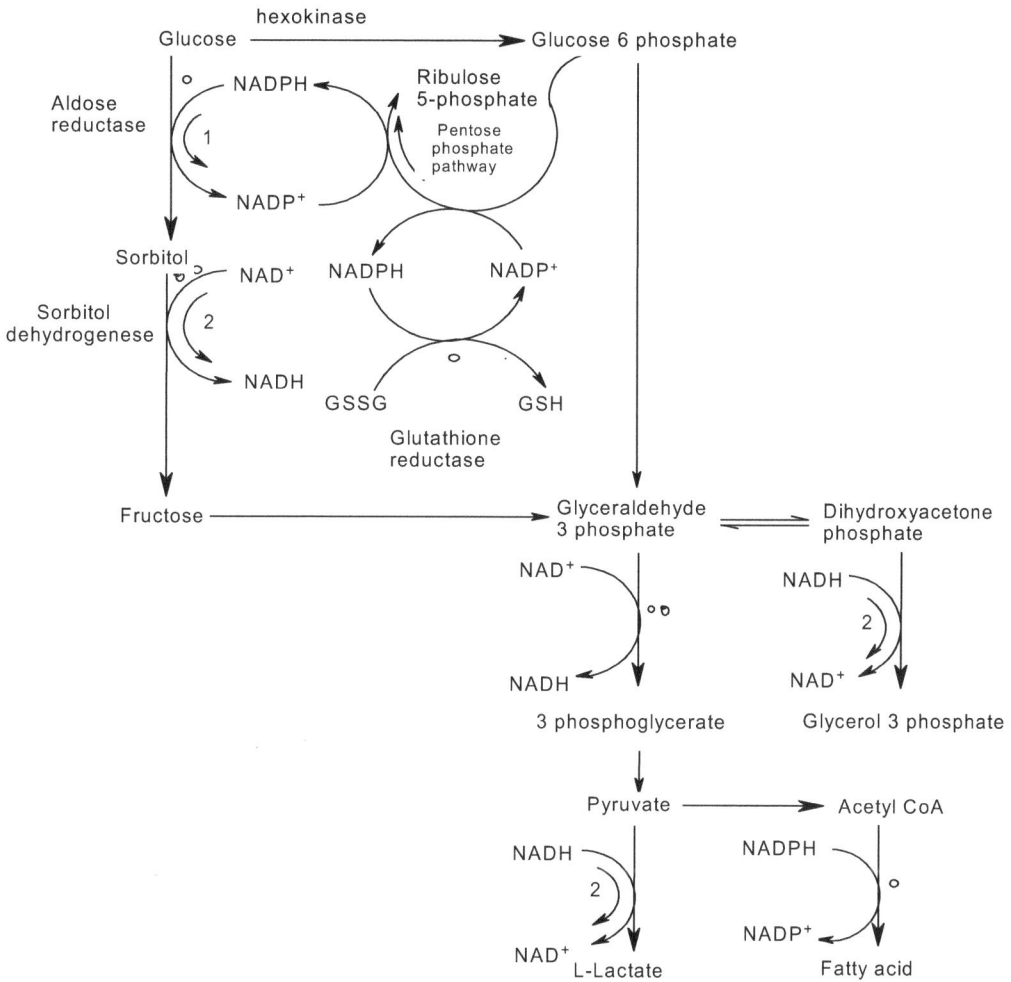

Figure 4: Sorbitol Pathway and its correlation with Glycolysis and Pentose Phosphate Pathway. The sorbitol pathway involves the conversion of glucose to sorbitol by *aldolase reductase* and sorbitol to fructose by *sorbitol dehydrogenase*. Reaction coupled to oxidation of NADPH are shown by* and reactions coupled by NAD+ by**. *Aldose reductase* competes with *glutathione reductase* for NADPH while *sorbitol dehydrogenase* competes with *glyceraldehydes 3 phosphate dehydrogenase* for NAD+. 1. increased flux through *aldolase reductase* favours an increased activity of PPP and increased flux through *sorbitol dehydrogenase* favours increased conversion of dihydroxyacetone phosphate to glycerol 3-phosphate and decreased conversion of glyceraldehydes 3-phosphate to 3-phosphoglycerate (After Taylor and Agius, 1988 [29]).

oxidized to reduced glutathione, a powerful antioxidant which protects cellular components from oxidative damage, and for fatty acid and cholesterol biosynthesis. Earlier studies suggested that the tissue injury caused by increased sorbitol pathway may be due to: (i) the decreased availability of NADPH (required for maintenance of reduced glutathione) which is oxidized to $NADP^+$ through reduction of glucose to sorbitol by aldose reductase; (ii) the competition between aldose reductase and glutathione reductase for NADPH cofactor depletes reduced glutathione [48]. Interestingly GSH depletion can play a role in increased oxygen free radicals production, that lead to oxidative tissue damage; (iii) increased $NADH/NAD^+$ ratio mediated oxidation of sorbitol to fructose by NAD^+-dependent sorbitol dehydrogenase. Ceriello *et al.* 1996 [49] reported that NADH produced in the cytoplasm by oxidation of sorbitol to fructose is transported to the mitochondria for oxidation by respiratory chain generates superoxide radical and other oxygen reactive species. Thus, an increase in the cytosolic NADH may be accompanied by increased load of mitochondrial NADH, which in turn leads to increased oxygen radicals generation.

Auto-Oxidation of Glucose: Glucose is found to be auto-oxidized in a cell-free system under physiological conditions *via* enediol tautomer formation that generates hydrogen peroxide, hydroxyl and superoxide radicals, and ketoaldehydes [50, 51] when catalyzed by the transition metal iron [51]. Several reports indicated that glucose auto-oxidation occurred in diabetes and responsible for generation of increased oxygen radicals [52].

Non-Enzymatic Glycosylation of Proteins: Non-enzymatic glycation is a spontaneous chemical reaction between glucose and the amino groups of proteins forming reversible Shift bases and more stable Amadori products [53]. Further auto-oxidation of Amadori product produced advanced glycation end products (AGE) which bind to specific cellular receptors [54, 55], as found in receptor for AGEs on endothelial cells [56], monocytes/macrophages, mesangial cells, neurons and smooth muscle cells. Interaction of AGEs with endothelial surface receptor generates intracellular oxidative stress and therapy modulates cellular functions, even in presence of antioxidant mechanisms. This process is probably enhanced and amplified when antioxidant defense mechanisms are reduced [57].

MECHANISMS OF OXYGEN FREE RADICALS PRODUCTION IN INCREASED INSULIN PRODUCTION

Decline in physical fitness, increase in body fatness and upper body fat distribution are frequently associated with increased insulin production or hyperinsulinemia and insulin resistance. Several evidence indicates the relationship between hyperinsulinemia and free radical production. When human fat cells are exposed to insulin a time-and dose-dependent accumulation of hydrogen peroxidase occur by bypassing the receptor kinase step. In addition, increased insulin concentration in experimental animals, following *i.p.* injection of dextrose, is found to be associated with increased free radical production. Since fasting hyperinsulinemia is considered to be a hallmark of insulin resistance, a relationship between insulin resistance and plasma free radical concentration cannot be excluded [58]. Therefore, the genesis of free radical concentration in insulin resistant conditions might be due to: (i) an insulin-mediated over activity of the sympathetic nervous system and increase free radical production through higher metabolic rate and auto-oxidation by catecholamines; and (ii) the elevation in plasma non-esterified fatty acid concentration, as insulin resistance is associated with elevated fasting plasma non-esterified fatty acid concentration. The imbalance in generation and scavenging of free radicals is important in determining diabetic tissue damage. The primary cellular damage resulting from free radical is lipid peroxidation, along with changes in cellular lipid structures [59], due to peroxidative deterioration of unsaturated fatty acids of membrane phospho-lipids. The net effect is the generation of highly toxic peroxyl radicals (ROO⁻) that produce lipid hydroperoxides due to their closeness with other lipids of the biomembranes [60]. While hypoinsulinemia increases the activity of fatty acyl-CoA oxidase that indicates 3-oxidation of fatty acids resulting in increased production of H_2O_2.

CHANGES IN ANTIOXIDANT ENZYME ACTIVITIES

Studies on the tissue levels of the antioxidant enzymes in diabetes revealed varying results. In experimental diabetes only the catalase activity was increased in vascular tissues but not the superoxide dismutase and glutathione peroxidase, though Wohaieb and Godin (1987) [61] showed increased activities of catalase (CAT) and superoxide dismutase (SOD) in the pancreas of diabetic rats, while the liver showed a generalized decrease in CAT, SOD and glutathione peroxidase (GSH-Px) activities. Earlier, the increase in the activities of both CAT and SOD occurred in the tissue with the lowest antioxidant enzymatic activities (pancreas) before onset of diabetes, suggesting a compensatory response to an increase in endogenous oxidant radicals in pancreas by diabetes. A decrease in reduced glutathione (GSH) has been observed in erythrocytes from diabetic subjects, due to decreases in activities of the enzymes involved in GSH synthesis (such as γ-glutamycystein synthetase) or in the transport rate of oxidized glutathione from erythrocytes [62] and enhanced sorbitol pathway [48]. In addition a decrease in the activity of glutathione reductase that reduces glutathione has also been reported [63]. Kazuhiro *et al.* (1989) [64] and Matkovics *et al.* (1998) [65] elucidated that glutathione reductase activity decreased in erythrocyte hemolysates of diabetic rats due to decrease enzyme glycation by the uncontrolled hyperglycemia. Dominguez *et al.* (1998) [66] reported a significant decrease of erythrocyte peroxidase activity in diabetic children and adolescents compared with control, due to a decline in blood glutathione content, since GSH is a substrate and cofactor for this enzyme. Therefore, low GSH content indicates low peroxidase activity, which may produce increased oxidative stress. Moreover, enzyme inactivation either through glycation or of increased oxidative stress might contribute to low GSH-Px activity [67].

OXIDATIVE STRESS IN DIABETES

Both radical and non-radical oxidants induce lipid peroxidation particularly of unsaturated fatty acid containing lipoproteins. The reaction between a superoxide anion and nitric oxide produces peroxynitrite, a powerful oxidant of low-density lipoproteins [68]. The evidence for oxidative damage in diabetes was first reported in 1979 [69] that the average level of lipid peroxides in plasma is higher in diabetic patients, and much higher in patients with diabetic angiopathy, than in normal people. This high level of lipid peroxide in plasma may cause an increased peroxide levels in the blood vessel to initiate atherosclerosis. Recent studies reported similar oxidation of plasma low density lipoprotein (LDL) from diabetic patients and found auto-antibodies against oxidatively modified LDL in type I diabetic patients, suggesting that LDL oxidation occurs *in vivo* in diabetes [70]. Lipid peroxidation is thought to be responsible for the pathogenesis of many degenerative disorders including naturally occurring and chemically induced DM [71]. Lipid hydroperoxides (LHP) produced from a variety of long-chain polyunsaturated fatty acid precursors *via* intermediate radical reactions, involve oxygen and metal cations (iron and copper). The combined reactions generate highly reactive and cytotoxic lipid radicals, which in turn generate new LHP, which then transported in the systemic circulation by low- and high-density lipoproteins. When released locally, LHP produce structural damage [72]. This peroxidative regulation occurs through lipid and water-soluble antioxidants, as well as by antioxidant enzymes, *i.e.*, dioxide (1-) dismutase, peroxidase and catalase.

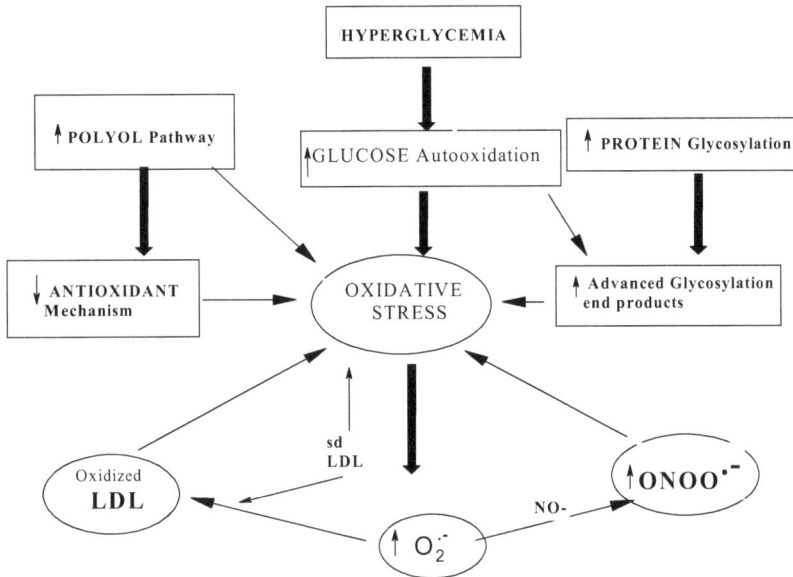

Figure 5: Pathogenesis of hyperoxidative stress in non-insulin dependent diabetes. Major mechanisms directly related to hyperglycaemia (shown in boxes), and some others that result from the reaction of free radicals with lipoproteins (e.g. small dense LDL, sd LDL) and nitric oxide (NO), oxidised LDL, oxidized LDL- ONOO, and peroxynitrite (in circle) (After Ahmaed, 2005[92]).

Moreover, increased generation of free radicals (oxidative stress) in diabetes was observed from *in vitro* experiments [39, 73]. The primary causal factor is hyperglycaemia which operates through several mechanisms (Fig. **5**), although the individual contribution of each mechanism to hyperoxidative stress remains undefined, as does the dose response relationship between hyperglycaemia and overall oxidative stress. Glycoxidation of glucose generates ROS, such as superoxide, hydrogen peroxide and hydroxyl radical [39] that accelerate the formation of advanced glycosylation end-products (AGEs) which in turn generate more free radicals [39, 53]. Increased cellular uptake of glucose stimulates protein kinase C activity which also activates peroxidase enzymes and the cyclooxygenase (COX) pathway [74, 75], resulting in overproduction of oxidative molecules. By elevating endothelial calcium level, hyperglycaemia stimulates the synthesis of nitric oxide [76], which can be converted into the highly potent oxidant peroxynitrite (ONOO⁻) [77]. Impaired antioxidant defences and decreased tissue concentrations of antioxidants vitamin E, SOD and CAT contribute to net oxidative stress. Although it is extremely difficult to measure free radicals *in vivo*, but some reports of increased oxidative stress in diabetes and coronary heart disease have been derived from diabetic patients [78, 79]. Increased oxidative stress provides a plausible pathobiological basis for the direct association between hyperglycaemia and increased cardiovascular risk in diabetes [80]. In spite of some evidence [81], definitive clinical proof for the role of oxidative stress in the pathogenesis of atherosclerosis remains outstanding. Insulin resistance and increased oxidative stress observed in obese Type 2 diabetic patients [82], suggest a relationship between insulin action and oxidative stress [83]. A decrease of oxidative stress could therefore improve insulin action in insulin resistance subjects. Hence, the drugs or dietary components acting like free radical scavengers are promising tool in the treatment of patients with increased oxidative stress.

On the other hand, plasma lipid peroxide levels of diabetics are found to be significantly higher than healthy individuals [84]. Furthermore, an increase in thiobarbituric acid reaction in poorly controlled diabetic and diabetic angiopathy is considered as a cause of organ or tissue degeneration. In adult diabetic patients significantly higher level of thiobarbituric acid reactive substances (TBARS) provide an indirect measurement of lipid peroxidation and decreased erythrocyte antioxidant enzyme activities [85, 86]. Hence, TBARS is considered as an indicator of free radical production. An increase in TBARS level in liver may therefore be due to increased oxidative stress that promotes DNA and protein alterations including changes in the enzyme activities implicated in lipid metabolism and free radicals scavenging process [87]. Also, increased oxidative stress in DM may be a reason for such decrease in erythrocytes count and hyperglycemia that burden the cells with extra free radicals [88]. This, coupled with reduced GSH in diabetic erythrocytes [89] can cause peroxidative breakdown of phospholipids fatty acids in the erythrocytes membrane. This is supported by the fact that erythrocytes of diabetic patients are more susceptible to lipid peroxidation when treated with hydrogen peroxide *in vitro* [90]. In addition, the decrease in hematocrit (PCV) percentage may be attributed to the reduction in the total RBC count and the failure in blood osmoregulation and plasma osmolarity [91].

OXIDATIVE MODIFICATION OF PROTEINS AND LIPOPROTEINS

Oxidative damage to biological macromolecules occurs by non-radical oxidants (hydrogen peroxide, hypochlorous acid or singlet oxygen), and by ROS (superoxide anion, hydroxyl radicals). These oxidants attack the double bonds in unsaturated fatty acids resulting in the formation of lipid peroxides. Oxygen radicals, particularly the very aggressive hydroxyl radical, can also oxidize apolipoproteins and other plasma proteins. The decrease in the total proteins concentration in serum of diabetic animals ascribed to (i) decreased amino acids uptake [93], (ii) greatly decreased concentration of essential amino acids [94], (iii) increased conversion of glycogenic amino acids to CO_2 and H_2O [95] and (iv) reduction in protein synthesis and availability of mRNA [96]. Furthermore, in diabetes, the decrease of albumin concentration is evident in experimental condition. Thus regular dietary supply of nine essential amino acids to diabetic patients can be helpful to reduce the long term damage.

THE RELATION BETWEEN ATHEROGENESIS AND OXIDATIVE STRESS

Several observations revealed additional mechanisms relevant to atherogenesis both in type 2 diabetes and obese. These patients (type 2 diabetes and/or obesity) have an increased oxidative stress and inflammation. Increased oxidative stress is indicated by an increase in ROS generation by circulating mononuclear cells, increased lipid peroxidation, protein carbonylation [97], nitro-tyrosine formation [98], and DNA damage. Increased oxidative stress was also demonstrated in the obese, as reflected in increased lipid peroxidation, protein carbonylation, and ortho-tyrosine and meta-tyrosine formation. These changes reversed after caloric restriction to 1,000 calories/day for 4 weeks, as did ROS generation by leukocytes [99]. Similarly, glucose and macronutrient intake set up a state of oxidative stress and inflammation [100, 101]. Thus, there is a close link between type 2 diabetes and macronutrient intake, oxidative stress, inflammation, and obesity.

DISORDERS OF CARBOHYDRATE METABOLISM

Carbohydrates are polymers of simple (monosaccharide) and complex sugars (di, oligo and polysaccharides). Disaccharide like sucrose (cane sugar) consists of two monosaccharides glucose and fructose, while lactose (milk sugar) contains glucose and galactose. Both sucrose and lactose is broken down into their component sugars by enzymes before the body absorb and use them. The carbohydrates of foods are broken down by the body, and if the enzyme needed to process a certain sugar is missing, the sugar can accumulate in the body, causing problems. Table **3** represents the types and characteristics of glycogen storage diseases.

Table 3: Types and Characteristics of Glycogen Storage Diseases.

Type	Affected Tissues or Cells	Symptoms
O	Liver or muscle	Hypoglycemia episodes occur during fasting
IA (von Gierke's disease)	Liver, kidney	Enlarged kidney and liver, slow growth, very low blood sugar, abnormally high levels of acid, fats, uric acid
IB	Liver, WBC	Same but less severe than IA, Low WBC, recurring infections, inflammatory bowel disease
II Pompe's disease	All organs	Enlarged heart and liver, muscle weakness
III Forbes' disease	Liver, muscle, heart	Cirrhosis or enlarged liver, low blood sugar, damage muscle and heart, weak bones
IV Andersen's disease	Liver, muscle, tissues	Cirrhosis, muscle damage, delayed growth
V McArdle disease	Muscle	Weakness, Muscle cramps
VI Hers' disease	Liver	Low blood sugar, enlarged liver or no symptoms
VII Tarui's disease	RBC, Skeletal muscle	Hemolysis, muscle cramp.

1. Glycogen storage diseases or *glycogenoses* occur when there is a defect in the enzymes that are involved in the metabolism of glycogen, resulting in growth abnormalities, weakness, and confusion. These diseases are caused by lack of an enzyme needed to convert glucose into glycogen and break down glycogen into glucose. Typical symptoms include weakness, sweating, confusion, kidney stones, and stunted growth. The diagnosis is made by biopsy and the treatment depends on the type of disease that usually involves the regulation of carbohydrate intake. The glucose is the main source of energy for the muscles, heart and brain, and any unused glucose is reserved as glycogen in the liver, muscles, and kidneys and released when needed by the body. Glycogen consists straight (amylase) and branched chains (amylopectins) of many glucose molecules and there are many different glycogen storage diseases identified by Roman numeral (I-VII), which are caused by a hereditary lack of one of the essential enzymes of glucose into glycogen

and breaking down glycogen into glucose pathways. About 1 in 20,000 infants has some form of glycogen storage disease. The specific symptoms, age at which symptoms start and their severity vary considerably among these diseases. For types II, V and VII, the main symptom is weakness, while for I, III and VI, symptoms are low levels of blood sugar and protrusion of the abdomen (as excess or abnormal glycogen enlarge the liver). Low levels of sugar in the blood cause weakness, sweating, confusion, and sometimes seizures and coma. Other consequences are stunted growth, frequent infections, or sores in the mouth and intestines. Glycogen storage diseases tend to cause uric acid (a waste product) to accumulate in the joints (cause gout), and in the kidneys (cause kidney stones). In type I glycogen storage disease, kidney failure is common in the second decade or later life. The specific type of glycogen storage disease is diagnosed by biopsy of the affected tissue and treatment depends on the type of disease. For most types, eating many small carbohydrate-rich meals daily (taking uncooked cornstarch every 4 to 6 hours around the clock) helps prevent blood sugar levels from dropping. Sometimes it is necessary to supply carbohydrate solutions through a stomach tube all night to prevent low blood sugar levels from occurring at night.

2. Galactosemia or a high blood level of galactose is caused by lack of one of the enzymes necessary for metabolizing galactose (a sugar in lactose, fruits and vegetables). A deficient enzyme or liver dysfunction can alter the metabolism, leading to high levels of galactose in the blood (galactosemia). There are different forms of galactosemia, but in classic galactosemia a toxic metabolite to the liver and kidneys builds up, that damages the eye lens, causing cataract. Symptoms include vomiting, jaundice, diarrhoea, and abnormal growth. The diagnosis is based on a blood test, but even with adequate treatment, affected children develop mental and physical problems. Treatment involves complete elimination of milk and milk products from the diet.

3. Fructose intolerance, is a hereditary disorder caused by lack of the enzyme needed to metabolize fructose. As a result, a by-product of

fructose accumulates in the body, blocking the formation of glycogen and its conversion to glucose for use as energy. *Very small amounts of fructose cause low blood sugar (hypoglycemia) that leads to kidney and liver damage with sweating, confusion, sometimes seizures and coma.* Children who continue to eat fructose containing foods develop kidney and liver damage, resulting in jaundice, vomiting, mental deterioration, seizures, and death. Chronic symptoms include poor eating, failure to thrive, digestive symptoms, liver failure, and kidney damage. Early diagnosis and dietary restrictions can help to prevent serious problems and diagnosis is made by chemical examination of liver tissue to determine the missing enzyme. Treatment involves excluding fructose (sweet fruits), sucrose, and sorbitol (a sugar substitute) from the diet.

4. *Mucopolysaccharidoses*, are a group of hereditary disorders when complex sugar molecules are not broken down normally due to the lack of necessary enzymes responsible for its break down and storage, leading to its accumulation in harmful amounts in the tissues. Thus, results are a characteristic facial appearance and abnormalities of the bones, eyes, liver, and spleen, or even by intellectual disability. Typical symptoms are short stature, hairiness, stiff finger joints, and coarseness of the face. The diagnosis is based on symptoms and a physical examination. Usually a normal life span is possible, but some types cause premature death.

PYRUVATE METABOLISM DISORDERS

Pyruvate metabolism disorders are caused due to lack one of the enzymes involved in its metabolism. The symptoms include seizures, intellectual disability, muscle weakness, and coordination problems. It can be controlled by diets that are either high in fat and low in carbohydrates or high in carbohydrates and low in protein. Pyruvate formed during the carbohydrates and proteins breakdown serves as an energy source. This problem therefore, limits the cell's ability to produce energy and allows a build up of lactic acid. A hereditary deficiency in any one of these enzymes results in one of a variety of disorders, depending on which enzyme is missing. Symptoms may develop any time between early infancy and late adulthood. Exercise and infections can worsen symptoms, leading to severe lactic acidosis, diagnosed by measuring enzyme activity in cells from the liver or skin.

Pyruvate dehydrogenase complex *deficiency* disorder is caused by the lack of a group of enzymes required to breakdown pyruvate, resulting in a variety of symptoms from mild to severe. Some newborns with this deficiency have brain malformations; others appear normal at birth but develop symptoms like weak muscles, seizures, poor coordination, and a severe balance problem later with intellectual disability. This disorder cannot be cured, but sometimes helped by a diet that is high in fat and low in carbohydrates.

Absence of pyruvate carboxylase enzyme causes a very rare condition that interferes with or blocks the production of glucose from pyruvate. Lactic acid and ketones build up in the blood with a variety of neurologic abnormalities. Often it is fatal, and children who survive have seizures and severe intellectual disability. There is no cure, but can be controlled by providing frequent carbohydrate-rich meals and restricting dietary protein.

HYPERTENSION

Hypertension or high blood pressure (BP) is the man made ailment caused by overeating, with refined grains, sugar, oils, margarine, inactivity, stress and smoking, as it was unknown in primitive cultures that eat diet of unprocessed foods. *Vicious Cycle*: high blood pressure is often accompanied with high level of insulin, which in turn may cause high blood pressure and make weight loss more difficult.

Nutritional Factors that Affect Blood Pressure

Sugar: Refined sugar raises insulin levels, which in turn may raise blood pressure. Sugar stresses the organ and glands that control blood pressure, and depletes many nutrients needed to lower BP.

Salt: Sodium salt leads to imbalances in many minerals and cause calcium depletion. It also increases the risk of hardening arteries and promotes stomach cancer.

Cadmium: It raises blood pressure, induces aggressive behaviour, and depletes blood pressure lowering minerals. The people with family history of diabetes can take the optimal amount of niacinamide, chromium, and essential fatty acids for prevention [102].

Several botanicals like *Garlic* (lower blood pressure); *Celery* (release smooth muscle of blood vessel lining and thereby reduces blood pressure); *Fish Oil* (reduces high blood pressure slowly at 2gm EPA/day when taken with calcium, magnesium, potassium, garlic, onion for better effect); *Vitamin C* (lowers high diastolic pressure, as with 1gm/day in their diet had the lowest blood pressure); *Calcium-Magnesium* (calcium (1000 mg) and magnesium (600 mg) together can lower blood pressure).

Potassium: low level of potassium raises blood pressure and calcium excretion. However, potassium depletion helps to retain more sodium that can increase blood pressure. Thus, potassium supplementation can lower blood pressure in long term with magnesium. The natural source of which is whole unprocessed foods like vegetable, fruits, fresh meat, fresh vegetable juice.

Chromium picolinate (controls sugar cravings, lowers insulin level, increases weight loss and leans tissue growth. It help to lower blood pressure and losing weight at 200-600 µg/day).

Taurine (an amino acid at 1-3 gm/day helps insulin be more effectively taken up by the body).

Co-Q10: high BP people are deficient in CoQ10. At 50-75 mg/day, it can lower blood pressure and protect against the damaging effect of high blood pressure. It also helps in weight loss and thereby reduces BP.

It is necessary to check blood pressure regularly and take medication because high BP should not be allowed to persist, as it is highly damaging to several organs. Patient can follow nutrition and lifestyle changes for controlling BP but it will take time to regulate the blood pressure. The ideal is to lose weight 1-2 pounds per week; regulate the BP regulating minerals like magnesium, potassium. Hypertension with overweight should restrict carbohydrates to grains, beans, legumes, fruits (40% of diet) and have to eliminate salty food, processed food, caffeinated beverages, sugar, margarine, fried food, refined flours, rice, oils, and stimulant like alcohol, kola, *Ephedra etc.* [102, 103].

RELATIONSHIP BETWEEN DIABETES AND HYPERTENSION

The relationship between diabetes and hypertension is complex and poorly understood. The information suggests that metabolic factors related to the obese state are importantly involved. The pertinent observations showed that (i) diet influences sympathetic nervous system activity (fasting suppresses, but carbohydrate and fat diet stimulate sympathetic activity); (ii) dietary-induced changes in sympathetic activity contribute to the changes in metabolic rate that accompany changes in dietary intake; (iii) insulin-mediated glucose metabolism in the hypothalamus provides a link between dietary intake and sympathetic nervous system activity; and (iv) hyperinsulinemia, a consequence of insulin resistance, is associated with hypertension. These observations have suggested that hyperinsulinemia results in sympathetic stimulation which drives thermogenic mechanisms, thereby increasing metabolic rate [104]. The net result is a restoration of energy balance at the expense of hyperinsulinemia and increased sympathetic activity. Hypertension is thus an unfortunate consequence of hyperinsulinemia, which increases renal sodium reabsorption, and sympathetic stimulation of the heart, kidney, and vasculature [104]. The pathophysiological significance of those observations lies in the findings that insulin has mitogenic properties and can potentiate vascular smooth muscle growth, promote structural changes in vessels and atherosclerosis. Insulin could also promote high blood pressure *via* its effect in increasing sodium reabsorption and sympathetic nervous system activity.

Obesity is an increasing global problem, among both children and adults, as about 20 percent or more of adults are classified as obese, and thus many suffers from related health problems. The major health problem that goes hand in hand with obesity is diabetes and in turn hypertension. Diabetes can occur as a result of a disease, or genetics or poor diet, while hypertension usually caused by genetics, diet and stress. Individuals with abnormal glucose and insulin metabolism have a higher incidence of hypertension; and untreated hypertension has higher than normal plasma insulin, are resistant to insulin-stimulated glucose uptake and often with lipid disorders [105].

Cause and Effect: The cause of type 1 diabetes is unknown, but is usually attributed to genetic predisposition, environmental factors and a viral trigger; occur at any age anywhere in the world, when the immune system attacks the beta cells in the pancreas. The beta cells produce insulin, responsible for distribution of glucose into cells to be used for energy. **Effects**: Once the beta cells are attacked, the pancreatic cells become inactive, or produce very little insulin (known as the honeymoon period), leading to the dangerous levels of glucose within the bloodstream.

A variety of therapies is available for treatment of hypertension in patients with metabolic complications. *Lifestyle modification* is considered to be the initial approach, with weight management the most important component. Although diuretics and β-blockers have a proven record in reducing morbidity and mortality, they may have adverse effects on glucose, insulin and lipids and should be used with caution in hypertensive subjects with metabolic risks, α-adrenergic blockers have favorable effects on lipids and glucose. Calcium antagonists have no adverse effects on glucose or insulin in patients with essential hypertension or diabetic patients with hypertension. ACE inhibitors, on the other hand, have neutral or beneficial effects on glucose, insulin and lipid metabolism, improving insulin sensitivity, insulin secretion, potassium balance and intermediary metabolism. Finally, oral hypoglycemic agents, which improve glucose metabolism and insulin sensitivity, can reduce blood pressure in obese, hypertensive subjects [105].

PHYSICAL AND STATISTICAL RELATIONSHIP

Statistically speaking, individuals with diabetes are at a much greater risk for developing hypertension than are individuals who do not have diabetes. Hypertension is twice as common in those with diabetes as in nondiabetic individuals. It is theorized that diabetes raises the risk of hypertension because diabetes causes hyperinsulinemia, *i.e.*, the increased amount of absorbable sodium by the body. It also promotes the stimulation of the sympathetic nervous system. This is due to the changes in blood vessel structure, which affects the function of the heart and blood pressure. Vascular problems that occur as a result of diabetes are made worse when blood pressure is elevated from sources such as poor diet or lack of exercise. Metabolism is related to obesity, which is related to diabetes, and diabetes is related to hypertension. Reducing weight can often lower blood pressure. This lowering of hypertension symptoms is associated with a decrease in the symptoms of diabetes. An individual thus can treat diabetes by treating their hypertension and *vice versa*.

There are several ways to address the dual conditions hypertension and diabetes, but diet is by far the easiest way. Eating a well-balanced diet low in sodium is beneficial for the reduction of symptoms of both conditions, though both can be treated through medications, as well. Exercise is recommended as it affects metabolic rates and thus in turn diabetes and moreover, weight loss can lower blood pressure levels too.

Insulin Therapy: Diabetes mellitus is typically treated through daily self-maintenance with synthetic insulin shots made from rDNA to compensate for the pancreas's inability to produce insulin on its own. These shots are administered by a syringe, insulin pen or an insulin delivery pump. This synthetic insulin is used in two forms: a fast-acting insulin to cover carbohydrates and glucose corrections, and a slow-acting insulin to cover a 12 to 24 hours period.

Carbohydrates: The management of insulin therapy in relation to carbohydrate can be tricky. Typically a ratio is established during the beginning of the onset of diabetes to determine the body's carb-to-unit dosage. Carbohydrates are a key component of self-maintenance for diabetes, and are initiators of increased blood sugar, as breakdown of carbohydrates into glucose finally produced ATP, or energy, in the cells with the aid of insulin. Too little insulin causes an excess of unconverted glucose causing hyperglycemia, and too much insulin causes hypoglycemia, or low blood sugar. Carbohydrates are necessary when a diabetic is experiencing hypoglycemia to compensate for the excess insulin in the blood stream, which can lead to serious consequences, such as seizure or even death.

CONCLUSION

Till date some questions about the biochemical basis of diabetes remain unanswered. In particular, hormone insensitivity, the reversal of such insensitivity, metabolic interactions between tissues and the pathogenesis of chronic complications are areas of very uncertain knowledge. On the other hand, obesity is considered one of the main cause of the worldwide increase in the prevalence of type 2 diabetes [17, 18] and hyperglycaemia is largely due to increased hepatic gluconeogenesis [106]. The medial hypothalamus is considered to integrate nutritional and hormonal signals [17, 18, 107], and thus play a major role in the regulation of energy balance and the modulation of liver glucose output [108, 109]. This bidirectional changes in hypothalamic insulin signaling result in parallel changes in energy balance [110, 111] and glucose metabolism [110]. Recent report on activation of ATP-sensitive potassium (K_{ATP}) channels [19] in the mediobasal hypothalamus lower blood glucose levels through inhibition of hepatic gluconeogenesis and any alteration within central nervous system/liver circuit can contribute to diabetic hyperglycaemia. On the basis of the current therapeutic development insulin-replacement therapies will dominate the market for T1D over the next decade. However, in the long term novel tolerogenic, antigen-specific and β-cell-specific regenerative agents could provide a promising platform for the development of disease-modifying therapies. Although single-agent therapies are likely to reach the market first, combination therapies could be most effective in delivering the long-sought cure of this biochemical pandemic. Further research on these questions will provide a basis for advances both in understanding and therapy of diabetes and hypertension.

ACKNOWLEDGEMENTS

The authors extend their thanks to Bentham Science Publishers.

DECLARATION OF CONFLICT OF INTEREST

No conflict of interest was declared by the authors.

REFERENCES

[1]   Wild S, Roglic G, Green A, Sicree R, King H. Global prevalence of diabetes: estimates for 2000 and projections for 2030. Diabetes Care 2004; 27(5): 1047-53.
[2]   Tanner J. High Blood Sugar can cause serious damage to the body if untreated. EzineArticles.com. 2009. Accessed 8 Mar2010http://ezinearticles.com/?High-Blood-Sugar-Can-Cause-Serious-Damage-to-the-Body-If-Untreated&id=2847825.
[3]   McPhee SJ, Papadakis MA. Current medical Diagnosis and Treatment. International edition. 2002, New York: Lange Medical Books/McGraw-Hill. pp. 1203-1215.
[4]   Rother KI. Diabetes treatment-bridging the divide. New England J Med 2007; 356(15): 1499-1501.
[5]   Klein R and Klein BEK. Blood pressure control and diabetic retinopathy. Br J Ophthalmol 2002; 86:365-367.
[6]   Alwakeel JS, Suwaida AA, Isnani AC, Harbi AA, Alam A. Concomitant macro and microvascular complications in diabetic nephropathy. Saudi journal of kidney diseases and transplantation 2009; 20(3): 402-409.
[7]   Nakhoul FM, Lotan RM, Awaad H, Asleh R, Levy AP. Hypothesis-haptoglobin genotype and diabetic nephropathy. Nature Reviews Nephrology 2007; 3: 339-344.
[8]   Insel PM, Roth WT. Cardiovascular Disease and Cancer. In: Core Concepts in Health, 9th edition, 2004. Boston: McGraw-Hill.
[9]   Kokubo Y, Kamide K, Okamura T, Watanabe M, Higashiyama A, Kawanishi K, Okayama A and Kawano Y. Impact of High-Normal Blood Pressure on the Risk of Cardiovascular Disease in a Japanese Urban Cohort: The Suita Study. Hypertension 2008; 52: 652-659.

[10]   Cooke DW, Plotnick L. Type 1 diabetes mellitus in pediatrics. Pediatr Rev 2008; 29(11): 374-384.

[11]   Huppmann M, Dipsocsc AB, Ziegler A-G, Bonifacio E. Neonatal Bacille Calmette-Guerin Vaccination and Type 1 Diabetes. Diabetes Care 2005; 28(5): 1204-1206.

[12]   Daneman D. Type 1 diabetes. Lancet 2006; 367(9513): 847-58.

[13]   Shehadeh N, Shamir R, Berant M, Etzioni A. Insulin in human milk and the prevention of type 1 diabetes. Ped Diab 2001; 2(4): 175-177.

[14]   Virtanen SM, Knip M. Nutritional risk predictors of beta cell autoimmunity and type 1 diabetes at a young age. American J Clin Nutr 2003; 78(6): 1053-1067.

[15]   Hyppönen E, Läärä E, Reunanen A, Järvelin MR, Virtanen SM. Intake of vitamin D and risk of type 1 diabetes: a birth-cohort study. Lancet 2001; 358(9292): 1500-1503.

[16]   Elliott RB, Pilcher CC, Fergusson DM, Stewart AW. A population based strategy to prevent insulin-dependent diabetes using nicotinamide. J Ped Endocrinol & Metab; 1969; (5): 501-509.

[17]   International Diabetes Federation. Diabetes Atlas 3rd Edn., 2007 (IDF, Brussels).

[18]   Dabelea D. The accelerating epidemic of childhood diabetes. Lancet 2009; 373: 1999-2000.

[19]   Burn P. Type 1 Diabetes. Nat Rev D Disc 2010; 9: 187-188 doi: 10.1038/nrd 309.

[20]   Risérus U, Willett WC, Hu FB. Dietary fats and prevention of type 2 diabetes. Progress in Lipid Res 2009; 48 (1): 44–51.

[21]   Eberhart MS, Ogden C, Engelgau M, Cadwell B, Hedley AA, Saydah SH. Prevalence of overweight and obesity among adults with diagnosed diabetes - United States, 1988-1994 and 1999-2002. Morb Mort Weekly Report CDC 2004; 53(45): 1066-1068.

[22]   Camastra S, Bonora E, Del Prato S, Rett K, Weck M, Ferrannini E. Effect of obesity and insulin resistance on resting and glucose-induced thermogenesis in man. Int J Obes Relat Metab Disord 1999; 23(12): 1307-1313.

[23]   Rosenbloom A, Silverstein JH. Type 2 Diabetes in Children and Adolescents: A Clinician's Guide to Diagnosis, Epidemiology, Pathogenesis, Prevention, and Treatment. American Diabetes Association, US.2003, pp. 1. ISBN 978-1580401555.

[24]   Mozaffarian D, Kamineni A, Carnethon M, Djoussé L, Mukamal KJ, Siscovick D. Lifestyle risk factors and new-onset diabetes mellitus in older adults: the cardiovascular health study. Archives Inter Med 2009; 169(8): 798-807.

[25]   National Institute of Diabetes and Digestive and Kidney Diseases (NIDDK) Recent Advances & Emerging Opportunities: Diabetes, Endocrinology, and Metabolic Diseases 15-45.   NIH   Publication   No.   09-3873   November   2008. www.diabetes.niddk.nih.gov/dm/pubs/statistics.

[26]   Gallivan J, Brown C, Greenberg R, Clark CM, Jr. Predictors of Perceived Risk of the Development of Diabetes. Diabetes Spectrum 2009; 22(3): 163-169.

[27]   Lawrence JM, Contreras R, Chen W, Sacks DA. Trends in the prevalence of pre-existing diabetes and gestational diabetes mellitus among a racially/ethnically diverse population of pregnant women, 1999–2005. Diabetes Care 2008; 31(5): 899-904.

[28]   DeFronzo RA, Gunnarsson R, Björkman O, Olsson M, Wahren J. Effect of insulin on peripheral and splanchnic glucose metabolism in noninsulin-dependent (type II) diabetes mellitus. J Clin Invest 1985; 76: 149-155.

[29]   Taylor R, Agius L. The biochemistry of diabetes. Biochem J 1988; 250: 625-640.

[30]   Pehling G, Tessari P, Gerich J, Haymond M, Service F, Rizza R. Abnormal carbohydrate deposition in insulin dependent diabetes; relative contributions of endogenous glucose

production and initial splanchnic uptake and effect of intensive insulin therapy. J Clin Invest 1984; 74: 991-995.

[31] Pocai A, Lam Tony KT, Gutierrez-Juarez R, Obici S, Schwartz GJ, Bryan J, Aguilar-Bryan L, Rossetti L, Nature 2005; 434, 1026-1031.

[32] Malaisse WJ. Insuline release: the fuel concept. Diab & Metabol 1983; 9: 313-320.

[33] Gopaul NK, Änggård EE, Mallet AI, Betteridge DJ, Wolff SP, Nourooz-Zadeh J. Plasma 8-epi-prostaglandin F2α levels are elevated in individuals with non-insulin dependent diabetes mellitus. FEBS Lett 1995; 368: 225-229.

[34] Paolisso G, D'Amore A, Volpe C, Balbi V, Saccomanno F, Galzerano D, Giugliano D, Varricchio M, D'Onofrio F. Evidence for a relationship between oxidative stress and insulin action in non-insulin-dependent (type II) diabetic patients. Metabol 1994; 43: 1426-1429.

[35] Oberley LW. Free radicals and diabetes. Free Radical Biol Med 1988; 5: 113-124.

[36] Hunt JV, Bottoms MA, Mitchinson MJ. Ascorbic acid oxidation: A potential cause of the elevated severity of altherosclerosis in diabetes mellitus. FEBS Lett 1992; 311: 161-164.

[37] Low PA, Nickander KK, Tritschler HJ. The roles of oxidative stress and antioxidant treatment in experimental diabetic neuropathy. Diabetes 1997; 46: S38-S42.

[38] Roussel A-M, Kerkeni A, Zouari N, Mahjoub S, Matheau J-M, Anderson RA. Antioxidant Effects of Zinc Supplementation in Tunisians with Type 2 Diabetes Mellitus. Journal of American College of Nutrition 2003; 22(4): 316-321.

[39] Giugliano D, Ceriello A, Paolisso G. Oxidative stress and diabetic vascular complications. Diabetes Care 1996; 19: 257-267.

[40] Grisham MB, McCord JM. Chemistry and cytotoxicity of reactive oxygen metabolites. In: Physiology of oxygen radicals. Ed by Taylor AE, Matalon S, Ward P. Bethesda MD: American Physiology Society, 1986, pp 1-19.

[41] Katusic ZS. Superoxide anion and endothelial regulation of arterial tone. Free Radical Biol Med 1996; 20: 443-446.

[42] Jang YY, Song JH, Shin YK, Han ES, Lee CS. Protective effect of boldine on oxidative mitochondrial damage in streptozotocin-induced diabetic rats. Pharmacol Res 2000; 42: 361-371.

[43] Mullarkey CJ, Edelstein D, Brownlee M. Free radical generation by early glycation products: a mechanism for accelerated atherogenesis in diabetes. Biochem Biophys Res Commun 1990; 173: 932-939.

[44] Kawamura M, Heinecke JW, Chait A. Pathophysiological concentrations of glucose promote oxidative modification of low density lipoprotein by a superoxide dependent pathway. J Clin Invest 1994; 94: 771-778.

[45] Hicks M, Delbridge L, Yue DK, Reeve TS. Increase in cross linking of nonenzymatically glycosylated collagen induced by products of lipid peroxidation. Arch Biochem Biophys 1989; 268: 249-254.

[46] Miyata T, van Ypersele de Strihou C, Kurokawa K, Baynes JW. Origin and significance of carbonyl stress in long-term uremic complications. Kidney International 1999; 55: 389-399.

[47] Matteucci E, Giampietro O. Oxidative stress in families of type 1 diabetic patients. Diabetes Care 2000; 23: 1182-1186.

[48] Ciuchi E, Odetti P, Prando R. Relationship between glutathione and sorbitol concentrations in erythrocytes from diabetic patients. Metabolism 1996; 45(5): 611-613.

[49] Ceriello A, Russ P, Amstael P, Cerutt P. High glucose induces antioxidants enzymes in humans endothelial cells in culture: Evidence linking hyperglycemia and oxidative stress. Diabetes 1996; 45: 471-477.

[50]   Brownlee M, Cerami A, Vlassara H. Advanced glycation end products in tissue and biochemical basis of diabetic complication. N Engl J Med 1988; 318: 1315-1322.

[51]   Packer L. The role of antioxidant treatment in diabetes mellitus. Diabetologia 1993; 36: 1212-1213.

[52]   Santini SA, Marra G, Giardina B, Cotrono P, Mordenter E, Mortorana GE, Manto A, Ghirlanda G. Defective plasma antioxidant defenses and enhanced susceptibility to lipid peroxidation in uncomplicated IDDM. Diabetes 1997; 46: 1853-1858.

[53]   Vlassara H, Bucala R, Striker L. Pathogenetic effects of advanced glycosylation: Biochemical, biologic and clinical implications for diabetes and aging. Lab Invest 1994; 20: 138-151.

[54]   Schmidt AM, Hori O, Brett J, Van SD, Wautier JL, Stern D. Cellular receptors for advanced glycation end products: Implications for induction of oxidant stress and cellular dysfunction in the pathogenesis of vascular lesions. Anterioscler Thromb 1994; 14: 1521-1528.

[55]   Vlassara H, Li YM, Imani F, Wojcie chowicz D, Yang Z, Liu FT, Cerami A. Identification of galectin-3 as a high affinity binding protein for advanced glycation end products: A new member of the AGE-receptor complex. Mol Med 1996; 1: 634-646.

[56]   Ritthaler U, Deng Y, Zhang Y, Greten J, Abel M, Sido B, Allenberg J, Otto G, Roth H, Bierhaus A, Ziegler R, Schmidt AM, Waldherr R, Wahl P, Stern DM, Nawroth PP. Expression of receptors for advanced glycation end products in peripheral occlusive vascular disease. American J Pathol 1995; 146: 688-694.

[57]   Bierhaus A, Chevion S, Chevion M, Hofman M, Quehenberger B, Illmer T, Lutber T, Nawroth PP. Advanced glycation end product-induced activation of NF-KB is suppressed by α-lipoic acid in cultured endothelial cells. Diabetes 1997; 46: 1481-1490.

[58]   Ceriello A. Oxidative strees and glycemic regulation. Metabolism 2000; 49: 27-29.

[59]   Betteridge DJ. What is oxidative stress? Metabolism 2000; 49(2): 3-8.

[60]   Kajanachumpol S, Komindr S, Mahaisiriyodom A. Plasma lipid peroxide and antioxidant levels in diabetic patients. J Med Assoc Thai 1997; 80(6): 372-377.

[61]   Wohaieb SA, Godin DV. Alterations in free radical tissue-defense mechanisms in streptozotocin-induced diabetes in rat: Effects of insulin treatment. Diabetes 1987; 36: 1014-1018.

[62]   Murakami K, Kondo T, Ohtsuka Y. Impairment of glutathione metabolism in erythrocytes from patients with diabetes mellitus. Metabolism 1989; 38: 753-758.

[63]   Tagami S, Kondo T, Yoshida K, Hirokawa J, Ohtsuka Y, Kawakam Y. Effect of insulin on impaired antioxidant activities in aortic endothelial cells from diabetic rabbits. Metabolism 1992; 11: 1053-1058.

[64]   Kazuhiro M, Takahito-Kondo Y, Ohsuka Y, Fujiwara MS, Yoshikazu K. Impairment of glutathione metabolism in erythrocytes from patients with diabetes mellitus. Metabolism 1989; 8: 753-758.

[65]   Matkovics B, Kotorman M, Varga ISz, Hai DQ, Varga Cs. Oxidative stress in experimental diabetes induced by streptozotocin. Acta Physiologica Hungarica 1998; 85(1): 29-38.

[66]   Dominguez C, Ruiz E, Gussinye M, Carrascosa A. Oxidative stress at onset and in early stages of type I diabetes in children and adolescents. Diabetes Care 1998; 21(10): 1736-1742.

[67]   Lyons TJ. Oxidized low density lipoproteins: A role in the pathogenesis of atherosclerosis in diabetes. Diabetic Med 1991; 8: 411-419.

[68]   Violi F, Marino R, Milite MT, Lofrredo L. Nitric oxide and its role in lipid peroxidation. Diabetes Mefab Res Rev 1999; 15: 283-288.

[69]   Sato Y, Hotta N, Sakamoto N, Matsuoka S, Ohishi N, Yagi K. Lipid peroxide level in plasma of diabetic patients. Biochem Med 1979; 21: 104.

[70]   Jain SK, McVie R, Jaramillo JJ, Chen Y. Hyperketonemia (acetoacetate) increases the oxidizability of LDL $^+$ VLDL in type 1 diabetic patients. Free Rad Biol Med 1998; 24(1): 175-181.

[71]   Armstrong D, Sohal R, Cutler R, Slater T. Free radicals in molecular biology and aging. New York: Raven Press, 1982.

[72]   Berdanier C. Role of membrane lipids in metabolic regulation. Nutr Rev 1988; 46: 145-149.

[73]   Wolff SP. Diabetes mellitus and free radicals. Free radicals, transition metals and oxidative stress in the aetiology of diabetes mellitus and complications. Brit Med Bull 1993; 49: 642-652.

[74]   Lee TS, Saltsman KA, Ohashi H, King GL. Activation of protein kinase C by elevation of glucose concentration: proposal for a mechanism in the development of diabetic vascular complications. Proc Natl Acad Sci USA, 1989; 86: 5141-5145.

[75]   Feener EP, King GL. Vascular dysfunction in diabetes mellitus. Lancet 1997; 350: 9-13.

[76]   Poston L, Taylor PD. Endothelium-mediated vascular function in insulin-dependent diabetes mellitus. Clin Sci 1995; 88: 245-255.

[77]   Beckman JS, Beckman TW, Chen J, Marshall PA, Freeman BA. Apparent hydroxyl radical production by peroxynitrite: implications for endothelial injury from nitric oxide and superoxide. Proc Natl Acad Sci USA, 1990; 87: 1620-1624.

[78]   Nourooz-Zadeh J, Rahimi A, TajadamT, Sarmadi J, Tritschler H, Rosen P, Halliwell B. Relationships between plasma measures of oxidative stress and metabolic control in NIDDM. Diabetologia 1997; 40: 647-653.

[79]   Griffin ME, Mclnerney D, Fraser A, Johnson AH, Collins PB, Owens GH. Autoantibodies to oxidized low density lipoprotein: the relationship to two density lipoprotein fatty acid composition in diabetes. Diabet Med 1997; 14: 741-747.

[80]   Lehto S, Rönneman T, Haffner SM, Pyörälä K, Kallio V, Laakso M. Dyslipidaemia and hyperglycaemia predict coronary heart disease events in middle-aged patients with NIDDM. Diabetes 1997; 46: 1254-1359.

[81]   Griendling KK, Alexander RW. Oxidative stress and cardiovascular disease. Circulation 1997; 96: 3264-3265.

[82]   Skrha J, Hodinar A, Kvasnicka J, Hilgertova J. Relationship of oxidative stress and fibrinolysis in diabetes mellitus. Diabetic Med 1996; 13: 800-805.

[83]   Paolisso G, Giugliano D. Oxidative stress and insulin action: is there a relationship? Diabetologia 1996; 39: 357-363.

[84]   Kaji H, Kurasak M, Ito K. Increased lipoperoxide value and glutathione peroxidase activity in blood plasma of type 2 (noninsulin dependent) diabetic women. Klin Wochenschr 1985; 63: 765-768.

[85]   Arai K, Magushi S, Fujii S. Glycation and inactivation of human CuZn superoxide dismutase: Identification of the *in vitro* glycated sites. J Biol Chem 1987; 262: 16969-16972.

[86]   Sharma A, Kharb S, Chug SN, Kakkar R, Singh GP. Elevation of oxidative stress before and after control of glycemia and after vitamin E supplementation in diabetic patients. Metabolism 2000; 49(2): 160-162.

[87]   Douillet C, Bost M, Accominotti M, Borson-Chazot F, Ciavatti M. Effect of selenium and vitamin E supplements on tissue lipids peroxides and fatty acid distribution in experimental diabetes. Lipids 1998; 33: 393-399.

[88]   Fujiwara Y, Kondo T, Murakamig K. Decrease of the inhibition of lipid peroxidation by glutathione dependent system in erythrocytes of non-insulin dependent diabetes. Klin Wochenschr 1989; 67: 336-341.

[89]   Jain SK, Me Vie R. Effect of glycemic control race (white *vs.* black), and duration of diabetes on reduced glutathione content in erythrocytes of diabetic patients. Metabolism 1994; 43: 306-309.

[90]   Uzel N, Sivas A, Uysal M, Oz H. Erythrocyte lipid peroxidation and glutathione peroxidase activities in patients with diabetes mellitus. Horm Metab Res 1987; 19: 89-90.

[91]   Wong EL, Davidosn RL. Raised coulter mean corpuscular volume in diabetic ketoacidosis and its underlying association with marked plasma hyperosmolarity. J Clin Pathol 1983; 36: 334.

[92]   Ahmed RG. The Physiological and Biochemical effects of Diabetes on the balance between Oxidative Stress and Antioxidant Defense System. Medical Journal of Islamic World Academy of Sciences 2005; 15: 31-42.

[93]   Garber AJ. The impact of streptozotocin-induced diabetes mellitus on cyclic nucleotide regulation of skeletal muscle amino acid metabolism in the rat. J Clin Invest 1980; 65: 478-487.

[94]   Brosnan JT, Man KC, Hall HE, Clobourne SA, Brosnan ME. Interorgan metabolism of amino acids in streptozotocin-diabetic rat. Am J Physiol 1984; 244: E151-E158.

[95]   Mortimore GE, Mandon CE. Inhibition of insulin of valine turnover in liver. J Biol Chem 1970; 245: 2375-2383.

[96]   Peavy DE, Taylor JM, Jefferson LS. Time course of changes in albumin synthesis and mRNA in diabetic and insulin treated diabetic rats. Am J Physiol 1985; 248: E656-E663.

[97]   Aljada A, Thusu K, Armstrong D, Nicotera T, Dandona P. Increased carbonylation of proteins in diabetes mellitus. Diabetes 1995; 44: 113A.

[98]   Aydin A, Orhan H, Sayal A, Ozata M, Sahin G, Isimer A. Oxidative stress and nitric oxide related parameters in type II diabetes mellitus: effects of glycemic control. J din Biochem 2001; 34: 65-70.

[99]   Dandona P, Mohanty P, Ghanim H, Aljada A, Browne R, Hamouda W, Prabhala A, Afzal A, Garg R. The suppressive effect of dietary restriction and weight loss in the obese on the generation of reactive oxygen species by leukocytes, lipid peroxidation, and protein carbonylation. J Clin Endocrinol Metab 2001; 86: 355-362.

[100]   Mohanty P, Hamouda W, Garg R, Aljada A, Ghanim H, Dandona P. Glucose challenge stimulates reactive oxygen species (ROS) generation by leucocytes. J Clin Endocrinol Metab 2000; 85: 2970-2973.

[101]   Mohanty P, Ghanim H, Hamouda W, Aljada A, Garg R, Dandona P. Both lipid and protein intakes stimulate increased generation of reactive oxygen species by polymorphonuclear leukocytes and mononuclear cells. American J Clin Nutr 2002; 75: 767-772.

[102]   Houston MC. Nutraceuticals, Vitamins, Antioxidants, and Minerals in the prevention and treatment of Hypertension. Prog Card Dis 2005; 47(6): 396-449.

[103]   Steffen LM. Eat your fruit and vegetables. Lancet 2006; 367: 278-279.

[104]   Landsberg L. Obesity, metabolism, and hypertension. Yale J Biol Med 1989; 62(5): 511-519.

[105] Cony DB, Tuck ML. Glucose and Insulin Metabolism in Hypertension. Am J Nephrol 1996; 16: 223-236.

[106] Pittenger GL. Taylor-Fishwick D, Vinik AI. A role for islet neogenesis in curing diabetes. *Diabetologia* 2009; **52**: 735-738.

[107] Suarez-Pinzon WL. Power RF, Yan Y, Wasserfall C, Atkinson M, Rabinovitch A. Combination therapy with glucagon-like peptide-1 and gastrin restores normoglycemia in diabetic NOD mice. Diabetes 2008; **57**: 3281-3288.

[108] Suarez-Pinzon WL, Cembrowski GS, Rabinovitch A. Combination therapy with a dipeptidyl peptidase-4 inhibitor and a proton pump inhibitor restores normoglycaemia in non-obese diabetic mice. Diabetologia 2009; **52**, 1680-1682.

[109] Fleming A. What will it take to get therapies approved for type 1 diabetes? Immunology of diabetes V. Ann NY Acad Sci 2008; **1150**: 25-31.

[110] Ringholm Nielsen L, Rehfeld JF, Pedersen-Bjergaard U, Damm P, Mathiesen ER. Pregnancy-induced rise in serum C-peptide concentration in women with type 1 diabetes. Diabetes Care 2009; **32**: 1052-1057.

[111] Gates C, Wong D, Dreyfus J. Type 1 Diabetes 1-147, 2008 (Decision Resources, Waltham, Massachusetts).

CHAPTER 3

Diabetes, Hypertension and Cardiovascular Disease-An Unsolved Enigma

Arpita Chakraborty and Maitree Bhattacharyya*

Department of Biochemistry, University of Calcutta, 35, Ballygunge Circular Road, Kolkata-700019, India

Abstract: Diabetes is a major public health problem that is approaching epidemic proportions globally. Worldwide, the prevalence of chronic, non-communicable diseases is increasing at an alarming rate. Cardiovascular diseases (CVDs) are the major cause of mortality in persons with diabetes, and many factors, including hypertension, contribute to this high prevalence of CVD. Hypertension is approximately twice as frequent in patients with diabetes compared with patients without the disease. Conversely, recent data suggest that hypertensive persons are more predisposed to the development of diabetes than are normotensive persons. Co-existence of diabetes mellitus and hypertension increases the risk of macro- and micro-vascular complications. In this review, an attempt has been made to explore the risk factors which can be helpful to prevent hyperglycemia and the related manifestation of Type 2 diabetes. Both biochemical and genetic diagnostic markers identified till now have been catalogued to describe the status of pathogenesis in hyperglycemic subjects.

Keywords: Type 2 Diabetes, Cardiovascular Disease, Hypertension, Biochemical risk factors, Genetic susceptibility.

INTRODUCTION

The Diabetes Epidemic: A Few Snapshots

Diabetes is a condition primarily defined by the level of hyperglycaemia giving rise to risk of microvascular damage (retinopathy, nephropathy and neuropathy) as well as macrovascular complications (ischaemic heart disease, stroke and peripheral vascular disease).

Diabetes, a chronic disease marked by elevated blood glucose levels, affects 6.4% of the global adult population.

*Address correspondence to Maitree Bhattacharyya: Department of Biochemistry, University of Calcutta, 35, Ballygunge Circular Road, Kolkata-700019, India; Tel: +91-33-24614712, 09830306307; Fax: +91-33-24614849; E-mail: bmaitree@gmail.com

Mohamed Eddouks and Debprasad Chattopadhyay (Eds)
All rights reserved-© 2012 Bentham Science Publishers

Type 2 diabetes is emerging at an alarming rate due to increased urbanization, high prevalence of obesity, sedentary lifestyle and other stress related factors.

Complications from diabetes, such as coronary artery and peripheral vascular disease, stroke, diabetic neuropathy, amputations, renal failure and blindness are resulting in increasing disability, reduced life expectancy and enormous health costs for virtually every society.

Diabetes affects 285 million people worldwide and is expected to affect some 438 million by 2030.

Each year, 38 Lacs deaths are linked directly to diabetes- related causes including cardiovascular disease made worse by diabetes-related lipid disorders and hypertension.

India has the largest diabetes population in the world with an estimated 50.8 million people, amounting to 6% of the adult population.

Cardiovascular disease is the major cause of death in diabetes, accounting for some 50% of all diabetes fatalities and much disability. People with type 2 diabetes are over twice as likely to have a heart attack or stroke as people who do not have diabetes. The economic costs for diabetes are high and will continue to rise. The identification of effective new strategies for the control and management of diabetes and its complications is a public health priority.

The Diabetes Epidemic: Genes and Environment Interaction

"Type 2 Diabetes Mellitus is a heterogeneous, multifactorial, polygenic disease characterized by a defect in insulin's secretion (the beta cell secretory defect) and action (insulin resistance)" [1].

Diabetes mellitus (DM) is a multi-systemic metabolic disorder characterized by certain abnormalities in carbohydrate, fat, electrolyte and protein metabolism, which ultimately lead to several acute and chronic complications. Diabetes mellitus is classically classified into Insulin Dependent Diabetes Mellitus (IDDM) or (**type I**) and Non-insulin dependent Diabetes Mellitus (NIDDM) or (**type II**) [2]. In this article the discussion has been restricted within the problem, risk factors and management of Type 2 Diabetes, earlier know as NIDDM.

Type 2 is the most common form of diabetes, accounting to 90-95% of all diabetes cases, in developed countries. This is adult-onset diabetes, resulting from a combination of insulin resistance and inadequate secretion of insulin [3-5]. Type 2 diabetes is characterized by hyperglycemia leading to long-term complication [6] with the occurrence of severe secondary complications such as neuropathy, nephropathy, retinopathy and accelerated macrovascular disease [7]. Vascular disease particularly coronary heart disease (CHD) is the major cause of morbidity and mortality in diabetic patients [8].

The problem of diabetes is growing in epidemic proportions and is taking a toll of millions of lives worldwide. The number of people with diabetes is increasing due to population growth, aging, urbanization, and increasing prevalence of obesity and physical inactivity. Traditional genetic research, including twin, adoption, and family studies, consistently supports the fact that type 2 diabetes has strong genetic component. During past decades, extensive efforts have been made to detect the underlying genetic structure for type 2 diabetes. However, until very recently, the genes involved are poorly understood. Using new technology in the form of a 'genome-wide chip' that genotypes up to hundreds of thousands of single nucleotide polymorphism (SNPs), genome-wide association (GWA) studies have recently led to the discovery of a group of novel genes that are reproducibly associated with diabetes risk [9, 10]. It is now believed that the genetic factors may not only directly affect the susceptibility but also interplay with environment *(e.g.*, diet and lifestyle) in determining disease risk. Our modern environment causes diabetes in at least three ways: stress, barriers to physical activity, and unhealthy food. Major lifestyle changes resulting from industrialization are contributing to a rapid rise in diabetes worldwide [11].

However, little is known about the precise pattern of gene-environment interaction in predicting diabetes risk [12]. Since Type 2 diabetes essentially did not exist 100 years ago, it is obvious that environmental modification has a lot of influence for emergence of the disease, but genetic susceptibility is definitely another additional component. Environmental and lifestyle factors combine to unmask the genetic factors and these combined interactions only become successful to create diabetes.

Prevalence of Cardiovascular Complications in Patients with Type 2 Diabetes

Cross sectional epidemiological studies have firmly reflected the association among type 2 diabetes and prevalence of CVD and hypertension for last few decades [13, 14]. Cardiovascular disease is very often contemplated as complication of type 2 diabetes, but genetic and environmental history of the disease is more or less same and both should be considered as condemnation of metabolic disorder.There are bundle of risk factors for CVD that assemble in diabetes, including stress, aging, sedentary lifestyle, hypertension, BMI, dyslipidemia and microalbuminuria. Among those, hypertension is frequent and populous in CVD attacked diabetes patients compared to CVD patients without diabetes, even patients with the feature of hypertension are prone to have diabetes. Occurrences of association of cardiovascular events, including cardiovascular death, myocardial infarction, stoke and hypertension in type 2 diabetes patients is positively correlated [15, 16]. Large number of epidemiological studies revealed the fact that the unfavorable distribution of diabetes associated CVD and hypertension are never restricted to any specific race, age and sex. Prospective studies have shown the evidence that the people with CVD and HPT account for 80% mortality in type 2 diabetes patients.

The perception of metabolic syndrome is possibly the most momentous development in the management of CVD and hypertension in last 15 years [17], before that, physician often treated diabetes CVD and hypertension as separate diseases. Obesity, basal metabolic index, waist circumference and lipid profile always reflect divergent datasheet among type 2 diabetes patients. Simultaneously, nontraditional risk factors like advance glycation end product, advance oxidation protein product, reactive oxygen species and inflammatory product have also been identified which are not less significant components for the expression of hypertension and CVD in diabetics. The importance and role of these traditional as well as nontraditional risk factors can be discussed in the following sections:

Stress

The risk of type 2 diabetes is suggested to be enhanced for individuals exposed to stress. Recent research indicates that prolonged stress can be an underlying cause of metabolic syndrome by upsetting the hormonal balance of the hypothalamic-pituitary-adrenal axis (HPA-axis). An activation of the hypo thalamo-pituitary-adrenal (HPA) axis and the central sympathetic system has been proposed to be responsible for the development of endocrine perturbations, leading to obesity and type 2 diabetes. Hence, psychosocial stress causes insulin resistance *via* psychoendocrine pathways. In addition, increased levels of stress hormones, *e.g.*, catecholamine and glucocorticoids, may impair insulin secretion [18]. The risk is specifically evident in genetically susceptible individuals exposed to perceived environmental psychological stress. A baseline study was conducted by Stockholm Diabetes Prevention Program consisting of 4,821 Swedish women [19]. This study demonstrates that self-reported low decision latitude at work and low SOC were associated with type 2 diabetes. All babies in Southeast Sweden (ABIS) project were conducted from 1 October 1997 to 1 October 1999, all parents-to-be in southeast Sweden were invited to participate in the study, yielding a sample of 17,055 families at birth. This project found that high parenting stress, experiences of serious life events, foreign origin of the mother, and low socioeconomic status to be associated with beta cell-related autoimmunity in young children.

Aging

Type 2 diabetes mellitus (T2DM), classically a diagnosis restricted to adults, became increasingly recognized in children and adolescents worldwide over the last two decades. Several complex and interrelated factors are at work in bringing about the rise in T2DM prevalence. It is most common among the elderly in the developed countries, while in the developing world the prevalence rates are increasing particularly quickly among comparatively young and productive populations. Furthermore, traditional lifestyles and dietary patterns giving way to a sedentary lifestyle and a high-fat diet are important risk factors. The age dependency of the syndrome's prevalence is seen in most populations around the world. In the United States, between 2002 and 2003, the proportion of physician-classified T2DM among newly diagnosed diabetes cases in the 10 to 19 years age group ranged from 14.9% in non Hispanic whites to 46.1% in Hispanics, 57.8% in African Americans and 86.2% in American Indians [20]. The rates are lower in Europe, where T2DM accounts for 1% to 2% of young-onset diabetes mellitus cases [21]; higher in Taiwan, where T2DM accounts for 54.2% of newly diagnosed diabetes mellitus cases in school age children [22]. The increase in T2DM cases in youth has paralleled the epidemic increase in childhood obesity and an increase in the prevalence of adult T2DM [23].

Sedentary Lifestyle

The rise in diabetes is largely endorsed with the sedentary lifestyle as well as unhealthy dietary habits [24] and is considered as the major contributor to the rising epidemic of diabetes across various ethnic and age groups. Many components of metabolic syndrome are associated with a sedentary lifestyle, including increased adipose tissue (predominantly central); reduced HDL cholesterol; and a trend toward increased triglycerides, blood pressure, and glucose in the genetically susceptible individuals. Sedentary lifestyle and hyper caloric diet leading to obesity, is one of the sources of the rising occurrence of diabetes among adults and more terrifyingly among adolescents. To assess the impact of diet and physical activity on the risk of type 2 diabetes mellitus (T2DM) in the Kingdom of Saudi Arabia a case-control study was conducted among 498 patients from September to November 2009 [25]. The study has shown a strong association between diabetes and lack of exercise, and dietary habits. Healthy diet and active lifestyle may considerably decrease the risk of T2DM in spite of having a family history of diabetes. The Diabetes prevention program (DPP) trial in US enrolled 3,234 subjects with pre-diabetes, defined as an IFG or IGT, randomized to intensive lifestyle modification program, metformin (850 mg twice a day), or matching placebo [26]. An obvious benefit of lifestyle changes led to the premature discontinuation of the study with a relative risk reduction of progression to diabetes at 3 years of 58% in the lifestyle changes group and 31% in the metformin group when compared with placebo and NNT of 6.9 and 13.9, respectively (cumulative incidence of DM of 28.9%, 21.7%, and 14.4% in the placebo, metformin, and lifestyle intervention groups, respectively). Lifestyle changes were significantly more effective than metformin and were consistent in men and women across ages and ethnic groups. In a 10-year follow-up of the DPP study published in 2009, all participants were offered group-implemented lifestyle changes and were followed for additional 5.7 years [27]. In one study, those who had high levels of physical activity, a healthy diet, did not smoke, and consumed alcohol in moderation had an 82% lower rate of diabetes. When a normal weight was included the rate was 89% lower. In this study a healthy diet was defined as one high in fiber, with a high polyunsaturated to saturated fat ratio, and a lower mean glycemic index [28].

Obesity

Obesity is a key feature of metabolic syndrome, reflecting the fact that the syndrome's prevalence is driven by the strong relationship between body mass index (BMI) and increasing adiposity. There has been some debate regarding not only the connection of obesity with CVD and hypertension [29], but regarding whether or not it should be included as a feature of the metabolic syndrome. Today, more than 1.1 billion adults worldwide are overweight, and 312 million of them are obese. Given its meticulous association with cardiovascular atherosclerotic disorder, hypertension, and diabetes [30], researchers have attempted to discriminate the contribution that obesity makes to stroke incidence with variable results [31-33]. More than 300,000 deaths per year are occurred due to obesity. It doubles the risk of death from all causes [34-36]. An association of BMI and risk of stroke has been noted in studies of specific subpopulations, such as middle-aged, Korean, or nonsmoking Japanese men [37-39]. The Nurses' Health Study demonstrated a noticeable association with BMI, such that subjects with BMI 27-28.9 kg/m^2 had an RR of 1.8 (95% CI 1.2-2.6), subjects with BMI 29-31.9 kg/m^2 had an RR of 1.9 (1.3-2.8), and subjects with BMI < 32 kg/m^2 had an RR of 2.4 (1.6-3.5) compared with those with BMI 25 kg/m^2 [40]. In the Physician's Health Study the risk increased by 6% for each unit increase in BMI, [41]. These studies recommend that obesity is a significant risk factor for ischemic stroke [42]. Hepatic glucose production is increased in obesity, reflecting chronic increases in endoplasmic reticulum (ER) stress that promote insulin resistance. It has been predictable that the reductions in diabetes, hypertension, and hyperlipidemia associated with a 10% weight loss could lead to reduction of stroke of up to 13 per 1,000 people [43].

Apart from obesity and abnormal lipid profile type 2 diabitic patients show an abdominal fat deposition feature, known as visceral obesity. It is now well established that regional adiposity plays a greater role in the development of diabetic CVD. This concept is not entirely new; Vague first described it in 1956. Several studies have demonstrated a clear relationship between central obesity and hypertension. Waist-to hip ratio (WHR), while highly correlated with BMI, better represents abdominal obesity and therefore may provide additional information on stroke risk [44].

Dyslipidemia

Type 2 diabetes is an important cardiovascular risk factor. A significant component of the risk associated with type 2 diabetes is thought to be because of its characteristic lipid "triad" profile of raised small dense low-density lipoprotein levels, lowered high-density lipoprotein, and elevated triglycerides (TGs). Trials of statins and fibrates have included substantial numbers of patients with diabetes and indicate that lipid lowering reduces cardiovascular event rates in these patients. However, statins alone do not always address all the lipid abnormalities of diabetes.

Diabetic patients who have suffered a stroke are more expected to have hyperlipidemia than those without diabetes (16 % *vs.* 8%, respectively, *P*<0.0001 in the GCNKSS) [45, 46]. The contribution of hyperlipidemia alone to stroke incidence is controversial [47-52]. In addition to obesity people with diabetes reflect a pattern of dyslipidemia characterized by elevated Triglyceride, low level of HDL and high level VLDL and LDL which are important markers for development of diabetic CVD and hypertension. The Collaborative Ato Rvastatin Diabetes Study (CARDS), evaluated the involvement of hyperlipidemia to stroke risk in the diabetic population without known CAD [53]. The Helsinki Heart Study and Scandinavian Simvastatin Survival Study evaluated cholesterol reduction as primary or secondary prevention of cardiovascular disease. The Heart Protection Study, in contrast, did not support this difference, evaluating that risk reduction did not vary with diabetic status [54].

Microalbuminuria

Microalbuminuria is an important indicator of cardiovascular disease and is strongly connected with hypertension [55, 56]. The normal rate of albumin excretion is less than 20 mg/day (15 µg/min); persistent albumin excretion between 30 and 300 mg/day (20 to 200 µg/min) is called microalbuminuria and, in patients with diabetes (particularly type 1 diabetes), is often indicative of early diabetic nephropathy, unless there is some coexistent renal disease [57].

Microalbuminuria is an important clinical marker in patients with diabetes because of its well-established association with progressive renal disease. It is also becoming increasingly recognized as an independent risk factor for cardiovascular disease in patients with hypertension and diabetes and also in the general population. Microalbuminuria has recently been recognized as one of the most significant factors for predicting morbidity and mortality in people with cardiovascular and peripheral vascular disease. It is noticed in diabetic patients more than nondiabetic patients [56] and may also contribute to the increased risk of stroke. In the EPIC-Norfolk Study conducted among 23,630 individuals aged 40-79 years, microalbuminuria conferred a significantly increased risk of total and ischemic stroke in multivariate modeling (hazard ratio [HR] 1.49 [95% CI 1.13-2.14] and 2.01 [1.29 -3.31], respectively) [58].

Potential Diagnostic Markers for Increased Atherosclerosis and Hypertension in Type 2 Diabetes

The search for improved molecular markers for diagnosis and prediction is a challenge for which recent time researches show great promise. As is becoming increasingly clear, diabetes mellitus is a perpetually-evolving, highly multi-factorial disease and it's liaison with hypertension and atherosclerosis is really a mystery. The ability to develop clinically useful molecular markers is very important for diagnosing and estimating the status of the disease and designing sophisticated analytical tools that synthesize high-throughput data into meaningful reflections of cellular states.

A 2 to 4 fold excess in coronary artery disease mortality among diabetic individuals has been noted in a number of prospective studies encompassing a variety of ethnic and racial groups. The increased risk of CVD and hypertension in Type 2 diabetes is partly explained by clustering of different diagnostic markers including advanced glycation end product (AGE), advanced oxidation protein product (AOPP), reactive oxygen species (ROS), inflammatory markers like C reactive protein, nitrosative stress markers, homocystiene and protein markers in membrane.

Advanced Glycation End Product (AGE)

Advanced glycation end products are modifications of proteins or lipids that become non-enzymatically glycated and oxidized after contact with aldose sugars [59]. Early glycation and oxidation processes result in the formation of Schiff bases and Amadori products. Glycation of proteins and lipids causes molecular rearrangements which lead to the generation of AGEs [60]. AGEs may fluoresce, produce reactive oxygen species (ROS), bind to specific cell surface receptors, and form cross-links. 1,3 AGEs form *in vivo* in hyperglycemic environments and during aging and contribute to the pathophysiology of vascular disease in diabetes. 4-7 AGEs accumulate in the vessel wall, where they may perturb cell structure and function. AGEs have been implicated in both the microvascular and macrovascular complications of diabetes. According to Brownlee, [61] AGEs may modify the action of hormones, cytokines, and free radicals *via* engagement of cell surface receptors; and have impact on the function of intracellular proteins. Key factors crucial to the formation of AGEs include the rate of turnover of proteins for glycoxidation, the degree of hyperglycemia, and the extent of oxidative stress in the environment. If one or more of these conditions is present, both intracellular and extracellular proteins may be glycated and oxidized [62].

Diabetes mellitus is related with enhanced non-enzymatic glycation [63], oxidative stress [64] imbalance between free radicals and reactive oxygen and nitrogen species), antioxidants in favor of free radicals, and carbonyl stress (increase of reactive carbonyl compounds caused by their enhanced formation and/or decreased degradation or excretion) [65]. Non enzymatic glycation accelerates the production of advanced glycation end-products which accumulates in the body and gradually biologically important compounds are damaged due to its toxic effects [66]. AGEs can modify proteins, directly damage the structure and metabolism of extracellular matrix or act *via* their specific receptors [67]. AGE-RAGE interaction activates nuclear factor NF-κB, stimulates the transcription of genes for cytokines, growth factors and adhesive molecules, induces migration of macrophages and has further toxic effects [68]. In addition to circulation in the blood, AGEs accumulate in tissues and thus take part in the development of diabetic complications. nephropathy, neuropathy, retinopathy and angiopathy. They cause damage to biological membranes and the endothelium. Moreover, they modify LDL particles and together with vascular damage, they are involved in the acceleration of atherosclerosis.

Advanced Oxidation Protein Products (AOPP)

Recently a new marker of protein oxidation, advanced oxidation protein products (AOPP), has begun to call the attention of the investigators. Advanced oxidation protein products were described by Witko-Sarsat *et al.* [69] for the first time.They are formed during oxidative stress [70] by the action of chlorinated oxidants, mainly hypochlorous acid and chloramines [69]. AOPP seems to be considered as a useful marker to estimate the degree of oxidative protein damage in diabetic patients. AOPP are elevated in patients with diabetes where they correlated with markers of oxidative stress. They are supposed to be structurally similar to AGE-proteins and to exert similar biological activities as AGEs, *i.e.* induction of proinflammatory cytokines and adhesive molecules. It is now established that the patients with diabetes had decreased antioxidative system and increased products of oxidative damage *versus* control subjects. Therefore, the measurement of products of oxidative stress rather than antioxidative enzymes seems to be the best biomarkers for diabetic complication and assessment of oxidative stress in diabetic patients may be important for the prediction and prevention of diabetic complications.

Reactive Oxygen Species (ROS)

Reactive oxygen species (ROS) are produced in the living cells in general metabolic pathway. Over production and insufficient scavenging of Reactive oxygen species cause oxidative stress situation in the cell. ROS are basically free radicals or super oxides, which cause contraction of vascular smooth muscles and endothelial dysfunction. In diabetic hypertensive patients the production of free radicals is much higher and antioxidant pathway is totally disrupted, consequently, micro and macro vascular complication arises [71]. ROS generation can also hamper the antioxidant defence mechanism in living system. Imbalanced ROS production is involved in the pathogenesis of hypertension and CVD in Type 2 patients [72]. Type 2 diabetes mellitus is associated with multiple metabolic derangements that result in the excessive production of reactive oxygen species and oxidative stress. These reactive oxygen species set in motion a host of redox reactions which can result in unstable nitrogen and thiol species that contribute to additional redox stress. The ability of a cell to deal with reactive oxygen species and oxidative stress requires functional chaperones, antioxidant production, protein degradation and a cascade of intracellular events collectively known as the unfolded protein response. Multiple evidence have suggested that ROS induced glucose autoxidation, elevated levels of free fatty acids, reduced antioxidant defences platelet aggregation, leucocytes adhesion and endothelial cell dysfunction are common among hyperglycemic subjects [73]. All these events appear to be involved in pathophysiology of diabetes-associated heart disease.

Glycated Hemoglobin (HbA$_{1c}$)

Hyperglycemia promotes non-enzymatic attachment of glucose to protein molecules (protein glycation). Glucose-protein adducts are transformed further in a sequence of nonenzymatic reactions collectively known as the Maillard reaction [63]. Amino acid residues involved include the α-amino terminal amino acid and ε-amino groups of lysine residues. First, a labile Schiff base is formed. This spontaneously transform to ketoamine through the Amadori rearrangement. Glycated hemoglobin, Hemoglobin A$_{1C}$ (HbA$_{1C}$) is one the most important Amadori product. The term glycohemoglobin refers to hemoglobin that has been modified post ribosomally by the attachment of glucose to the polypeptide chain [74]. This nonenzymatic glycation is a condensation reaction between the carbohydrate and free amino group at the amino terminus. The study of hemoglobin glycation serves as a model system for many proteins undergoing nonenzymatic glycation. Glycated haemoglobin (HbA$_{1c}$), a marker of average glycaemia, is a predictor of macro and microvascular complications in diabetic individuals. Glycated hemoglobin values reflect the 2 to 3 months average endogenous exposure to glucose, including postprandial spikes in the blood glucose level, and have low intra individual variability. These characteristics may contribute to the superiority of glycated hemoglobin over fasting glucose for long-term macrovascular risk stratification [75, 76]. In community-based study population glycated hemoglobin was superior to fasting glucose for assessment of the long-term risk of subsequent cardiovascular disease, especially at values above 6.0% [77]. Thus such prognostic data add to the evidence supporting the use of glycated hemoglobin as a diagnostic test for diabetes.

C-Reactive Protein (CRP)

The acute-phase protein, C-reactive protein (CRP), is an exquisitely responsive systemic marker of T2DM [78]. Recently, considerable attention has been focused on the association between cardiovascular disease and C-reactive protein (CRP) in patients with diabetes. CRP levels serve as an inflammatory marker that reflects underlying disease processes such as cardiovascular disease and diabetes. An elevated CRP level is also a risk factor for these and other illnesses; researchers now believe that this protein plays a role in the disease processes, although the mechanism is not understood. Inflammation, the key controller of CRP synthesis, plays a important role in atherothrombotic cardiovascular disease. There is a powerful predictive link between increased serum CRP values and the outcome of acute coronary syndromes and future atherothrombotic events in healthy individuals. The presence of CRP within most acute myocardial infarction lesions, binding of CRP to lipoproteins and its capacity for pro-inflammatory complement activation, suggests that CRP may contribute to the pathogenesis and complications of cardiovascular disease [79].

Nitric Oxide (NO)

Nitric oxide plays an important role in the physiological system. It is an imperative regulator and mediator in nervous, immune and cardiovascular systems [80]. Nitric oxide level has been observed to be lower in diabetic subjects compared to control. Nitric oxide is produced from L-arginine due to the enzymatic activity of nitric oxide synthase (NOS), a pH dependent enzyme is produced from L-arginine due to the enzymatic activity of nitric oxide synthase (NOS). In diabetes, reduced production of nitric oxide is evidenced. Oxygen is a cofactor for the activity of NOS. In absence of sufficient oxygen, the functioning of the enzyme NOS becomes affected and consequently, less nitric oxide is produced. Circulation of oxygen in the blood flow is highly impaired in diabetic patients [81]. Nitric oxide plays a major role in preventing the development of atherosclerosis. Any decrease of NO production or level may results in the promotion of this process. The extent of atherosclerosis in human arteries correlates with the impairment of endothelium dependent vasodilatation. Vascular disease in diabetes is accompanied by decreased levels of the vasodilators, nitric oxide (NO) and prostacyclin, and increased levels of vasoconstrictor eicosanoids, which enhance the progression of the disease. The vascular dysfunction caused by short term exposure to elevated glucose and the long term effects of diabetes are similar, suggesting that the alteration in endothelial factors in diabetes primarily results from exposure of endothelial cells to elevated glucose, undoubtedly hyperlipidaemia contributes as well. A significant negative correlation ($p<0.01$) was found when serum nitric oxide was associated with serum glucose and HbA_{1c} levels in diabetic normotensive and diabetic hypertensive patients. These findings suggest that the constellation of disturbed glycemic control and formation of advanced glycosylation end products like HbA_{1c} critically contribute to anomalies of NO metabolism or *vice versa* and may help to explain frequent clinical coexistence of diabetes and hypertension [82].

Homocysteine (Hcy)

Plasma Hcy, a sulfhydryl-containing amino acid formed during the metabolism of methionine, is associated with endothelial damage and hypertension. Elevated Hcy levels may be associated with functional abnormalities in the small arteries and/or arterioles, leading to increased stiffness of these arteries and contributing to delay in the recovery of systemic vascular resistance. Substantial evidence is accumulating suggesting that hyperhomocysteinemia (HHcy) may be a risk factor for ischemic stroke. Over the last decade, evidence has accumulated that elevated plasma or serum concentrations of total homocysteine (tHcy) is associated with an increased risk of atherosclerosis, cardiovascular disease, and ischemic stroke [83]. Numerous experimental studies have demonstrated that high plasma concentrations of tHcy may cause vascular damage and alteration in the coagulation process [84-110]. Observational studies available mainly over the last decade have revealed that an elevated total plasma tHcy concentration is also associated with thrombogenic and cardiovascular disorders in the general population [111-147]. This connection seems to be independent from other known risk factors in cross-sectional and case control studies. The findings are less consistent in some of the prospective studies [148-155]. Important information is found in the meta-analysis of Boushey *et al.*, an increase of 5 micro mol/l in serum homocysteine enhanced the risk for CVD by 1.6- to 1.8-fold [156]. Thus, clinical, experimental, and epidemiological evidence all tend to suggest a link between plasma tHcy and CVD. Despite the 4-6-fold increase in CVD risk found in diabetic patients compared with their non-diabetic counterparts, a clear relationship between Hcy levels and diabetes has not yet been established. Plasma Hcy in diabetes varies depending on the presence or absence of nephropathy with levels being normal or even lower when there is no nephropathy and higher when there is nephropathy. Many studies have shown an association between HHcy and decreased renal function in patients with Type 2 diabetes [157]. Nevertheless, the highest level of homocysteine was associated with the lowest level of glomerular filtration rate. Taking into account the fact that plasma homocysteine concentration is closely related to renal function, the significance of plasma homocysteine should be considered with great caution. A recent growing interest has been focused on the association of HHcy with diabetes mellitus and with chronic renal failure. Interactions of homocysteine with insulin, metformin and cyclosporine have been proposed [158].

Dynamic and Electro Kinetic Parameters in Erythrocyte Membrane

It is now commonly believed that the cell cytoskeleton, by virtue of its interaction with the plasma membrane not only regulates the membrane function but also control the membrane structure. Several dynamic processes like cell motility, cell-cell interactions, membrane deformability, endocytosis, lateral diffusibility of membrane integral proteins, *etc.*, seem to be governed by the cytoskeleton-membrane interactions [159]. The osmolarity at which cells lyses are related to their shape, deformability, surface area/volume ratio and intrinsic membrane properties; and varies in different pathological conditions. The osmotic fragility of erythrocytes in diabetic and diabetic CVD subjects was studied as an index of the integrity of the red blood cell membrane. Sulfhydryl oxidation, carbonyl groups and glycated protein levels showed statistically significant differences between the diabetic and control groups for both the plasma and the erythrocyte membrane proteins [160]. However, less is known about the content and quality of membrane proteins which may contribute to abnormalities in membrane dynamic and decreased erythrocyte deformability. It has been reported that erythrocyte rigidity and plasma and whole blood viscosities were significantly higher in type 2 diabetes samples compared to controls. SDS-PAGE revealed that the band 5 corresponding to actin was weaker while band 4.5 corresponding to integral membrane proteins (glycophorin A, B and C) disappeared. Also, band 4.9, which is composed of dematin (a protein with actin-bundling capacity), was lost. This indicated the observed abnormalities in membrane proteins might play a role in reduced erythrocyte deformability associated with diabetes mellitus. Alterations in rheological properties and erythrocyte membrane proteins in cats with diabetes mellitus [161].

Zeta potential is widely used for quantification of the magnitude of the electrical charge at the double layer of erythrocyte membrane and is derived by measuring the mobility distribution of dispersion of charged particles subjected to an electric field. The membrane surface charge and the morphological and mechanical properties of erythrocytes were estimated according to the Zeta potential in normal and diabetic physiological conditions. Alteration in Zeta potential value indicated the extent of injury of red blood cell membrane in hyperglycemic state. Osmotic fragility experiment reveals erythrocytes of diabetic CVD patients to be more fragile compared to diabetic and control subjects [162]. Changes in Zeta potential values of the red blood cell membrane are consistent with the decreased membrane fluidity in diseased erythrocytes. It is evident, from the experimental data that for very low values of Zeta potential of bilayer membrane (*i.e.*, in diabetic CVD), blood begins to coagulate; a condition known as intravascular coagulation arises. Erythrocyte membrane is a supra molecular matrix and many molecules like spectrin, ankyrin, band 4.1 to band 3 are organized through noncovalent interaction into a higher order structure having emergent properties. SDS-PAGE of membrane protein reveals ankyrin level to be significantly decreased in case of diabetic and diabetic CVD [162]. This significant reduction of ankyrin protein obviously affects the rigidity of the cytoskeleton and may also lead to cellular deformability as a result of increased membrane rigidity that may lead to disease pathogenesis. It can be attributed to the fact that quantitative changes of the membrane proteins in erythrocyte cytoskeleton negatively influence normal membrane organization and stable function of erythrocyte. This is highly significant as these parameters can be efficiently used as diagnostic markers to find a correlation between diabetes and cardiovascular disease.

Platelet Aggregation

Platelets, one of the important blood components are known to play a pivotal role not only in the formation of arterial thrombosis but also in the progression of atherosclerotic disease. Insulin resistance is a uniform finding in type 2 diabetes, as are abnormalities in the microvascular and macrovascular circulations. These complications are associated with dysfunction of platelets and the neurovascular unit. Intact healthy vascular endothelium is central to the normal functioning of smooth muscle contractility as well as its normal interaction with platelets. The role of hyperglycemia is not clear in the functional and organic microvascular deficiencies and platelet hyperactivity in individuals with diabetes. The entire coagulation cascade becomes dysfunctional in diabetes. Platelets in type 2 diabetic individuals adhere to vascular endothelium and aggregate more readily than those in healthy people. Loss of sensitivity to the normal restraints exercised by prostacyclin (PGI2) and nitric oxide (NO) generated by the vascular endothelium presents as the major defect in platelet function. Insulin is a natural antagonist of platelet hyperactivity. It sensitizes the platelet to PGI2 and enhances endothelial generation of PGI2 and NO. Thus, the defects in insulin action in diabetes create a milieu of disordered platelet activity conducive to macrovascular and microvascular events [163]. Increased platelet activity is critically involved in the increased thrombogenic potential among diabetic patients. Several humoral factors like, prostacyclin, nitric oxide or insulin inhibits platelet aggregation to obtain homeostasis under physiological conditions. While enhanced platelet aggregation may predispose the system to the development of thrombotic disorders, the inhibition of platelet aggregation has been reported to result in the prevention of these conditions. The poor outcome of patients with diabetes and coronary artery disease including aggressive atherosclerosis [164, 165], abnormal endothelial function, impaired fibrinolysis, platelet hyperactivity [166] and a propensity to form neointima following arterial injury involves a numerous pathophysiological mechanisms. Inhibition of platelet thrombosis within the arterial circulation for therapeutic strategies are at present used: GPIIb-IIIa antagonists (*i.e.* eptifibatide, abciximab and tirofiban), P2Y12 receptor antagonists (ticlopidine and clopidogrel), anticoagulants (heparin, low molecular weight heparin, hirulog), and a COX-1 inhibitor (aspirin). An array of antiplatelet agents acting on various target points in platelets have been developed, but they do not appear to reduce completely the heightened thrombotic potential, even in combination regimes. Furthermore, there remains the uphill task of balancing clinical efficacy against bleeding risk. Large randomised trials specifically designed to study these aspects in the population with diabetes, are lacking. Despite better understanding of the pathophysiological processes underlying platelet activation and therapeutic advancements, the morbidity and mortality from atherothrombosis in type 2 diabetes remain unacceptably high. This dictates that accelerated research on platelet and search for more potent antiplatelet agents is urgently needed.

Non Genetic Lifestyle Factors Associated with CVD and HPT in Type 2 Diabetes

Food Habbit

The prevalence of type 2 diabetes has increased rapidly during the past decades. From 1990 to 2001, the prevalence of self-reported diabetes nearly doubled within the group aged 30-39 y and increased by 83% within the group aged 40-49 y. Although lifestyle characteristics such as obesity, physical activity, and smoking are established risk factors for this disease, less is known about dietary factors. The center stage for the treatment of diabetes is always diet, irrespective of the absence or presence of dyslipidemia. Reduction in dietary saturated fat intake, along with reduced cholesterol consumption can lower the risk of CVD and hypertension [167]. During the past decade, several lines of evidence have collectively provided strong support for a relation between diets and diabetes incidence. In animals and in short-term human studies, a high intake of carbohydrates with a high glycemic index (a relative measure of the incremental glucose response per gram of carbohydrate) produced greater insulin resistance than did the intake of low-glycemic-index carbohydrates. In large prospective epidemiologic studies, both the glycemic index and the glycemic load (the glycemic index multiplied by the amount of carbohydrate) of the overall diet have been associated with a greater risk of type 2 diabetes in both men and women [168]. In summary, both metabolic and epidemiologic evidence suggests that replacing high-glycemic-index forms of carbohydrate with low-glycemic-index carbohydrates will reduce the risk of type 2 diabetes and reduce hypoglycemic episodes among those treated with insulin. This low-risk dietary pattern has also been associated with reduced incidence of coronary heart disease [169]. A diet rich in fruits, vegetables, legumes, whole grains, and healthy sources of protein (poultry and fish), and containing unsaturated vegetable fats as the main source of fat, but that is low in red and processed meats, refined grains, and sugar-sweetened beverages can offer significant protection against type 2 diabetes. Such diets, with favorable fatty acid composition and high amounts of fiber and micronutrients, may be beneficial also in weight maintenance [170].

Exercise

Strong epidemiologic evidence indicates that diabetes is associated with lifestyle. People who migrate to Westernized countries, with their more sedentary lifestyles and "Westernized" diets, have greater risk of developing type 2 diabetes than do their counterparts, who remain in the native countries [171]. Diabetic individuals are less likely to participate in regular physical activity than nondiabetic individual. Exercise can increase glucose uptake as much as 20 fold, and as exercise continues, fat rather than carbohydrate becomes the predominant fuel that is burned. Exercise alone without weight loss has variable effects on lipid profile in type 2 patients [172]. Physical activity reduces diabetes risk by helping to maintain a healthy body weight and by improving insulin sensitivity. Even moderate activities, *e.g.*, regular walking, offer substantial benefits. Sedentary behaviors like TV watching, in contrast, promotes weight gain and diabetes risk. A healthy diet, together with regular physical activity, maintenance of a healthy body weight, consumption of moderate amounts of alcohol, and avoidance of sedentary behaviors and smoking, is likely to prevent most type 2 diabetes cases.

Addiction (Smoking/Alcohol)

Smoking and alcohol addiction have detrimental effects on microvascular diseases [173]. Several prospective studies have demonstrated that smoking is associated with a modestly increased risk of developing diabetes [174]. Although smoking cessation is associated with a modest increase in weight, it increases insulin sensitivity and improves the lipoprotein profile. Prospective studies clearly demonstrated that the beneficial effects of smoking cessation on diabetes risk outweigh the adverse effects on weight gain [175].

Moderate alcohol consumption (1-3 drinks/day) has been consistently associated with lower incidence of diabetes compared with abstinence or occasional alcohol consumption [176]. Most studies have observed a U-shaped association, with heavy alcohol consumption being associated with increased risk compared with moderate consumption. One study with 51 postmenopausal women showed a significant increase in insulin sensitivity after 8 weeks of moderate alcohol consumption [177].

Genetic Susceptibility for Type 2 Diabetes and associated CVD and HPT

DM is probably the best example of a multifactorial disease. This condition is the result of a complex interplay between genetic and environmental factors [178] where the latter play a major role in the clinical expression of the disease. Although evidence for a genetic component in type 2 is high, only 10% of the genetic risk factors for this DM have been identified compared with ~ 65% in case of type 1 diabetes. DM may be considered as a syndrome linked to several genetic variants with clinically defined subtypes, which are however dependent upon environmental factors. Many genes, interacting with environmental factors, are predicted to affect disease predisposition. Because of its complexity, with both gene-gene and gene-environment interactions impacting on disease risk, genetic influences have been difficult to elucidate and identification of genes involved has not been easily achieved. In recent years there has been increasing support for the idea that genes involved in monogenic forms of diabetes may play a wider role in type 2 diabetes predispositions. The candidate genes that are involved in increasing risk for type 2 diabetes are few listed below:

The genetic contribution is likely to comprise several gene variants, each with relatively modest effect, which acts in combination with each other and with lifestyle and behavioral factors to cause the disease. Several lines of evidence suggest that aetiopathogenesis of the common form of T2DM and its intrinsically related features of impaired insulin secretion associated with decreased insulin sensitivity include a strong genetic component. The familial clustering of the disease implicates the role of genetics in the development of diabetes [179].

Research indicates that in most cases of type 2 diabetes, there is more than one gene involved and that the gene combinations may differ between families. In addition, the genes may have only slight variations, and it is possible that the variations are common in the human population. There have been several different regions of the human genome associated with susceptibility to Type 2 diabetes. The first type 2 diabetes susceptibility locus, was discovered in Mexican-Americans from Starr Country, Texas, and was localized to D2S125- D2S140 region on chromosome 2 [180]. To date only two genes, calpain 10 (CAPN10) and hepatocyte nuclear factor 4 alpha (HNF4A), have been identified as diabetes susceptibility genes, by whole-genome linkage studies method. Calpain 10 is a calcium-activated enzyme that breaks down proteins. Discrepancy in the non-coding region of the CAPN10 gene is allied with a threefold increased risk of type 2 diabetes in Mexican Americans. Insulin secretion, insulin action, and the production of glucose by the liver may alter by genetic variantion of CAPN10 [181]. Mutations of HNF4A can ground an extremely rare form of diabetes, maturity onset diabetes in the young (MODY). Two studies, one of the Ashkenazi Jew population [182], and the other of the Finnish population [183], recognized four SNPs (named rs4810424, rs1884613, rs1884614, and rs2144908) of HNF4A gene that were linked with type 2 diabetes. Scientists can also use genetic information to predict the risk associated with type 2 diabetes caused by aberrant genes. Researchers have identified regions of genes that influence the development of CVD, which is related to type 2 diabetes. Population-based studies have shown that the relative risk of CVD in DM is several fold higher compared with those without DM (gene1, gene4). Genetic factors could contribute to differences in susceptibility to CVD among individuals with DM. One such factor is a functional allelic polymorphism in the haptoglobin gene. In different ethnic groups haptoglobin alleles diverge noticeably in their relative frequency [184]. The biophysical and biochemical properties of protein products of the two haptoglobin alleles (allele1 and 2) differ from each other. The protein product of the allele 1 is a more effective antioxidant compared with that produced by the 2 allele [185]. The Strong Heart Study, Munich Stent Study demonstrated that haptoglobin phenotype is predictive of development of microvascular complications in DM [186]. Over the last decade, tHcy has been identified as latent contributors for CVD. The plasma concentration of tHcy is determined by several factors, both genetic and acquired [187-196]. The most important genetic defects in the genes encoding for homocysteine metabolism are CBS and MTHFR. Mutated MTHFR (C677T) result in the substitution of an alanine residue by valine, as a result the enzyme become thermolabile and less active, which leads to an increase in tHcy levels especially in low folate conditions. T833C mutation and 844INS68 in the CBS gene in different ethnic backgrounds is a reliable index to predict CVD in type 2 patients [197]. KCNJ11 gene encodes potassium channels in the beta cells of the pancreas, activates the release of insulin. Cui N *et al.,* established that K_{ATP} channel-pore polymorphisms (P266T and R371H) have also been linked to sudden cardiac death [198] in Type 2 diabetes. A population based genomic study conducted among 1825 peoples (1460 men and 365 women) from Malaga, a city on the Mediterranean coast of southern Spain has shown that the genetic variants HindIII (rs320), S447X (rs328), D9N (rs1801177) and N291S (rs268) (*LPL*) are associated with TG levels [199], which is a common index of CVD in type 2 diabetes. In 785 Chinese subjects, of which about 60% had been diagnosed with early-onset type 2 diabetes (<40 years old) HindIII polymorphism was further investigated [200] and found that HindIII polymorphism of LPL is associated with coronary heart disease. Adiponectin is an insulin sensitizer in muscle and liver [201]. It is predictable that eight tagging SNPs in the ADIPOQ are in connection with serum adiponectin (R-Adiponectin gene). Association of hypoadiponectinemia with coronary artery disease in Japanese population was studied by Kumada M *et al.* [202]. Till date, intense efforts to identify genetic risk factors in type 2 diabetes mellitus induced CVD and hypertension have met with only limited success. Several whole-genome linkage studies are needed to find out the diabetes-cardiomyopathy susceptibility genes.

CONCLUSIONS

Diabetes is becoming the leading non communicable disease all over the world making a dent on personal and medical resources and it is high time an effective individualized strategy is devised for tackling the issue because it is a heterogeneous disorder in which both genetic and non genetic influences contribute to disease risk. Management of hyperglycemia, the hallmark metabolic abnormality associated with type 2 diabetes, has historically taken center stage in the treatment of diabetes, therapies directed at other coincident features, such as dyslipidemia, hypertension, hypercoagulability, obesity, and insulin resistance, have also been a major focus of research and therapy. However, current studies have failed to demonstrate a beneficial effect of intensive diabetes therapy on CVD in type 2 diabetes, although some management strategies are adopted to prevent diabetes and diabetes related CVD and hypertension. High economic and social costs of type 2 Diabetes and its rising prevalence emphasizes for its prevention. Intervention prior to the onset of type 2 Diabetes may be the only way of preventing the complications of Diabetes. Because of its chronic nature, the severity of its complications and the means required to control them, diabetes is a costly disease, not only for affected individuals and their families, but also for the health system itself. Developments in diabetes care and management have evolved over the last decade and include: the introduction of recombinant human insulin; the use of second generation oral agents; home glucose monitoring and glycohemoglobin monitoring; and a better understanding of the relationship between diabetic control and complications. Type 2 Diabetes can be prevented, but it will take enormous social and political will to make this a reality. Life is a journey, going on like a beautiful sparkling glass in spite of its imperfections and unstable character. The small steps one can take to delay or prevent the disease and live a long, healthy life will bring great rewards.

ACKNOWLEDGEMENTS

The authors extend their thanks to the Editors and Bentham Science Publishers.

DECLARATION OF CONFLICT OF INTEREST

No conflict of interest was declared by the authors.

REFERENCES

[1]   Hayden MR. Islet Amyloid, Metabolic Syndrome, and the Natural Progressive History of Type 2 Diabetes Mellitus. J Pancreas 2002; 3(5): 126-138.

[2]   Mahgoub MA and Abd-Elfattah AS. Diabetes mellitus and cardiac function. Molecul Cell Biochem 1998; 180:59-64.

[3]   Castano L and Eisenbarth GS. Type-I diabetes: a chronic autoimmune disease of human, mouse, and rat. Annu Rev Immunol 1990; 8: 647-679.

[4]   Reaven GM. Role of insulin resistance in human disease. Diabetes 1988; 37: 1595-1607.

[5]   Sacks DB and McDonald JM. The pathogenesis of type II diabetes mellitus: a polygenic disease. Am J Clin Pathol 1996; 105: 149-156.

[6]   Taylor SI. Deconstructing type 2 diabetes. Cell 1999; 97:9-12.

[7]   Baynes JW and Thorpe SR. The role of oxidative stress in diabetic complications. Curr Opin Endocrinol 1996; 3: 277-284.

[8]   Grundy SM. Current Medicine, 4th edition. Philadelphia: LLC, 2005; 11: 212.

[9]   Sladek R, Rocheleau G, Rung J, Dina C, Shen L, Serre D, Boutin P, Vincent D, Belisle A, Hadjadj S, Balkau B, Heude B, Charpentier G, Hudson TJ, Montpetit A, Pshezhetsky AV, Prentki M, Posner BI, Balding DJ, Meyre D, Polychronakos C, and Froguel P. A genome-wide association study identifies novel risk loci for type 2 diabetes. Nature 2007; 445: 881-885.

[10] Scott LJ, Mohlke KL, Bonnycastle LL, Willer CJ, Li Y, Duren WL, *et al.* A genome-wide association study of type 2 diabetes in Finns detects multiple susceptibility variants. Science 2007; 316: 1341-1345.

[11] Narayan KMV, Gregg EW, Fagot-Campagna A, Engelgau MM, and Vinicor F. Compliance and adherence are dysfunctional concepts in diabetes. Diabetes Res Clin Pract 2000; 50: 77-84.

[12] Hunter DJ. Gene-environment interactions in human diseases. Nat Rev Genet 2005; 6: 287-298.

[13] Maahs D M, Kinney GL, Wadwa P, S-Bergeon JK, Dabelea D, Jhokanson J, Ehrlich J, Garg S, Eckel RH, Rewers MJ. Hypertension prevalence, awareness, treatment, and control in an adult type1 diabetes population and a comparable general population. Diabetes Care 2005; 28: 301-306.

[14] Hajjar I, Kotchen TA: Trends in prevalence, awareness, treatment, and control of hypertension in the United States, 1988-2000. JAMA 2003; 290: 199-206.

[15] Khot UN, Khot MB, Bajzer CT, Sapp SK,Ohman EM, Brener SJ, Ellis SG, Lincoff AM, Topol EJ: Prevalence of conventional risk factors in patients with coronary heart disease. JAMA 2003; 290: 898-904.

[16] Berlowitz DR, Arlene S, Hickey EC, Glickman M, Friedman R, Kader B. Hypertension management in patients with diabetes. Diabetes Care 2003; 26: 355-359.

[17] Creely SJ, Aresh J, Anware J, Kumar S. The metabolic syndrome and vascular disease. Editted by Michael T Johnstone, Veves A. Second edition, Human press. Totowa, New Jersey.

[18]   Sepa A, Wahlberg J, Vaarala O, Frodi A, Ludvigsson J. Psychological Stress May Induce Diabetes-Related Autoimmunity in Infancy. Diabetes Care 2005; 28: 290-295.

[19]   Agardh EE, Ahlbom A, Andersson T, Efendic S, Grill V, Hallqvist J, Norman A, Gorano Stenson C. Work stress and low sense of coherence Is associated with type 2 diabetes in middle-aged swedish women. Diabetes Care 2003; 26: 719-724.

[20]   Dabelea D, Bell RA, D'Agostino RB, Imperatore G, Johansen JM, Linder B, Liu LL, Loots B, Marcovina S, Mayer-Davis EJ, Pettitt DJ, Waitzfelder B. Writing Group for the SEARCH for Diabetes in Youth Study Group. Incidence of diabetes in youth in the United States. JAMA 2007; 297(24): 2716-24.

[21]   Rotteveel J, Belksma EJ, Renders CM, Hirasing RA, Delemarre-Van de Waal HA. Type 2 diabetes in children in the Netherlands: the need for diagnostic protocols. Eur J Endocrinol 2007; 157(2): 175-80.

[22]   Wei JN, Sung FC, Lin CC, Lin RS, Chiang CC, Chuang LM. National surveillance for type 2 diabetes mellitus in Taiwanese children. JAMA 2003; 290(10): 1345-50.

[23]   Dabelea D, Pettitt DJ, Jones KL, Arslanian SA. Type 2 diabetes mellitus in minority children and adolescents. An emerging problem. Endocrinol Metab Clin North Am 1999; 28(4): 709-29.

[24]   Jocelyne G. Karam & Samy I. McFarlane. Update on the Prevention of Type 2 Diabetes Curr Diab Rep DOI 10.1007/s11892-010-0163-x 2010.

[25]   Midhet FM, Al-Mohaimeed AA, Sharaf FK. Lifestyle related risk factors of type 2 diabetes mellitus in Saudi Arabia. Saudi Med J. 2010; 31(7): 768-74.

[26]   Knowler WC, Barrett-Connor E, Fowler SE, *et al.* Reduction in the incidence of type 2 diabetes with lifestyle intervention or metformin. N Engl J Med 2002; 346: 393-403.

[27]   Knowler WC, Fowler SE, Hamman RF. 10-year follow-up of diabetes incidence and weight loss in the Diabetes Prevention Program Outcomes Study. Lancet 2009; 374 (9702): 1677-1686.

[28]   Mozaffarian D, Kamineni A, Carnethon M, Djoussé L, Mukamal KJ, Siscovic, D. "Lifestyle risk factors and new-onset diabetes mellitus in older adults: the cardiovascular health study". Archives of Internal Medicine 2009; 169(8): 798-807.

[29]   Garrow J. Importane of obesity. BMJ 1991; 303: 704-706.

[30]   Wilson PW, D'Agostino RB, Sullivan L, Parise H, Kannel WB. Overweight and obesity as determinants of cardiovascular risk: the Framingham experience. Arch Intern Med 2002; 162: 1867-1872.

[31]   Kurth T, Gaziano JM, Rexrode KM, Kase CS, Cook NR, Manson JE, Buring JE. Prospective study of body mass index and risk of stroke in apparently healthy women. Circulation 2005; 111: 1992-1998.

[32]   Folsom AR, Rasmussen ML, Chambless LE, Howard G, Cooper LS, Schmidt MI, Heiss G. Prospective associations of fasting insulin, body fat distribution, and diabetes with risk of ischemic stroke: the Atherosclerosis Risk in Communities (ARIC) Study Investigators. Diabetes Care 1999; 1077-1083.

[33]   Suk SH, Sacco RL, Boden-Albala B, Cheun JF, Pittman JG, Elkind MS, Paik MC. Abdominal obesity and risk of ischemic stroke: the Northern Manhattan Stroke Study. Stroke 2003; 34: 1586-1592.

[34]   Centers for Disease Control (CDC): The Surgeon General's 1989 report on reducing the health consequences of smoking: 25 years of progress. MMWR Morb Mortal Wkly Rep 38 1989; (Suppl. 2): 1-32.

[35]   Mokdad AH, Marks JS, Stroup DF, Gerberding JL: Correction: actual causes of death in the United States 2000. JAMA 2005; 293: 293-294.

[36]   Mokdad AH, Marks JS, Stroup DF, Gerberding JL: Actual causes of death in the United States, 2000. JAMA 2004; 291: 1238- 1245.

[37]   Jood K, Jern C, Wilhelmsen L, Rosengren A. Body mass index in mid-life is associated with a first stroke in men: a prospective population study over 28 years. Stroke 2004; 35: 2764-2769.

[38]   Song YM, Sung J, Davey Smith G, Ebrahim S. Body mass index and ischemic and hemorrhagic stroke: a prospective study in Korean men. Stroke 2004; 35: 831- 836.

[39]   Abbott RD, Behrens GR, Sharp DS, Rodriguez BL, Burchfiel CM, Ross GW, Yano K, Curb JD: Body mass index and thromboembolic stroke in nonsmoking men in older middle age. the Honolulu Heart Program. Stroke 1994; 25: 2370-2376.

[40]   Rexrode KM, Hennekens CH, Willett WC, Colditz GA, Stampfer MJ, Rich- Edwards JW, Speizer FE, Manson JE. A prospective study of body mass index, weight change, and risk of stroke in women. JAMA 1997; 277: 1539-1545.

[41]   Kurth T, Gaziano JM, Berger K, Kase CS, Rexrode KM, Cook NR, Buring JE, Manson JE. Body mass index and the risk of stroke in men. Arch Intern Med 2002; 162: 2557-2562.

[42]   Lu M, Ye W, Adami HO, Weiderpass E. Prospective study of body size and risk for stroke amongst women below age 60. J Intern Med 2006; 260: 442-450.

[43]   Oster G, Thompson D, Edelsberg J, Bird AP, Colditz GA. Lifetime health and economic benefits of weight loss among obese persons. Am J Public Health 1999; 89: 1536-1542.

[44]   Ellen L. Air, Brett M. Kissela Diabetes, the Metabolic Syndrome, and Ischemic Stroke diabetes care 2007; 30:12.

[45]   Kissela BM, Khoury J, Kleindorfer D, Woo D, Schneider A, Alwell K, Miller R, Ewing I, Moomaw CJ, Szaflarski JP, Gebel J, Shukla R, Broderick JP. Epidemiology of ischemic stroke in patients with diabetes: the Greater Cincinnati/ Northern Kentucky Stroke Study. Diabetes Care 2005; 28: 355-359.

[46]   Jorgensen H, Nakayama H, Raaschou HO, Olsen TS. Stroke in patients with diabetes: the Copenhagen Stroke Study. Stroke 1994; 25: 1977-1984.

[47]   Iso H, Jacobs DR Jr, Wentworth D, Neaton JD, Cohen JD. Serum cholesterol levels and six-year mortality from stroke in 350,977 men screened for the multiple risk factor intervention trial. N Engl J Med 1989; 320: 904-910.

[48]   Laws A, Marcus EB, Grove JS, Curb JD. Lipids and lipoproteins as risk factors for coronary heart disease in men with abnormal glucose tolerance: the Honolulu Heart Program. J Intern Med 1993; 234: 471- 478.

[49]   Kagan A, Popper JS, Rhoads GG. Factors related to stroke incidence in Hawaii Japanese men: the Honolulu Heart Study. Stroke 1980; 11: 14-21.

[50]   Shahar E, Chambless LE, Rosamond WD, Boland LL, Ballantyne CM, McGovern PG, Sharrett AR. Plasma lipid profile and incident ischemic stroke: the Atherosclerosis Risk in Communities (ARIC) study. Stroke 2003; 34: 623-631.

[51]   Harmsen P, Rosengren A, Tsipogianni A, Wilhelmsen L. Risk factors for stroke in middle-aged men in Goteborg, Sweden. Stroke 1990; 21: 223-229.

[52]   Prospective Studies Collaboration. Cholesterol, diastolic blood pressure, and stroke: 13,000 strokes in 450,000 people in 45 prospective cohorts. Lancet 1995; 346: 1647-1653.

[53]   Colhoun HM, Betteridge DJ, Durrington PN, Hitman GA, Neil HA, Livingstone SJ, Thomason MJ, Mackness MI, Charlton- Menys V, Fuller JH. Primary prevention of

cardiovascular disease with atorvastatin in type 2 diabetes in the Collaborative Atorvastatin Diabetes Study (CARDS): multicentre randomised placebo- controlled trial. Lancet 2004; 364: 685-696.

[54]   Collins R, Armitage J, Parish S, Sleigh P, Peto R: MRC/BHF Heart Protection Study of cholesterol-lowering with simvastatin in 5963 people with diabetes: a randomised placebo-controlled trial. Lancet 2003; 361:2005-2016.

[55]   Ravera M, Ratto E, Vettoretti S, Viazzi F, Leoncini G, Parodi D, Tomolillo C, Del Sette M, Maviglio N, Deferrari G, Pontremoli R. Microalbuminuria and subclinical cerebrovascular damage in essential hypertension. J Nephrol 2002; 15: 519-524.

[56]   Gerstein HC, Mann JF, Yi Q, Zinman B, Dinneen SF, Hoogwerf B, Halle JP, Young J, Rashkow A, Joyce C, Nawaz S, Yusuf S. Albuminuria and risk of cardiovascular events, death, and heart failure in diabetic and nondiabetic individuals. JAMA 2001; 286: 421-426.

[57]   Eknoyan G, Hostetter T, Bakris GL, Hebert L, Levey AS, Parving HH, Steffes MW, Toto R. Proteinuria and other markers of chronic kidney disease: a position statement of the national kidney foundation (NKF) and the national institute of diabetes and digestive and kidney diseases (NIDDK). Am J Kidney Dis. 2003; 42: 617-22.

[58]   Yuyun MF, Khaw KT, Luben R, Welch A, Bingham S, Day NE, Wareham NJ. Microalbuminuria and stroke in a British population: the European Prospective Investigation into Cancer in Norfolk (EPIC-Norfolk) population study. J Intern Med 2004; 255: 247-256.

[59]   Ahmed N, babaei-jadidi R, Howell SK, Thornalley PJ, Beisswenger PJ. Glycated and Oxidized Protein Degradation Products Are Indicators of Fasting and Postprandial Hyperglycemia in Diabetes. Diabetes Care 2005; 28: 2465-2471.

[60]   Nishikawa T, Edelstein D, Du X, Yamagishi S, Matsumura T, Kaneda Y, Yorek M, Beebe D, Oates P, Hammes H, Giardino I, Brownlee M: Normalizing mitochondrial superoxide production blocks three pathways of hyperglycemic damage. Nature 2000; 404: 787-790.

[61]   Brownlee M. Biochemistry and molecular cell biology of diabetic complications. Nature 2001; 414: 813-820.

[62]   Hink U, Li H, Mollnau H, Oelze M, Matheis E, Hartmann M, Skatchkov M, Thaiss F, Stahl RA, Warnholtz A, Meinertz T, Griendling K, Harrison DG, Forstermann U, Munzel T. Mechanisms underlying endothelial dysfunction in diabetes mellitus. Circ Res 2001; 88:14-22.

[63]   Maillard LC. Action des acides amines sur les sucres; formation des melaniodines par voie methodique. C R Acad Sci 1912; 154: 66-68.

[64]   Arindam Saha, Sangeeta Adak, Subhankar Chowdhury, Maitree Bhattacharyya.Enhanced oxygen releasing capacity and oxidative stress in diabetes mellitus and diabetes mellitus-associated cardiovascular disease: A comparative study. Clinica Chimica Acta 2005; 361: 141-149.

[65]   Miyata T, Van Ypersele De Strihou C, Kurokawa K, Baynes JW. Alterations in nonenzymatic biochemistry in uremia: origin and significance of.carbonyl stress. in long-term uremic complications. Kidney Int 1999; 55: 389-399.

[66]   Witko-Sarsat V, Friedlander M, Capeillere-Blandin C, Nguyen-Khoa T, Nguyen AT, Zingraff J, Jungers P, Deschamps-Latscha B. Advanced oxidation protein products as a novel marker of oxidative stress in uraemia. Kidney Int 1996; 49: 1304-1313.

[67]   Kalousová M, KRHA J, ZIMA T. Advanced Glycation End-Products and Advanced Oxidation Protein Products in Patients with Diabetes Mellitus. Physiol Res 2002; 51: 597-604.

[68]   Bierhaus A, Hofmann MA, Ziegler R, Nawroth PP. AGEs and their interaction with AGE-receptors in vascular disease and diabetes mellitus. I. The AGE concept. Cardiovasc Res 1998; 37: 586-600.

[69]   Witko-Sarsat V, Friedlander M, Nguyen-Khoa T, Capeillere-Blandin C, Nguyen AH, Canterloup S, Drayer JM, Jungers P, Drueke T, Deschamps-Latscha B. Advanced oxidation protein products as novel mediator of inflammation and monocyte activation in chronic renal failure. J Immunol 1998; 161: 2524-2532.

[70]   Arpita Chakraborty, Subhankar Chowdhury, Maitree Bhattacharyya. Effect of metformin on oxidative stress, nitrosative stress and inflammatory biomarkers in type2 diabetes patients. Diabetes Research and Clinical Practice 2010. In press.

[71]   Antonio C. Possible role of oxidative stress in the pathogenesis of hypertension diabetes care 2008; 31; 2.

[72]   Ehud Grossman. Does Increased Oxidative Stress Cause Hypertension? Diabetes care 2008; 31: 2.

[73]   Camici GG, Schiavoni M, Francia P, Bachschmid M, Martin-Padura I, Hersberger M *et al.* Genetic deletion of p66 (Shc) adaptor protein prevents hyperglycemia-induced endothelial dysfunction and oxidative stress. Proc Natl Acad Sci USA 2007; 104(12): 5217-5222.

[74]   Peter Chase H, Lockspeiser T, Peery B, Shepherd M, Mackenzie T, Anderson J, Garg SK. The Impact of the Diabetes Control and Complications Trial and Humalog Insulinon Glycohemoglobin Levels and Severe Hypoglycemia in Type 1 Diabetes. Diabetes Care 2001; 24: 430-434.

[75]   Selvin E, Crainiceanu CM, Brancati FL, Coresh J. Short-term variability in measures of glycemia and implications for the classification of diabetes. Arch Intern Med, 2007; 167: 1545-51.

[76]   Meigs JB, Nathan DM, Cupples LA, Wilson PW, Singer DE. Tracking of glycated hemoglobin in the original cohort of the Framingham Heart Study. J Clin Epidemiol 1996; 49: 411-7.

[77]   Selvin E, Steffes M, Zhu H, Matsushita K, Wagenknecht L, Pankow PHJ., Coresh J, Brancati FL.Glycated Hemoglobin, Diabetes, and Cardiovascular Risk in Nondiabetic Adults, N Engl J Med 2010; 362: 800-11.

[78]   Danesh J, Collins R, Appleby P, Peto R. Association of fibrinogen, C-reactive protein, albumin, or leukocyte count with coronary heart disease. J Am Coll Cardiol 1998; 279: 1477-82.

[79]   Lagrand WK, Visser CA, Hermens WT, Niessen HWM, Verheugt FWA, Wolbink G-J, Hack CE. C-reactive protein as a cardiovascular risk factor. More than an epiphenomenon? Circulation 1999; 100: 96-102.

[80]   Loscalzo J, Welch G. Nitric oxide and its role in the cardiovascular system. Pro Car Disease 1995; 38, 87-104.

[81]   Nitric oxide and its role in health and diabetes. Available from http://www.diabetesincontrol.com/burkearchive/nitricoxide.shtml accessed 2008.

[82]   Shahid SM, Mahboob T. Diabetes and Hypertension: Correlation Between Glycosylated Hemoglobin (HbA1c) and Serum Nitric Oxide (NO). Australian Journal of Basic and Applied Sciences 2009; 3(2): 1323-1327.

[83]   Tayama J, Munakata M, Yoshinaga K, Toyota T. Higher plasma homocysteine concentration is associated with more advanced systemic arterial stiffness and greater blood pressure response to stress in hypertensive patients. Hypertens Res 2006; 29: 403-409.

[84]   McDonald L, Bray C, Field C, Love F, Davies B. Homocystinuria, thrombosis and the blood platelets. Lancet 1964;1: 745-6.

[85]   Harker LA, Slichter SJ, Scott CR, Ross R. Homocysteinemia. Vascular injury and arterial thrombosis. N Engl J Med 1974; 291(11): 537-43.

[86]   Harker LA, Ross R, Slichter SJ, Scott CR. Homocystine-induced arteriosclerosis. The role of endothelial cell injury and platelet response in its genesis. J Clin Invest 1976; 58(3): 731-41.

[87]   Wall RT, Harlan JM, Harker LA, Striker GE. Homocysteine induced endothelial cell injury *in vitro*: a model for the study of vascular injury. Thromb Res 1980; 18(1-2): 113-21.

[88]   Graeber JE, Slott JH, Ulane RE, Schulman JD, Stuart MJ. Effect of homocysteine and homocysteine on platelet and vascular arachidonic acid metabolism. Pediatr Res 1982; 16(6): 490- 3.

[89]   Harker LA, Harlan JM, Ross R. Effect of sulfinpyrazone on homocysteine-induced endothelial injury and arteriosclerosis in baboons. Circ Res 1983; 53(6): 731-9.

[90]   Harman LS, Mottley C, Mason RP. Free radical metabolites of L-cysteine oxidation. J Biol Chem 1984; 259(9): 5606-11.

[91]   Starkebaum G, Harlan JM. Endothelial cell injury due to copper-catalyzed hydrogen peroxide generation from homocysteine. J Clin Invest 1986; 77(4): 1370-6.

[92]   Heinecke JW, Rosen H, Suzuki LA, Chait A. The role of sulfur-containing amino acids in superoxide production and modification of low density lipoprotein by arterial smooth muscle cells. J Biol Chem 1987; 262(21): 10098-103.

[93]   Parthasarathy S. Oxidation of low-density lipoprotein by thiol compounds leads to its recognition by the acetyl LDL receptor. Biochim Biophys Acta 1987; 917(2): 337-40.

[94]   Rodgers GM, Conn MT. Homocysteine, an atherogenic stimulus, reduces protein C activation by arterial and venous endothelial cells. Blood 1990; 75(4): 895-901.

[95]   Lentz SR, Sadler JE. Inhibition of thrombomodulin surface expression and protein C activation by the thrombogenic agent homocysteine. J Clin Invest 1991; 88(6): 1906-14.

[96]   Blom HJ, Engelen DP, Boers GH, Stadhouders AM, Sengers RC, de Abreu R *et al.* Lipid peroxidation in homocysteinemia. J Inherited Metab Dis 1992; 15: 419-22.

[97]   Ueland PM, Brattstrom L, Refrim H. Plasma homocysteine and cardiovascular disease. In: Francis RB Jr, editor. Atherosclerotic cardiovascular disease, hemostasis and endothelial function. New York: Marcel Dekker, 1992: 183-235.

[98]   Lentz SR, Sadler JE. Homocysteine inhibits von Willebrand factor processing and secretion by preventing transport from the endoplasmic reticulum. Blood 1993; 81(3): 683-9.

[99]   Stamler JS, Osborne JA, Jaraki O *et al.* Adverse vascular effects of homocysteine are modulated by endothelium-derived relaxing factor and related oxides of nitrogen. J Clin Invest 1993; 91(1): 308-18.

[100]   Tsai JC, Perrella MA, Yoshizumi M, Hsieh CM, Haber E, Schlegel R *et al.* Promotion of vascular smooth muscle cell growth by homocysteine: a link to atherosclerosis. Proc Natl Acad Sci USA 1994; 91: 6369-73.

[101]   Blom HJ, Kleinveld HA, Boers GHJ *et al.* Lipid peroxidation and susceptibility of low-density lipoprotein to *in vitro* oxidation in hyperhomocysteinemia. Eur J Clin Invest 1995; 25: 149-54.

[102]   Blundell G, Jones BG, Rose FA, Tudball N. Homocysteine mediated endothelial cell toxicity and its amelioration. Atherosclerosis 1996; 12: 163-72.

[103]   Halvorsen B, Brude I, Drevon CA, Nysom J, Ose L, Christiansen EN *et al.* Effect of homocysteine on copper ioncatalysed, azo compound-initiated, and mononuclear cell-

mediated oxidative modification of low density lipoprotein. J Lipid Res 1996; 37: 1591-600.

[104]   Lentz SR, Sobey CG, Piegors DJ *et al.* Vascular dysfunction in monkeys with diet-induced hyperhomocyst(e)inemia. J Clin Invest 1996; 98(1): 24-9.

[105]   Tsai JC, Wang H, Perrella MA, Yoshizumi M, Sibinga NE, Tan LC *et al.* Induction of cyclin A gene expression by homocysteine in vascular smooth muscle cells. J Clin Invest 1996; 97: 146-53.

[106]   Woo KS, Chook P, Lolin YI, *et al.* Hyperhomocyst(e)inemia is a risk factor for arterial endothelial dysfunction in humans. Circulation 1997; 96(8): 2542-4.

[107]   Tawakol A, Omland T, Gerhard M, Wu JT, Creager MA. Hyperhomocyst(e)inemia: is associated with impaired endothelial- dependent vasodilatation in humans. Circulation 1997; 95: 1119-21.

[108]   Majors A, Ehrhart LA, Pezacka EH. Homocysteine as a risk factor for vascular disease. Enhanced collagen production and accumulation by smooth muscle cells. Arterioscler Thromb Vasc Biol 1997; 17(10): 2074-81.

[109]   Chambers JC, Obeid O, McGregor A, Powell-Tuck J, Boustead L, Kooner JS. The relationship between hyperhomocysteinemia and endothelial dysfunction is concentration-dependant, and present even at physiological levels. Circulation 1998; 98:1-192.

[110]   Al-Obaidi MK, Philippou H, Stubbs PJ, *et al.* Relationship between homocysteine, Factor VIIa, and thrombin generation in acute coronary syndromes. Circulation 2000; 101: 372-7.

[111]   Malinow MR, Kang SS, Taylor LM, *et al.* Prevalence of hyperhomocyst(e)inemia in patients with peripheral arterial occlusive disease. Circulation 1989; 79(6): 1180-8.

[112]   Genest J Jr, McNamara JR, Salem DN, Wilson PF, Schaefer EJ, Malinow MR. Plasma homocyst(e)ine levels in men with premature coronary artery disease. JACC 1990; 16: 1114-9.

[113]   Malinow MR. Hyperhomocyst(e)inemia. A common and easily reversible risk factor for occlusive atherosclerosis. Circulation 1990; 81(6):2004-6 Published erratum appears in Circulation 1990; 82(4): 1547.

[114]   Coull BM, Malinow MR, Beamer N, Sexton G, Nordt F, de Garmo P. Elevated plasma homocyst(e)ine concentration as a possible independent risk factor for stroke. Stroke 1990; 21(4): 572-6.

[115]   Stampfer MJ, Malinow MR, Willett WC *et al.* A prospective study of plasma homocyst(e)ine and risk of myocardial infarction in US physicians. JAMA 1992; 268(7): 877-81.

[116]   Brattstrom L, Lindgren A, Israelsson B *et al.* Hyperhomocysteinaemia in stroke: prevalence, cause, and relationships to type of stroke and stroke risk factors. Eur J Clin Invest 1992; 22(3): 214-21.

[117]   Rees MM, Rodgers GM. Homocysteinemia: association of a metabolic disorder with vascular disease and thrombosis. Thromb Res 1993; 71(5): 337-59 Review.

[118]   Malinow MR, Nieto FJ, Szklo M, Chambless LE, Bond G. Carotid artery intimal-medial wall thickening and plasma homocyst(e)ine in asymptomatic adults. The Atherosclerosis risk in communities study. Circulation 1993; 87(4): 1107-13.

[119]   von Eckardstein A, Malinow MR, Upson B, Heinrich J, Schulte H, Schonfeld G *et al.* Effects of age, lipoproteins, and hemostatic parameters on the role of homocyst(e)inemia as a cardiovascular risk factor in men. Arterioscler Thromb 1994; 14(3): 464.

[120] Malinow MR, Stampfer MJ. Role of plasma homocyst(e)ine in arterial occlusive diseases. Clin Chem 1994; 40(6): 857-8 Editorial.

[121] Selhub J, Jacques PF, Bostom AG *et al.* Association between plasma homocysteine concentrations and extracranial carotidartery stenosis. N Engl J Med 1995; 332(5): 286-91.

[122] Perry IJ, Refsum H, Morris RW, Ebrahim SB, Ueland PM, Shaper AG. Prospective study of serum total homocysteine concentration and risk of stroke in middle-aged British men. Lancet 1995; 346(8987): 1395-8.

[123] Nygard O, Vollset SE, Refsum H, *et al.* Total plasma homocysteine and cardiovascular risk profile. The Hordaland Homocysteine Study. JAMA 1995; 274(19): 1526-33.

[124] Dalery K, Lussier-Cacan S, Selhub J, Davignon J, Latour Y, Genest J Jr. Homocysteine and coronary artery disease in French Canadian subjects: relation with vitamins B12, B6, pyridoxal phosphate, and folate. Am J Cardiol 1995; 75(16): 1107- 11.

[125] Arnesen E, Refsum H, Bonaa KH, Ueland PM, Forde OH, Nordrehaug JE. Serum total homocysteine and coronary heart disease. Int J Epidemiol 1995; 24(4): 704-9.

[126] Boushey CJ, Beresford SA, Omenn GS, Motulsky AG. A quantitative assessment of plasma homocysteine as a risk factor for vascular disease. Probable benefits of increasing folic acid intakes. JAMA 1995; 274(13): 1049-57.

[127] Hopkins PN, Wu LL, Wu J, Hunt SC, James BC, Vincent GM, *et al.* Higher plasma homocyst(e)ine and increased susceptibility to adverse effects of low folate in early familial coronary artery disease. Arterioscler Thromb Vasc Biol 1995; 15(9): 1314-20.

[128] Robinson K, Mayer EL, Miller DP *et al.* Hyperhomocysteinemia and low pyridoxal phosphate. Common and independent reversible risk factors for coronary artery disease. Circulation 1995; 92(10): 2825-30.

[129] Selhub J, Jacques PF, Bostom AG, *et al.* Relationship between plasma homocysteine, vitamin status and extracranial carotidartery stenosis in the Framingham study population. J Nutr 1996; 126: 1258-65.

[130] Malinow MR, Ducimetiere P, Luc G, *et al.* Plasma homocyst(e)ine levels and graded risk for myocardial infarction: findings in two populations at contrasting risk for coronary heart disease. Atherosclerosis 1996; 126(1): 27-34.

[131] Malinow MR. Plasma homocyst(e)ine: a risk factor for arterial occlusive diseases. J Nutr 1996; 126(Suppl 4): 1238S-43S Review.

[132] van den Berg M, Stehouwer CD, Bierdrager E, Rauwerda JA. Plasma homocysteine and severity of atherosclerosis in young patients with lower-limb atherosclerotic disease. Arterioscler Thromb Vasc Biol 1996; 16: 165-71.

[133] Petri M, Roubenoff R, Dallal GE, Nadeau MR, Selhub J, Rosenberg IH. Plasma homocysteine as a risk factor for atherothrombotic events in systemic lupus erythematous. Lancet 1996; 348(9035): 1120-4.

[134] Nygard O, Nordrehaug JE, Refsum H, Ueland PM, Farstad M, Vollset SE. Plasma homocysteine levels and mortality in patients with coronary artery disease. N Engl J Med 1997; 337(4): 230-6.

[135] Graham IM, Daly LE, Refsum HM *et al.* Plasma homocysteine as a risk factor for vascular disease. The European concerted action project. JAMA 1997; 277(22): 1775-81.

[136] Aronow WS, Ahn C, Schoenfeld MR. Association between plasma homocysteine and extracranial carotid arterial disease in older persons. Am J Cardiol 1997; 79(10): 1432-3.

[137] Aronow WS, Ahn C. Association between plasma homocysteine and coronary artery disease in older persons. Am J Cardiol 1997; 80(9): 1216-8.

[138] Konecky N, Malinow MR, Tunick PA *et al.* Correlation between plasma homocyst(e)ine and aortic atherosclerosis. Am Heart J 1997; 133(5): 534-40.

[139] Alfthan G, Aro A, Gey KF. Plasma homocysteine and cardiovascular disease mortality. Lancet 1997; 349(9049): 39 Letter.

[140] Joubran R, Asmi M, Busjahn A, Vergopoulos A, Luft FC, Jouma M. Homocysteine levels and coronary heart disease in Syria. J Cardiovasc Risk 1998; 5(4): 257-61.

[141] Omenn GS, Beresford SA, Motulsky AG. Preventing coronary heart disease: B vitamins and homocysteine. Circulation 1998; 97: 421-4.

[142] Wald NJ, Watt HC, Law MR, Weir DG, McPartlin J, Scott JM. Homocysteine and ischemic heart disease: results of a prospective study with implications regarding prevention. Arch Intern Med 1998; 158(8): 862-7.

[143] Robinson K, Arheart K, Refsum H *et al.* Low circulating folate and vitamin B6 concentrations: risk factors for stroke, peripheral vascular disease, and coronary artery disease. European COMAC group. Circulation 1998; 97(5): 437-43.

[144] Refsum H, Ueland PM, Nygard O, Vollset SE. Homocysteine and cardiovascular disease. Annu Rev Med 1998; 49: 31-62.

[145] Welch GN, Loscalzo J. Homocysteine and atherothrombosis. N Engl J Med 1998; 338(15): 1042-50 Review.

[146] Stehouwer CD, Weijenberg MP, van den Berg M, Jakobs C, Feskens EJ, Kromhout D. Serum homocysteine and risk of coronary heart disease and cerebrovascular disease in elderly men: a 10-year follow-up. Arterioscler Thromb Vasc Biol 1998; 18(12): 1895-901.

[147] Bostom AG, Silbershatz H, Rosenberg ICH *et al.* Nonfasting plasma total homocysteine levels and all-cause and cardiovascular disease mortality in elderly Framingham men and women. Arch Int Med 1999; 159: 1077-80.

[148] Booth GL, Wang EE. Preventive health care: 2000 update: screening and management of hyperhomocysteinemia for the prevention of coronary artery events. CMAJ 2000; 163(1): 21-9.

[149] Verhoef P, Hennekens CH, Malinow MR, Kok FJ, Willet WC, Stampfer MJ. A prospective study of plasma homocyst(e)ine and risk of ischemic stroke. Stroke 1994; 25: 1924 30.

[150] Alfthan G, Pekkanen J, Jauhiainen M, Pitkaniemi J, Karvonen M, Tuomilehto J *et al.* Relation of serum homocysteine and lipoprotein (a) concentrations to atherosclerosis disease in a prospective Finnish population based study. Atherosclerosis 1994; 106: 9-19.

[151] Chasan-Taber L, Selhub J, Rosenberg IH, Malinow MR *et al.* A prospective study of folate and vitamin B6 and risk of myocardial infarction in US physicians. J Am Coll Nutr 1996; 15: 136-43.

[152] Verhoef P, Hennekens CH, Allen RH, Stabler SP, Willet WC, Stampfer MJ. Plasma total homocysteine and risk of angina pectoris with subsequent coronary artery bypass surgery. Am J Cardiol 1997; 79: 799-801.

[153] Evans RW, Shaten BJ, Hempel JD, Cutler JA, Kuller LH. Homocysteine and risk of cardiovascular disease in the multiple risk factor intervention trial. Arterioscler Thromb Vasc Biol 1997; 17: 1947-53.

[154] Folsom AR, Nieto FJ, McGovern PG *et al.* Prospective study of coronary heart disease incidence in relation to fasting total homocysteine, related to genetic polymorphisms, and b vitamins. The Atherosclerosis risk in communities (ARIC) study. Circulation 1998; 98: 204-10.

[155] Ubbbink JB, Fehily AM, Pickering J, Elwood PE, Hayward Vermaak WJ. Homocysteine and ischaemic heart disease in the Caerphilly cohort. Atherosclerosis 1998; 140: 349-56.

[156] Boushey CJ, Beresford SA, Omenn GS, Motulsky AG. A quantitative assessment of plasma homocysteine as a risk factor for vascular disease. Probable benefits of increasing folic acid intakes. JAMA 1995; 274(13): 1049-57.

[157] Davies L, Wilmshurst EG, McElduff A, Gunton J, Clifton-Bligh P, Fulcher GR. The relationship among homocysteine, creatinine clearance and albuminerea in patients with type 2 diabetes. Diabetes care 2001; 24: 1805-9.

[158] Socha MW, Polakowska MS, Socha-Urbanek K, Fiedor P. HHcy as a risk factor for cardiovascular diseases. The association of hyperhomocysteinemia with diabetes mellitus and renal transplant recipients. Ann Transplant 1999; 4: 11-19.

[159] Jain SK, Mohandas N, Clark MR, Shobel SB. Br J Haematol 1983; 53: 247-252.

[160] Resmi H, Pekçetin C, Güner G. Erythrocyte membrane and cytoskeletal protein glycation and oxidation in short-term diabetic rabbits. Clin Exp Med 2001; 1: 187-193.

[161] A A Kaymaz, S Tamer, I Albeniz, K Cefle, S Palanduz, S Ozturk, Nl Salmayenli˙ Alterations in rheological properties and erythrocyte membrane proteins in cats with diabetes mellitus. Clinical Hemorheology and Microcirculation 2005; 33: 81-88.

[162] Adak S, Chowdhury S, Bhattacharyya M. Dynamic and electrokinetic behavior of erythrocyte membrane in diabetes mellitus and diabetic cardiovascular disease. BBA Acta 2008; 1780: 108-115.

[163] Aaron I. Vinik, Tomris Erbas, Tae Sun Park, Roger Nolan, Gary L. Pittenger. Platelet Dysfunction in Type 2 Diabetes. Diabetes Care 2001; 24: 1476-1485.

[164] Ruderman NB, Haudenschild C. Diabetes as an atherogenic factor. Prog Cardiovasc Dis 1984; 26: 373-412.

[165] Aronson D, Bloomgarden Z, Rayfield EJ. Potential mechanisms promoting rest enosis in diabetic patients. J Am Coll Cardiol 1996; 27: 528-535.

[166] Colwell JA, Nesto RW. The platelet in diabetes: focus on prevention of ischemic events. Diabetes Care 2003; 26: 2181-2188.

[167] Bruckert E, Rosenbaum D. Lowering LDL-cholesterol through diet: potential role in the statin era. Curr Opin Lipidol. 2011; 22(1): 43-8.

[168] Willett W, Manson J, Liu S. Glycemic index, glycemic load, and risk of type 2 diabetes, American Journal of Clinical Nutrition 2002; 76: 274-280.

[169] Matthias B Schulze, Simin Liu, Eric B Rimm, JoAnn E Manson, Walter C Willett and Frank B Hu Glycemic index, glycemic load, and dietary fiber intake and incidence of type 2 diabetes in younger and middle-aged women, American Journal of Clinical Nutrition 2004; 80: 348-356.

[170] Diet, nutrition and the prevention of chronic diseases: report of a joint WHO/FAO expert consultation. WHO Tech Rep Ser No 916, Geneva, Switz 2002.

[171] Manson JE, Spelsberg A. Primary prevention of non-insulin-dependent diabetes mellitus. Am J Prev Med 1994; 10: 172-84.

[172] Seeger JP, Thijssen DH, Noordam K, Cranen ME, Hopman MT, Nijhuis-van der Sanden MW. Exercise training improves physical fitness and vascular function in children with type 1 diabetes. Diabetes Obes Metab 2011.

[173] Robert H, Fagard. Smoking Amplifies Cardiovascular Risk in Patients With Hypertension and Diabetes. Diabetes care 2009; 32: 2.

[174] Will JC, Galuska DA, Ford ES, Mokdad A, Calle EE. Cigarette smoking and diabetes mellitus: evidence of a positive association from a large prospective cohort study. Int J Epidemiol 2001; 30: 540-46.

[175] Wannamethee SG, Shaper AG, Perry IJ. Smoking as a modifiable risk factor for type 2 diabetes in middle-aged men. Diabetes Care 2001; 24: 1590-95.

[176] Wei M, Gibbons LW, Mitchell TL, Kampert JB, Blair SN. 2000. Alcohol intake and incidence of type 2 diabetes in men. Diabetes Care 2000;23:18-22.

[177] Davies MJ, Baer DJ, Judd JT, Brown ED, Campbell WS, Taylor PR. Effects of moderate alcohol intake on fasting insulin and glucose concentrations and insulin sensitivity in postmenopausal women: a randomized controlled trial. JAMA 2002; 287: 2559-62.

[178] Adak S,SenguptaS, Chowdhury S, Bhattacharyya M. Co-existence of risk and protective haplotypes of Calpain 10 gene to type 2 diabetes in the eastern Indian population Diabetes & Vascular Disease Research 2010; 7(1): 63-68.

[179] Bloomgarden Z. Cardiovascular Disease in Diabetes. Diabetes Care 2010; 3: 4.

[180] Hanis CL, Boerwinkle E, Chakraborty R, Ellsworth DL, Cocannon P, Stirling B, Morrison VA, Wapelhorst B, Spielman RS, Gogolin-Ewens KJ, Shepard JM, Williams SR, Risch N, Hinds D, Iwasaki N, Ogata M, Omori Y, Petzold C, Rietzch H, Schroder HE, Schulze J, Cox NJ, Menzel S, Bororaj VV, Chen X *et al.* A genome-wide search for human non-insulin-dependent (type 2) diabetes genes reveals a major susceptibility locus on chromosome 2. Nat Genet 1996; 13: 161-166.

[181] Horikawa Y *et al.* Genetic variation in the gene encoding calpain-10 is associated with type 2 diabetes mellitus. Nat Genet 2000; 26: 163-175.

[182] Love-Gregory L D, Wasson J, Ma J *et al.* A common polymorphism in the upstream promoter region of the hepatocyte nuclear factor-4 alpha gene on chromosome 20q is associated with type 2 diabetes and appears to contribute to the evidence for linkage in an Ashkenazi jewish population. Diabetes 2004; 53: 1134-1140.

[183] Silander K, Mohlke K L, Scott L J. *et al.* Genetic variation near the hepatocyte nuclear factor-4 alpha gene predicts susceptibility to type 2 diabetes. Diabetes 2004; 53: 1141-1149.

[184] Andrew P. Levy Irit Hochberg, Kathleen Jablonski, Helaine E. Resnick, Elisa T. Lee, Lyle Best, Barbara V. Howard. Haptoglobin phenotype is an independent risk factor for cardiovascular disease in individuals with diabetes the strong heart study Journal of the American College of Cardiology 2002; 40(11): 1984-1990.

[185] Melamed-Frank M, Lache O, Enav BI, Rickliss R, Levy AP. Structure/function analysis of the anti-oxidant properties of haptoglobin. Blood 2001; 98: 3693-8.

[186] Levy AP. Genetics of diabetic cardiovascular disease: identification of a major susceptibility gene. Acta Diabetol 2003; 330-333.

[187] Refsum H, Ueland PM, Nygard O, Vollset SE. Homocysteine and cardiovascular disease. Annu Rev Med 1998; 49: 31-62.

[188] Eikelboom JW, Lonn E, Genest J Jr, Hankey G, Yusuf S. Homocyst(e)ine and cardiovascular disease: a critical review of the epidemiologic evidence. Ann Intern Med 1999; 131(5): 363- 75.

[189] Sebastio G, Sperandeo MP, Panico M, de Franchis R, Kraus JP, Andria G. The molecular basis of homocystinuria due to cystathionine beta-synthase deficiency in Italian families, and report of four novel mutations. Am J Hum Genet 1995; 56(6): 1324-33.

[190] Selhub J. Homocysteine metabolism. Annu Rev Nutr 1999; 19: 217-46.

[191] Andersson A, Brattstrom L, Israelsson B, Isaksson A, Hamfelt A, Hultberg B. Plasma homocysteine before and after methionine loading with regard to age, gender, and menopausal status. Eur J Clin Invest 1992; 22(2): 79-87.

[192] Mudd S, Levy H, Skoby F. Disorders of transulfuration. In: Scriver C, Beaudet A, Sly W, Valle D, editors. The metabolic and molecular bases of inherited disease. New York: McGraw- Hill, 1995: 1279-327.

[193] Bostom AG, Shemin D, Lapane KL *et al.* Hyperhomocysteinemia and traditional cardiovascular disease risk factors in end stage renal disease patients on dialysis: a case-control study. Atherosclerosis 1995; 114(1): 93-103.

[194] Kang SS, Wong PW. Genetic and nongenetic factors for moderate hyperhomocyst(e)inemia. Atherosclerosis 1996; 119(2): 135-8.

[195] Kang SS, Wong PW, Susmano A, Sora J, Norusis M, Ruggie N. Thermolabile methylenetetrahydrofolate reductase: an inherited risk factor for coronary artery disease. Am J Hum Genet 1991; 48(3): 536-45.

[196] Frosst P, Blom HJ, Milos R, *et al.* A candidate genetic risk factor for vascular disease: a common mutation in methylenetetrahydrofolate reductase. Nat Genet 1995; 10(1): 111-3.

[197] Grazyna Chwatko, Godfried H. J. Boers, Kevin A. Strauss, Diana M. Shih, and Hieronim Jakubowski Mutations in methylenetetrahydrofolate reductase or cystathionine _-syntase gene, or a high-methionine diet, increase homocysteine thiolactone levels in humans and mice. The FASEB Journal; 1707-1713.

[198] Inagaki N, Gonoi T, Clement J T. *et al.* Reconstitution of IKATP: an inward rectifier subunit plus the sulfonylurea receptor. Science 2003; 270: 1166-1170.

[199] Ariza M-J, Sanchez-Chaparro M-A, Baron F-J, Hornos A-M, Bonacho EC, Rioja J, Valdivielso P, Gelpi JA, Gonzalez-Santos P. Effects of LPL, APOA5 and APOE variant combinations on triglyceride levels and hypertriglyceridemia: results of the ICARIA genetic sub-study. BMC Medical Genetics 2010; 11: 66.

[200] Ma Y Q, Thomas GN, Ng MC, *et al.* The lipoprotein lipase gene HindIII polymorphism is associated with lipid levels in early-onset type 2 diabetic patients. Metabolism. 2003; 52: 338-343.

[201] Goodarzi M O. Guo X, Taylor KD, *et al.* Lipoprotein lipase is a gene for insulin resistance in Mexican Americans. Diabetes 2004; 53: 214-220.

[202] Theodosios Kyriakou, Laura J. Collins, Nicola J. Spencer-Jones, Clare Malcolm, Xiaoling Wang, Harold Snieder, Ramasamyiyer Swaminathan, Keith A. Burling Deborah J. Hart, Tim D. Spector, Sandra D. O'Dell1Adiponectin gene ADIPOQ SNP associations with serum adiponectin in two female populations and effects of SNPs on promoter activity J Hum Genet 2008; 53(8): 718-727.

Send Orders of Reprints at reprints@benthamscience.org

CHAPTER 4

The Role of Phytotherapy in the Management of Diabetes Mellitus

Adeyemi O. Olufunmilayo[1,*] and Adeneye A. Adewale[1,2]

[1]*Department of Pharmacology, College of Medicine of The University of Lagos, Idi-Araba, Lagos State, Nigeria and* [2]*Department of Pharmacology, Faculty of Basic Medical Sciences, Lagos State University College of Medicine, Ikeja, Lagos State, Nigeria*

Abstract: Diabetes mellitus remains the most common endocrine disorder of carbohydrate metabolism, often associated with attendant complications with high morbidity and mortality. Despite the successes recorded with the use of conventional chemotherapy in the disease management, phytotherapy appears to have good prospects in the effective management of the disease course and prognosis. In this review we will examine the etiopathological basis (including the recent advancements in its pathology), diagnosis and monitoring of diabetes mellitus. The chapter provides information on the current conventional pharmacotherapy and supportive care as well as an in-depth and incisive analysis on the emerging trend in the use of herbal products. The evidence-based herbal pharmacotherapy that is currently employed in the management of the disease is discussed. In the concluding part of the chapter, the future prospects of the diverse anti-diabetic herbal remedies are also discussed.

Keywords: Diabetes, phytotherapy, medicinal plants, pharmacotherapy, herbal, metabolic, hyperglycemia, insulin, plasma levels, resistance.

INTRODUCTION

Historically, the word *diabetes* was coined from the Greek word meaning a *siphon* by the 2nd Century Greek physician, Aretus the Cappadocian. He used the word to connote a condition of passing water (urine) like a *siphon*. Later the Latin description *mellitus* meaning sweetened or honey-like was added. Put together, the term *diabetes mellitus* was literarily used to denote a disease condition which was associated with the persistent passage of sweetened urine [1].

In 1999, the World Health Organization described diabetes mellitus as a metabolic

*****Address correspondence to Adeyemi O. Olufunmilayo:** Department of Pharmacology, College of Medicine of The University of Lagos, Idi-Araba, Lagos State, Nigeria; Tel/Fax: +234-802-069-0946; E-mail: oadeyemi@unilag.edu.ng

Mohamed Eddouks and Debprasad Chattopadhyay (Eds)
All rights reserved-© 2012 Bentham Science Publishers

disorder of multiple aetiology characterized by chronic hyperglycaemia (the fasting blood glucose level equal or above 200 mg/dl taken at least twice, on different occasions) with disturbances of carbohydrate, fat and protein metabolism resulting from defects in insulin secretion, insulin action, or both. In fact, diabetes mellitus is a chronic disease with insidious onset in which the fasting blood glucose is persistently raised above the normal range values, between 60 to 120 mg/dl of blood [1]. It occurs either because of a lack of insulin (the hormone responsible for glucose metabolism), or due to the presence of certain factors opposing the action of insulin on the organs that are involved in glucose metabolism, particularly, the liver and the skeletal muscles. The consequence of insufficient insulin action is hyperglycaemia which may be associated with metabolic abnormalities like the development of hyperketonaemia resulting from disordered protein metabolism, and derangements in fatty acid or lipids metabolism. When the fasting blood glucose lies between 100 to 130 mg/dl, it is referred to as *Prediabetes* which is associated with an increased tendency or potential of developing *frank* diabetes. A fasting blood glucose of 140 mg/dl or higher is consistent with either type of diabetes mellitus, particularly, when accompanied by classic symptoms of diabetes [2].

CLASSIFICATION OF DIABETES MELLITUS

Basically, diabetes mellitus can be classified into two broad categories namely:

(i) Type 1 diabetes mellitus which is less common in terms of its prevalence. It often results from an absolute deficiency of insulin synthesis and secretion as a consequence of autoimmune destruction of the pancreatic β-cells.

(ii) Type 2 diabetes mellitus which is a more prevalent category, caused due to a combination of resistance to insulin action and an inadequate compensatory insulin secretory response.

Other forms of diabetes include:

(iii) Impaired glucose tolerance (IGT), a category of glucose intolerance when post-challenge values are between diabetic and normal. IGT is considered a strong risk factor for type 2 diabetes mellitus.

(iv) Gestational diabetes mellitus is defined as glucose intolerance that develops during pregnancy and returns to normal tolerance after child birth.

(v) Malnutrition-related diabetes which according to the WHO [3] can be divided into two types:

- protein-deficient pancreatic diabetes (PDPD)

- fibrocalculus pancreatic diabetes (FCPD)

According to Winter *et al.* (1987) [4] and Morrison (1981) [5], other atypical diabetes syndromes characterized by ketosis resistance and periods of normoglycaemic remission with subsequent hyperglycaemic relapse include:

- atypical maturity-onset diabetes of the young (MODY)

- the diabetic syndrome of phasic insulin dependence

(vi) Secondary diabetes mellitus can occur as a consequence of pancreatic disorders (such as pancreatitis, pancreatic trauma, pancreatic surgery, pancreatic tumors, cystic fibrosis and hemochromatosis) or other endocrinopathies (such as acromegaly, Cushing's disease, glucagonoma, phaeochromocytoma, somatostatinoma- and aldosteronoma-induced hypokalaemia).

EPIDEMIOLOGY AND PUBLIC HEALTH IMPLICATIONS OF DIABETES MELLITUS

Diabetes mellitus is a major non-communicable disease with a higher incidence in the developed countries [3]. The prevalence of diabetes for all age-groups worldwide was estimated to be 2.8% (171 million people) in the year 2000 but projected to increase to 4.4% (about 366 million) by the year 2030 [6]. This estimated exponential rise is attributable to the global increase in population number, increasing aged population, urbanization, better diagnostic tools and increasing prevalence of obesity and physical inactivity [6]. Considering its increasing prevalence, attendant complications (which are often associated with high mortality and morbidity) and the heavy economic and social burdens, diabetes mellitus is now considered a public health night mare.

In terms of age by sex, diabetes prevalence is similar in men and women but it is slightly higher in men less than 60 years of age and in women at older ages. Overall, across all age-groups diabetes prevalence is higher in men, but there are more women with the disease than men [6].

In the U.S. and other developed countries, diabetes affects 1 in every 16 people. In the U.S. alone, each year about 800,000 Americans are newly diagnosed and about 182,000 deaths are linked to complications of diabetes mellitus, making it the third largest killer disease in the country [7]. However, there is demonstrable evidence to show that the incidence is equally on the rise in the developing countries with prevalence estimates in Africa of 1% in rural areas and 5-7% in urban sub-Saharan Africa, while estimates of up to 13% has been reported in more developed areas in South Africa and Indian populations [8-10]. The burden of diabetes mellitus in Nigeria is similar to that obtainable in other parts of sub-Saharan Africa [11] and its prevalence varies between 1-8% depending on the area of the country that is surveyed [12]. For example in rural Nigeria, the prevalence of diabetes was estimated to be 2.8% [13] but in urban Nigeria it was reported to be as high as 6% [14].

AETIOPATHOPHYSIOLOGY/RISK AND PREDISPOSING FACTORS OF DIABETES MELLITUS

Genetic Predisposition: The Human Leucocyte Antigen (HLA) concept. Type 1 diabetes mellitus is known to arise as a consequence of selective destruction of the insulin-producing and secreting pancreatic β-cells, resulting in insulinopenia [15]. In the face of absolute insulinopenia, type 1 diabetic patients are predisposed to develop ketoacidosis. Generally the Type 1 diabetes is of early onset, usually within the first 2 decades of life, hence the name, *juvenile-onset diabetes mellitus*, but may occur at any stage of life. The prevalence of this type of diabetes among the Caucasians is 1 in every 300 persons [15].

Genetically, multiple loci have demonstrated close association or linkages to type 1 diabetes mellitus. Both human leukocyte antigen (HLA) and non-HLA genes contribute to diabetes susceptibility and the best and most studied of these susceptible genes are the insulin dependent diabetes mellitus 1 (IDDM1) HLA and *insulin dependent diabetes 2 (IDDM2) INS-VNTR*. Of these two, *IDDM1* appears to confer about 50% of genetic susceptibility to type 1 diabetes. The current concept in the aetiology of type 1 diabetes is that the pancreatic β-cells in predisposed individuals are destroyed by autoimmune response primarily mediated by T-lymphocytes that react secondarily to one or more β-cell proteins otherwise called auto-antigens. The onset of the disease is insidious and is marked by the presence of several immunological markers which include immunofluorescent islet cell auto-antibodies (ICA), insulin autoantibodies (IAA), glutamic acid decarboxylase auto-antibodies (GAD65) and transmembrane tyrosine phosphatase auto-antibodies (ICA512). This is accompanied by progressive and successive pancreatic β-cell function which is characterized by the loss of first-phase insulin response (FPIR) to an intravenous glucose tolerance test (IVGTT). With loss of about 70-90% of pancreatic β-cell population, chronic hyperglycaemia and typical clinical syndrome of type 1 diabetes begin to manifest. Overall, the onset of type 1 diabetes appears to be influenced by the net effect of genetic and environmental factors on immunoregulatory responses.

Type 2 diabetes mellitus is a heterogeneous metabolic disorder which is characterized by impaired and defective insulin secretion by the β-cell function, and/or defective sensitivity of peripheral tissues (such as the skeletal and hepatic tissues) to insulin action [16]. Based to the fact that the primary cause is not insulin deficiency, the type 2 diabetics do not require exogenous insulin for survival and as such are not prone to ketosis. Type 2 diabetes mellitus is the most common, accounting for over 90% of all diabetic cases. The disease has a strong hereditary component and genetic predisposition. However, factors contributing to its development include central obesity, sedentary lifestyle, and the sarcopenia of aging. Typically, the age onset of type 2 diabetes is usually in or after the 4th decade of life (thus the previous name, *adult-onset diabetes mellitus*) but could occur at any age. Similarly, type 2 diabetes has been linked to multiple genetic loci as in type 1 diabetes but the most important locus found so far has been traced to chromosome 2 (*NIDDM1*). However, it remains unclear which of the two defects: impaired insulin secretion or insulin resistance precedes which. However, it is generally accepted that both defects are present in type 2 diabetes. Furthermore, defects in insulin secretion can result in insulin resistance and *vice versa*. Deficiency in insulin secretion may manifest as decreased sensitivity of insulin response to glucose ("hyperglycaemia blindness", which is only selective for glucose), impaired first- and second-phases insulin response to glucose. Insulin resistance may co-exist with obesity, systemic hypertension, acromegaly or in patients on glucocorticoids and oestrogen therapy.

In maturity-onset diabetes of the young (MODY), there is an onset of mild hyperglycaemia at an early stage of life (usually before the age of 25 years) which is characterized by impaired insulin secretion with minimal or no defects in insulin action. This type of diabetes is inherited in an autosomal dominant pattern. To date, genetic mutations at three genetic loci on different chromosomes have been identified and these include: MODY1, resulting from mutations on chromosome 20q in a hepatic transcription factor (HNF-4α) gene region; MODY2, resulting from mutations in the *glucokinase* gene on chromosome 7p; and MODY3, resulting from mutations on chromosome 12 in a hepatic transcription factor (HNF-1α) gene region.

The Thrifty Gene Hypothesis: The thrifty gene hypothesis was first proposed by Neel, in 1962, as a way of explaining the type 2 diabetes in African- American and urban- African diabetics. In his hypothesis, Neel suggested that populations exposed to periodic famines (which occur more in developing tropical countries, particularly of the African continent) through natural adaptation mechanism, increase the expression of certain genetic trait(s), "thrifty genes", which would protect against starvation during time of famine [17]. These genes would allow for efficient energy preservation and fat storage during times of abundance. In circumstances of relative food abundance, the expression of these genes predisposes their carriers to the developing obesity and insulin resistance that ultimately result in development of type 2 diabetes.

Obesity: The positive correlation between type 2 diabetes mellitus and obesity has been established in many ethnic groups [18]. In most studies, obesity is either assessed and expressed as body mass index (BMI), which is a ratio of the body weight (in kg) to the corresponding height (in m^2) or as percent desirable weight

(PDW) based on the Metropolitan Life Insurance tables. The higher the BMI or PDW values than the normal value range obtained for the population under study, the higher the risk of developing type 2 diabetes. In addition to the degree or severity of obesity, regional body fat disposition (*vis-à-vis* central and peripheral fat distribution) is also strongly correlated to the increased predisposition, with individuals with central obesity at higher risk of developing type 2 diabetes [18].

Socioeconomic Status: In the U.S., an inverse relationship exists between socioeconomic status and the prevalence of diabetes in adults irrespective of race or ethnicity. It was reported that the prevalence of diabetes decreases with increasing level of education and family income [19]. However, when age and obesity are controlled for, the association of income and education with type 2 diabetes becomes significantly reduced [20]. Thus, the direct role of socioeconomic status in the aetiology of type 2 diabetes remains fuzzy.

Physical Inactivity: Physical inactivity as an independent risk factor for development of type 2 diabetes is well established [21]. As physical inactivity is closely associated with development of obesity and insulin resistance, so physical activity is considered a strong protective factor against the development of type 2 diabetes.

Insulin Resistance: High circulating free insulin levels is a strong predisposing factor in the development of type 2 diabetes [22]. Chronic hyperinsulinaemia has been reported to precede the eventual development of type 2 diabetes [23]. Type 2 diabetes resulting from insulin resistance is often characterized by progressive glucose tolerance impairment due to increasing desensitization of glucose transport systems by elevated levels of glucosamine, an alternative metabolic product of glucose metabolism in skeletal muscle and hepatic tissue to the hypoglycaemic effect of insulin (Cline *et al.*, 1997) [24]. Glucosamine has been shown to interfere with the translocation of glucose transporters subtypes 4 (GLU T4) in adipocytes *in vitro* and in rat muscle *in vivo* [24].

Impaired Glucose Tolerance: Impaired oral glucose tolerance is known to be a strong risk factor for type 2 diabetes. Its prevalence rates increase with age, especially for black men, white men and white women but they increase for black women older than 50 years [25].

Cigarette Smoking and Alcohol Consumption: Cigarette and alcohol are known to be converted to toxic metabolites in the body and these toxins are known to be injurious to the body tissues including the pancreatic tissues, causing pancreatitis and on long term, results in pancreatic insufficiency [26].

DIAGNOSIS AND MONITORING OF DIABETES MELLITUS

The aim of diagnosis of diabetes mellitus is the demonstration of persistent hyperglycaemia. Previous criterion was made mainly on the use of the oral glucose tolerance test (OGTT), which was discovered to be clinically inconvenient. As a result of this, in 1997, the fasting plasma glucose value equal or greater than 140 mg/dl (7.8 mmol/l) was adopted as the only diagnostic criterion of diabetes mellitus [7]. However, this cut-off point was soon to be confronted with two major challenges. The first was that this cut-off point was too high, based on the risk of retinopathy. The second was that the cut-off point did not correspond to the OGTT level. The latter short-coming left undiagnosed patients with the disease result in well-known attendant complications of diabetes mellitus. As a result of the associated short-comings, the American Diabetes Association (ADA) commissioned an *ad hoc* expert committee to evaluate the existing data and make recommendations that will make individuals with diabetes mellitus be screened and detected more easily in clinical practice. Based on the findings of the expert committee, a cut-off point of a fasting plasma glucose equal or greater than 126 mg/dl (7.0 mmol/l) was recommended, as most potential diabetic patients would easily become detected, without much risk of false-positive diagnosis. Consequently, 126 mg/dl (7.0 mmol/l) became a surrogate for an OGTT 2-hour value of 200 mg/dl (11.1 mmol/l). This change rather than increasing the number of people with diabetes mellitus, only increased the number of people with known diabetes.

The revised and adopted criteria for the diagnosis of diabetes mellitus include any or combination of:

a)   unequivocal and hallmark symptoms of diabetes mellitus (which include increased urine volume (polyuria), increased thirst (polydipsia), a progressive weight loss, frequent and recurrent infections and, in severe cases, drowsiness and coma; and a postprandial plasma glucose level equal or greater than 200 mg/dl (11.1 mmol/l);

b)   fasting (no caloric intake for at least 8 hours) plasma glucose equal or greater than 126 mg/dl (7.0 mmol/l);

c)   2-hours plasma glucose concentration equal or greater than 200 mg/dl (11.1 mmol/l) during an OGTT involving a single oral intake of 75 g glucose load [7].

Glycosylated haemoglobin (HbA_{1c}) measurement is currently not a good choice for the diagnosis of diabetes mellitus, although certain studies have reported that the frequency distribution for HbA_{1c} have similar characteristics to those of fasting plasma glucose and 2-hours plasma glucose. However, both HbA_{1c} and fasting plasma glucose have become the gold standard in the monitoring of treatment of diabetes mellitus [7].

THERAPEUTIC STRATEGIES

Chronic hyperglycaemia has consistently remained the principal cause of life threatening complications of diabetes mellitus. Thus, effective control of blood glucose remains the primary target towards preventing or reversing attendant complications of uncontrolled or poorly-controlled diabetes mellitus and in improving the quality of life in diabetics as unambiguously stipulated by the Diabetes Control and Complication Trial Research Group (1997) [2]. In the effective management of diabetes mellitus, various therapeutic strategies/options could be adopted which broadly can be categorized into:

a.   *Non-Pharmacological Approach*: this consists of various mechanical and nutritional therapies including regular aerobic physical exercise, nutritional modification particularly high fibre diets, cessation of smoking for smokers, abstinence from alcohol consumptions for alcoholics;

b.   *Pharmacological Interventions*: these involve use of various classes of oral hypoglycaemic agents such as biguanides (*e.g.* metformin), sulphonylureas (*e.g.* glibenclamide) which mediate their effects by augmenting insulin sensitivity of the skeletal and hepatic tissues, *alpha-glucosidase* inhibitors (*e.g.* acarbose), thiazolidinediones (*e.g.* rosiglitazone), and insulin injections (which could be short-acting, intermediate-acting or long-acting insulin prototype) [27].

HERBAL PHARMACOTHERAPIES

The discovery of the unbreakable relation between plants and human health has led to the launching of a new class of botanical therapeutic agents that includes plant-based pharmaceuticals, multi-component botanical drugs, dietary supplement *etc.*, as an alternative to the current conventional antidiabetic agents [28, 29]. In addition, in the last two to three decades, there has been an exponential growth in research into and utilization of medicinal plants, particularly, flora of the tropical rainforest [30]. Despite achievements recorded in drug discovery and development from plant sources, phytomedicine continues to be highly valuable for developing synthetic pharmaceuticals employed in the treatment of both human and animal diseases.

In the world today, there is a revolution in health care system, resulting in greater acceptance and trust in herbal medicine. According to the World Health Organization, about 80% of the world's population depends wholly or partly on plant-derived pharmaceuticals [31]. In most developing countries, there is a heavy dependence on herbal preparations for the treatment of human and animal diseases despite the availability of conventional pharmaceuticals [32]. This is because the exorbitant cost and associated intolerable side-effects of most conventional pharmaceuticals prevent most people from being able to acquire them. In this same vane, some diabetic patients resort to the use of alternative or complementary therapies such as vitamin supplements or herbal remedies either alone or as adjunct to their conventional anti-diabetic drugs. A landslide retrospective study conducted by Ernst (2000) [33] showed that over 90% of patients attending hospitals, clinics and any other health facilities would have taken or were still on one form of herbal products/supplements. This is borne out of the belief that *green medicine* is cheap, safe, more dependable and accessible than the costly synthetic drugs many of which are associated with intolerable effects [34, 35]. Associated with this increasing acceptance is the erroneous belief that there is no firm scientific evidence of the efficacy of these natural products. However, in the last half a century, there have been tremendous investigations into what dose, how, and what constituents of these herbal preparations treat disease and promote good health. Results of some of these investigations have not only validated the efficacies of these agents but have also promoted greater understanding of the role some of the natural products play in treating the disease process. Although some of these therapies may be helpful, others can be ineffective or out-rightly toxic for human use. It is therefore important that for the safety of any drug must be clearly determined before it is recommended for human consumption.

MONOHERBAL ANTIDIABETIC THERAPY

Trigonella foenum-graecum L. (Fenugreek)

Fenugreek is an erect annual legume native to southern Europe and Asia. It is now extensively cultivated in most parts of the world including northern Africa, United States, Canada, China, India and the Mediterranean. It is a common Indian spice and commonly used herbal remedy in Ayurvedic medicine. Historically, fenugreek was used for the treatment of a variety of health conditions, including menopausal symptoms, digestive problems and for inducing labour [36]. It was also used in the treatment of diabetes mellitus. In ancient China, herbalists used fenugreek seed to treat disorders of the kidney and male reproductive tracts [36].

Several independent clinical and experimental studies have confirmed the anti-diabetic effects of fenugreek seeds on both acute and long term uses [37]. In several animal and human studies, the antidiabetic effect of fenugreek seeds have been reported to be mediated *via* intestinal glucose uptake inhibition (by its gum fibre–*galactomannan*), hyperinsulinaemia, and enhanced peripheral glucose utilization [38]. The active principle was found to be abundant in the defatted portion of the seed. Daily administration of 1.5–2.0 g/kg of the defatted seed extract to both normal and drug-induced diabetic dogs significantly reduced the fasting blood and after-meal glucose, insulin, total cholesterol, and triglycerides, while significantly elevating plasma high density lipoprotein (HDL)-cholesterol levels [39]. In addition, clinical studies have shown that 50 g of the defatted seed powder to effectively lower the blood glucose levels and improve glucose tolerance test in insulin-dependent diabetic patients [40]. These reductions were associated with a significant reduction in the serum total cholesterol and triglyceride levels. In a similar study involving non-insulin (type 2) diabetics, significant postpandrial glycaemic control was achieved with 15 g of powdered fenugreek seed soaked in water [41]. Fenugreek seeds are rich in the amino-acids - trigonelline, lysine and L-tryptophan, steroidal saponins and fibres [42]. The steroidal saponins and fibres are speculated to account for the plant's hypocholesterolaemic and hypoglycaemic activities *via* modulation of activity of key hepatic enzymes that regulate carbohydrate and lipid metabolism [43-45]. Recently, the specific hepatic key enzymes which the plant extract modified by enhancing their activities were identified as the hepatic *glucokinase* and *hexokinase*. In fact, the aqueous seed extract of fenugreek, at a dose of 15 mg/kg body weight injected intraperitoneally to streptozotocin-diabetic BALB/cJ mice, enhanced the activities of hepatic *glucokinase* and *hexokinase* by 4.6 and 1.5 fold, respectively [29]. In another preclinical study conducted in Japan, fenugreek seed extract was found to reduce the body weight gain induced by a high-fat diet and also reduced plasma triglyceride. 4-hydroxyisoleucine was the isolated phytocompound responsible for these biological effects [46].

Possible side effects of fenugreek when taken orally include gastric irritation which may manifest as bloating and diarrhoea [47]. Given its historical use in inducing or augmenting labour, pregnant diabetic patients are strongly advised against using it [47].

Coccinia cordifolia

The herb *Coccinia cordifolia* which is widely abundant in India has a reputation in the traditional diabetes care. It is believed to effectively control blood sugar and other diabetes symptoms in the diabetes sufferers, particularly in type 2 diabetes subjects. In a randomized placebo controlled clinical trial conducted in Bangalore, India, involving 60 adult type 2 diabetics strictly only diet and lifestyle treatment, daily oral intake of an extract of the herb for 90 days was found to lower their fasting and postpandrial (after-meal) blood glucose and glycosylated haemoglobin (HbA$_{1c}$) levels, although the patients' free insulin levels were not studied.

Coccinia cordifolia was found to be more effective in lowering the blood glucose levels in patients with mild diabetes than those with severe form of the disease [48]. More studies would be needed to determine how it lowers the glucose and the active principles in it causing the observed effect.

Coccinia Indica (Ivy Gourd)

Coccinia indica, commonly called Ivy gourd, is a creeping plant which grows widely in many parts of India. It is reputed for treating diabetes in Ayurvedic medicine.

In a 6 week-randomized clinical trial conducted in India, the use of 500 mg/kg of the herbal powder obtained from the crushed dried leaves of the plant was reported to achieve good glycaemic control in type 2 diabetics [49]. The extract restored the activities of the enzyme *lipoprotein lipase* (LPL) that was reduced and *glucose-6-phosphatase* and *lactate dehydrogenase*, which were raised in untreated diabetics [50].

In another 12 week-well controlled clinical trial involving 70 type 2 diabetic subjects, dried herb pellets made from the plant fresh leaves were found to achieve comparable good glycaemic control as that of the oral hypoglycaemic agent, chlorpropamide, in the diabetic subjects [51].

Ginseng Species

Several different plant species are collectively referred to as ginseng. They include the Chinese or Korean ginseng (*Panax ginseng*), Siberian ginseng (*Eleutherococcus senticosus*), American ginseng (*Panax quiquefolius*), and the Japanese ginseng (*Panax japonicus*).

Hypoglycaemic effect of ginseng has been widely reported. Two longer-term trials involving the use of American ginseng on 36 and 24 patients lasting for 8 weeks, respectively, were reported to decrease the fasting blood glucose and HbA$_{1c}$ [52, 53]. Major components of ginseng are the triterpenoid saponin glycosides: *ginsenosides* or *panaxosides*. These phytocomponents are believed to induce hypoglycaemia by decreasing the rate of glucose absorption into the portal hepatic circulation, increased glucose transport and uptake mediated by nitric oxide, increased glycogen storage, and inducing hyperinsulinaemia [54].

Momordica Charantia (Bitter Melon)

This is commonly called bitter gourd, bitter melon, Karalla fruit, and balsam pear. It is a large trailing plant with wide leaves and tendrils traditionally employed in the treatment of diabetes mellitus in Africa, Southern America, India, and other Asian countries.

The main constituents of bitter melon include its steroidal saponin – *charantin*, triterpene glycosides and alkaloids. The antidiabetic activities of the extracts obtained from the plant fruit, seeds, leaves and whole plant have been widely reported. The protein, *polypeptide P*, which is abundant in the plant fruit and seeds, is being reported to behave like insulin when administered as subcutaneous injections to langurs monkey and humans [55]. In view of the plant's mechanism of inducing hypoglycaemia, it is popularly called "the plant-insulin". The use of the plant extract reduces the insulin requirements in type 1 diabetics. Also, in experimental animal models, ethanol extracts of *Momordica charantia* have been shown to possess hypoglycaemic and anti-hyperglycaemic effects in normal and streptozotocin-induced diabetic rats, respectively. These effects were reported to be mediated through the inhibition of hepatic *glucose-6-phosphatase* and *fructose-1,6-biphosphate* activities and stimulation of hepatic *glucose-6-phosphate dehydrogenase* activities [56], thus, exhibiting sulphonylurea-like activity. In addition, bitter melon has been reported to improve oral glucose tolerance by inhibiting intestinal glucose uptake [57].

Bitter melon has been reported to interact with insulin and conventional oral hypoglycaemic agents by potentiating their hypoglycaemic effects. Thus, diabetics on antidiabetic drugs who are willing to commence on bitter melon as an adjunct should closely monitor their blood glucose and adjust the dosages of their antidiabetic regimen appropriately to forestall hypoglycaemic complications [58]. However, the use of bitter melon is contraindicated in patients with existing liver diseases [59]. It is also contraindicated in pregnant and lactating women because of its emmenogogue and abortifacient side effects [58, 60].

Allium Species: *Allium Cepa* (Onion) and *Allium Sativum* (Garlic)

Allium cepa which is otherwise known as onions is traditionally employed in the management of diabetes mellitus. Various ether soluble and insoluble fractions of dried onion powder have been reported to exhibit hypoglycaemic, hypolipidaemic and antioxidant activities in several animal models [61, 62]. A sulphur-containing amino acid, S-methyl cysteine sulphoxide, which has been isolated from the plant bulb, has been implicated in its antidiabetic activities. Administration of 200 mg/kg of this isolate for 45 days to alloxanized diabetic rats has been reported to significantly control serum and tissue glucose and lipids and normalize the hepatic hexokinase, glucose-6-phosphatase and 3-Hydroxy-3-methylglutaryl coenzyme A (HMG-CoA) reductase activities [63, 64]. In a randomized clinical trial, oral administration of 50 g of onion juice to diabetic subjects significantly controlled their after-meal glucose levels [65]. In another small clinical study involving 6 non-diabetic volunteers, oral administration of allyl propyl disulphide extract capsule caused an acute decrease in the fasting blood glucose and increased the plasma free insulin levels [66].

Allium sativum, otherwise known as garlic, is a perennial herb belonging to the lily family. It is commonly used as condiment in cooking. *Allicin*, a sulphur-containing compound which is responsible for its pungent odour, has been shown to possess significant hypoglycaemic activity [67]. Oral administration of its aqueous extract to sucrose-fed rabbits for 60 days was associated with increased hepatic glycogen deposition and protein synthesis, decreased serum fasting blood glucose and triglyceride levels [68]. In addition, S-allyl cysteine sulphoxide, the precursor of *allicin* and volatile garlic oil, has been reported to effectively control lipid peroxidation complication of diabetes mellitus far better than the standard antidiabetic drugs. The S-allyl cysteine sulphoxide is known to enhance insulin secretion from isolated beta cells in pancreatic cell tissue culture [69]. In alloxanized diabetic rats, the isolate has been shown to cause moderate reductions in blood glucose but caused no effect in pancreatectomized rats [67, 70].

In a randomized clinical trial involving 60 healthy volunteers, capsulated extract of *Allium sativum* was found to significantly reduce the fasting glucose levels in the treated subjects [71].

Ocimum Sanctum (Holy Basil)

Ocimum sanctum (otherwise known as holy basil) is closely related to *Ocimum album* and *Ocimum basilicum*. Animal studies have shown the extracts of the plant to induce hypoglycaemia. Although the exact mechanism by which the extract induces hypoglycaemia remains unknown, its mechanism has been postulated to be mediated *via* enhanced beta cell function and insulin secretion [72].

A 4-week randomized placebo-controlled clinical trial involving 40 type 2 diabetics have shown the fresh leaf powder dissolved in water to cause a significant reduction in both fasting and after-meal glucose in the diabetic subjects [73].

Aloe Species: *Aloe Vera* and *Barbadensis*

Aloe is a popular household shrub which has an ancestral history in Asian folk medicine in the effective management of an array of human diseases including diabetes mellitus. *Aloe vera* is the most well-known species of aloe belonging to Lilacaea family. The dried sap of *Aloe vera* is traditionally used in the management of diabetes mellitus amongst the Arabians. The plant gel (mucilage) and latex (juice) have also been proven to possess oral hypoglycaemic activities in both normal and diabetic rats [74, 75]. The plant's hypoglycaemic phytoprinciple has been identified to be a lignan, *glucomannan* [54].

Two independent non-randomized clinical trials involving 40 and 76 diabetic patients treated with juice made from aloe gel for 6 weeks, was reported to significantly reduce the fasting blood glucose and HbA_{1c} in these subjects [76-78]. Also, prolonged oral treatment with the juice made from the blended fresh leaves of *Aloe barbadensis* has been documented to lower the blood glucose in alloxanized rats, an effect which was mediated through enhanced pancreatic stimulation [75].

Caesalpinia Bonducella

Caesalpinia bonducella is a tropical shrub ubiquitous to the tropical coastal regions including India. It is native to India where its traditional use in diabetes therapy can be traced to. Scientific evaluation of various extracts from the plant leaves have been shown to increase hepatic glycogenesis in the type 1 and 2 diabetic models in rats [79]. Some isolates from the plant extract have also been shown to stimulate insulin secretion in pancreatic tissue culture [79]. The aqueous and ethanol extracts of the plant have been reported to cause hypoglycaemic (*via* inhibition of intestinal glucose uptake) and hypolipidaemic effects in streptozotocin diabetic rats [80].

Opuntia Streptacantha (Prickly Pear Cactus)

This plant is native to Mexico and South-Western American countries where it is employed by the local inhabitants for the traditional management of diabetes mellitus. It has been reported to be rich in high soluble fibre and pectin contents and these are reported to inhibit intestinal glucose uptake acting like *alpha glucosidase* inhibitors [81]. Two Spanish randomized controlled clinical trials involving 14 and 32 diabetic patients have shown the plant fruit to reduce fasting blood glucose and insulin levels in type 2 diabetic patients, thereby increasing the peripheral tissue sensitivity to insulin action [82, 83].

Musanga Cecropioides

Musanga cecropioides, also known as the Umbrella tree is a tropical tree which is ubiquitous to the tropical rainforest of West Africa. In African traditional medicine, various parts of the plant are reputed for the treatment of various human diseases including diabetes mellitus. Water and alcoholic extracts of the plant stem bark, at the single, daily oral dose range of 250-1000 mg/kg for 14 days, have been reported to induce significant hypoglycaemic and antidiabetic activities in normal and alloxanized diabetic rats, respectively [84]. These biological activities were postulated to be mediated through increased peripheral glucose uptake mechanism, by any or combination of the flavonoids, alkaloids, and saponin which are abundant in the plant extract [84].

Citrus Species

Citrus is a perennial tropical plant which is widely distributed throughout the world, belonging to the family *Rutaceae*. There are several *Citrus* species and include *Citrus paradisi* Macfad (Grape fruit), *Citrus aurentifolia* (Christm.) Swingle (Lime), *Citrus limon* (L.) Burm. (Lemon), *Citrus sinensis* Osbek (Sweet orange), *Citrus aurantium* L. (Bitter Orange) and *Citrus aromaticum* [85]. *Citrus* juice, peel and seeds have been reported to have oral hypoglycaemic/antidiabetic and antihyperlipidaemic activities in both animals and humans. The alcoholic seed extract of *Citrus paradisi* Macfad, at the oral dose range of 100 - 600 mg/kg/day for 30 days, have been reported to have hypoglycaemic, hypolipidaemic and cardioprotective activities in an animal model [86]. These biological effects have been attributed to the abundant presence of flavonoids, alkaloids and saponins in the plant extracts [86].

Phyllanthus Species: *Phyllanthus Niruri and Amarus*

Phyllanthus niruri is a herbal shrub that is widely distributed in most tropical countries but most abundant in India. It has an ancestral history for its wide application in the traditional diabetes care. Several independent studies have reported its blood glucose lowering effect in animal studies. In an animal study, extract of *Phyllanthus niruri* was found to lower the blood glucose after glucose administration more than that produced by the standard drug, tolbutamide [87]. In another animal study, 120 and 240 mg/kg of the plant extract were orally administered to streptozotocin-induced diabetic rats for 14 days [88]. The doses were reported to significantly lower the plasma glucose concentrations in the treated rats in a dose related fashion. The hypoglycaemic effect was reported to possibly be mediated by the presence of flavonoids and alkaloids in the extract [88].

Phyllanthus amarus Schum and Thonn (Euphorbiaceae) is a small, erect annual herbal shrub, which is reputable for the traditional management of various human ailments including pain, swelling, hypertension, hepatic diseases and diabetes mellitus. Aqueous extract, prepared from the plant leaves and seeds, was found to lower blood glucose and cholesterol in experimental animal model [89]. The mechanism by which the extract induces hypoglycaemia was proposed to be mediated *via* either hyperinsulinaemia or enhanced peripheral utilization of glucose [89]. In another study, methanolic extract of the plant was reported to lower blood glucose returning it to about the normal levels in alloxan diabetic rats [90]. In humans, the aqueous extracts of *Phyllanthus amarus* have also been documented to attain good glycaemic haemostatic control in non-insulin dependent diabetic patients [91].

Coffee and Green Tea

Coffee is the most popular non-alcoholic beverage in the world. Regular consumption of several cups of coffee has been reported to reduce the risk of developing diabetes mellitus in the future. In a landslide 12 years prospective study involving 14, 629 Finnish people consisting of 6, 974 men and 7, 655 women aged 25–64 years with no existing heart disease, stroke or diabetes, daily consumption of 10 or more cups of coffee significantly prevented 97.4% of the studied subjects from developing diabetes mellitus [92]. Light coffee drinkers had the same risk as non-coffee drinkers [92]. In a similar study involving 17, 413 men and women in 25 communities across Japan, aged 40-65 years and with about half of the subjects being diabetics, it was found that the diabetes symptoms were significantly improved in subjects who drank 6 or more cups of green tea and 3 or more cups of coffee each day and about a third were less likely to develop diabetes [93]. In another larger study involving 41, 934 men and 84, 276 women, researchers found that daily intake of several cups of coffee or caffeine-containing drinks (*e.g.* soda and green tea) reduced the risk of developing type 2 diabetes mellitus by 95.7% [94]. However, caffeine appeared not to be the protective phytocomponents because in another study involving oral intake of caffeine concentrate in non-diabetic subjects, the plasma blood glucose and free insulin levels were elevated [95]. It was suggested that other phytocomponents present in coffee and caffeine-containing drinks could be responsible for the protective effects [95].

Eugenia Jambolana

Eugenia jambolana is a perennial tropical plant which is widely employed in Ayurvedic medicine in the management of diabetes mellitus, particularly decoctions made from its seed kernels. Extracts prepared from the lyophilized powdered sample of the plant have been reported to effectively control hyperglycaemia in different diabetic models of experimental animals [96]. The antihyperglycaemic effect of the plant extract was also reported to be mediated *via* increased skeletal and hepatic glycogen storage activities of the key enzymes involved in glycogen deposits in these organs [96]. Extract prepared from the pulp of the plant's fruit has also been reported to mediate hypoglycaemic and antihyperglycaemic effects in normal and streptozotocin diabetic rats, respectively, *via* enhanced hyperinsulinaemia (through increased insulin secretion and inhibited *insulinase* activity from the kidney and liver) [97]. Extracts made from the seed kernels have been documented to induce hypoglycaemia in diabetic rats [98] and alloxanized diabetic rabbits [99], in addition to its hypolipidaemic effect [98]. Flavonoids isolated from the kernel seeds were reported to stimulate 16% increase in insulin release *in vitro* from pancreatic islets. The hypolipidaemic action after this extract supplementation was confirmed by significant ($p<0.05$) decrease in the levels of low density lipoprotein (LDL)-cholesterol, triglycerides and increase in high density lipoprotein (HDL)-cholesterol over untreated diabetic rats. However, the hypolipidaemic action of the plant extract was found to be through reduced activity of *HMG-CoA reductase* in alloxan-diabetic rabbits [99] and in streptozotocin diabetic rats, through dual up regulation of both the peroxisome proliferators-activated receptors (PPAR-alpha and PPAR-gamma) up to about 3-4 folds (over control) [98].

Artemisia herba-alba

Artemisia herba-alba Asso (Asteraceae) is a medicinal plant that occurs around the Mediterranean basins of Egypt and Israel and stretching to Spain [100]. In a clinical study involving fifteen type 2 diabetic patients, treatment with *Artemisia herba-alba* extract (AHE) resulted in considerable lowering of elevated blood sugar and 14 out of 15 patients had good remission of diabetic symptoms with use of AHE [101].

Ficus Bengalensis

Ficus bengalensis Linn. is a large tropical plant with aerial roots and is known as Banya tree in English language and as Bargad in Hindu [102]. Different parts of the plant are attributed with diverse medicinal values.

The antidiabetic effect of a dimethoxy derivative of *perlargonidin 3-O-alpha-L rhamnoside* (250 mg/kg, single dose study and 100 mg/kg/day long term study) isolated from the bark of *Ficus bengalensis* Linn. in moderately diabetic rats has been reported [103]. The single dose glycoside treatment decreased fasting blood glucose by 19% and improved glucose tolerance by 29%. On one-month treatment the fasting blood glucose levels went down almost to half of the pre-treatment levels in both groups and their glucose tolerance improved by 41% in glibenclamide group and by 15% in glycoside treated group. Urine sugar decreased to traces in both groups and they appeared healthy. Furthermore, *in vitro* studies showed that insulin secretion by beta-cells was more in the presence of the *pelargonidin* derivative than in the presence of a *leucocyanidin* derivative, reported to be a good anti-diabetic agent [103]. Similarly, a *leucodelphinidin* derivative (a flavonoid) isolated from the bark of *Ficus bengalensis* Linn demonstrated hypoglycaemic action at a dosage of 250 mg/kg given both in normal and alloxan diabetic rats. Its action was closely similar to that of an effective dose of glibenclamide (2 mg/kg) tested under the same conditions [104]. In another study, the active biological principle of *Ficus bengalensis* inducing hypoglycaemia in normal and alloxan diabetic rabbit models was isolated and identified as *bengalenoside*, a glycoside [105]. More recently, another antidiabetic glycoside, *leucopelargonidin*, was isolated from the plant [106].

Apart from its hypoglycaemic activity, Shukla *et al.* (2004) [102] reported that the water extract of *Ficus bengalensis* decreased the serum cholesterol level by 59%, triacylglycerol by 54%, and low density lipoprotein (LDL)-cholesterol and very low density lipoprotein (VLDL)-cholesterol by 60% in rats fed with high cholesterol diet. In addition, treatment with this extract decreased lipid peroxidation, increased blood glutathione content and significantly increased the activities of antioxidant enzymes: *superoxide dismutase, catalase, glutathione peroxidase* and *glutathione reductase*. The antioxidant activity of the plant extract has been attributed to the presence of two flavonoid compounds: *5, 7-dimethyl ether* of *leucopelargonidin 3-0-alpha-L rhamnoside* and *5, 3'-dimethyl ether* of *leucocyanidin 3-0-alpha-D galactosyl cellobioside* obtained from the bark of *Ficus bengalensis* [107].

Tinospora cordifolia

Tinospora cordifolia (Wild.) Miers ex Hook. F. & Thomas is a rasayama drug from Ayurveda which is reputed and recommended for the treatment of a variety of diseases including diabetes mellitus and for promotion of health [108]. It is widely distributed in the tropics of Asia (such as India, Burma, Sri Lanka), tropics of Africa and Australia [109]. The antihyperglycaemic effects of extracts prepared from different parts of the plant have been reported. For example, the aqueous extract of the plant stem has been reported to decrease fasting blood glucose levels and increase oral glucose tolerance in normal rats [110] and alloxan-induced hyperglycaemic rats [111]. Similarly, oral treatment with 2500–7500 mg/kg of the aqueous root extract of the plant have also been documented to have significant hypoglycaemic effect in alloxanized diabetic rats, a biological effect that was comparable to that of 600 µg/kg of glibenclamide [112]. In addition to the oral hypoglycaemic effect of its methanol root extract [96, 113], 5000 mg/kg of the extract also caused pronounced decreases in the both the serum and tissue lipid levels [113]. Similar oral hypoglycaemic effect was reported for 250 mg/kg/day of the plant stem ethanol extract after one week of oral treatment of alloxanized diabetic rats [114]. However, the oral hypoglycaemic effects of the plant extracts were postulated to be predominantly due to stimulation of pancreatic β cells and not due to direct insulinomimetic action of the extract [108]. The oral hypoglycaemic effect of the plant extract in the diabetic rats was also reported to be mediated *via* increased glycolysis and glucose-6-phosphate concentration [96, 112].

POLYHERBAL ANTIDIABETIC FORMULAS

Many polyherbal formulations are currently sold in the market today for the traditional management of diabetes, either as monotherapy or as adjuvant to conventional antidiabetic agents. However, despite the abundance of varieties of herbal antidiabetic formulas, pre-clinical and clinical evaluations of their efficacies and safety are still lacking, although individual evaluation of some of the compositions have been conducted and reported. For the purpose of accurate scientific records, only scientifically validated oral hypoglycemic polyherbal formulas will be reviewed in this sub-section of the chapter, as the list of hypoglycaemic herbal formulas in current use is inexhaustible. However, it should be noted that these herbal formulations differ from one traditional medical system to another.

Diabecon (D-400)

Diabecon (D-400) is a tableted crude herbal extract of Ayurvedic polyherbal formulation consisting of *Eugenia jambolana, Tinospora cordifolia, Pterocarpus marsupium, Ficus glomerulata, Momordica charantia, Ocimum sanctum and Gymnema sylvestre* [115]. Preclinical studies have clearly shown Diabecon (D-400) to lack acute, chronic and teratogenicity toxicities and human studies have established its oral safety for long-term use [116]. Both animal and clinical trials have reported the oral hypoglycaemic effect of Diabecon (D-400). An animal study reported that oral administration of 1 g/kg body weight of the aqueous extract of Diabecon (D-400) to alloxan diabetic rats for 36 weeks significantly lowered the serum glucose, blood urea and serum creatinine in the Diabecon-treated rats [117].

In a small-size randomized, placebo-controlled clinical trial involving 43 maturity onset (type 2) diabetics, 12 weeks oral treatment Diabecon (D-400) was reported to be associated with significant reduction in both the fasting and postpandrial blood glucose in both newly diagnosed as well as those already on standard oral hypoglycaemic agents (with or without insulin), which was suggested to be mediated *via* reduction in the hepatic glycogenolysis and interference with the glucagons mechanism [116]. Other clinical trials have reported similar observations [118, 119]. In a more recent clinical study involving 21 (13 males and 8 females) adult type 2 diabetics, oral intake of 2 tablets thrice daily for 6 months resulted in significant reduction of the fasting and postpandrial blood and urine glucose, and glycosylated haemoglobin levels. Diabecon was also reported to have significantly increased the serum levels of free insulin and c-peptides [120].

Cogent db

Cogent db is a complex herbal drug derived from Ayurvedic plants with ancestral history in the effective management of diabetes mellitus. Preclinical studies have reported that oral administration of the aqueous extract to alloxanized diabetic rats for 40 consecutive days resulted in a significant reduction in the fasting blood glucose, glycosylated haemoglobin and increased plasma free insulin and total haemoglobin concentrations. The extract also exhibited antihyperlipidaemic effects, prevented body weight loss and improved oral glucose tolerance in the diabetic rats [121].

Diamed

Diamed is a herbal formulation composed of the aqueous extracts of *Azadirachta indica*, *Cassia auriculata* and *Momordica charantia*. Results from animal study showed that oral administration of various doses of *Diamed* to alloxan-induced diabetic rats for 30 days caused a significant reduction in blood glucose, glycosylated haemoglobin, and an increase in plasma insulin and total haemoglobin [122]. In addition, *Diamed* prevented a decrease in body weight and caused a significant improvement in the oral glucose tolerance in the *Diamed*-treated rats [122].

Episulin

Episulin derived from *Ptercarpus marsupium* and certain antidiabetic herbal plants with epicatechin content, is formulated and marketed by Swastik

Formulations Pvt. Ltd. (Uttar Pradesh, India). *Episulin* on prolonged study has been discovered to contain epicatechin, a *benzopyran*, as its active principle. Epicatechin, apart from promoting the pancreatic synthesis and release of insulin, is also insulinomimetic in its hypoglycaemic action. It also prevents and corrects other attendant nervous complications, such as neuropathy and retinopathy, which are often associated with unmanaged or poorly managed diabetic patients. A clinical trial involving type 2 diabetic patients which was conducted in India and designed to evaluate the efficacy of 1 capsule of *Episulin* taken twice daily before meal for 3 months showed the drug to cause significant reduction in fasting and postpandrial blood glucose, body mass index, serum total cholesterol and blood urea while causing a significant increase in the haemoglobin concentration in the diabetic subjects (Episulin.com) [123].

Dianex

Dianex is a polyherbal formulation consisting of the aqueous extracts of Gymnema sylvestre, *Eugenia jambolana, Momordica indica, Azadirachta indica, Cassia auriculata, Aegle marmelose, Withania somnifera and Curcuma longa.* Studies have shown Dianex (at the oral dose range of 100 to 500 mg/kg body weight) to cause hypoglycaemia and hypolipidaemia in normal and diabetic animals on acute and long-term studies [124]. Dianex also improved oral glucose tolerance in both normal and diabetic rats [124].

Okchun-San

Okchun-San is a Korean herbal medicine formula with an ancestral history of its wide use in the effective management of diabetes mellitus. It is composed of *Coicis semen* and *Oryzae semen*. Experimental study showed that the extracts of the dried plants significantly lowered the fasting blood glucose and improved the intraperitoneal glucose tolerance in diabetic C57BL/KsJ *db/db* mice [125].

Diasulin

Diasulin is an Ayuverdic polyherbal formulation composed of ethanolic extract of the flower of Tanner's cassia (*Cassia auriculata*, family: Ceasalpinaceae), fruit of Little gourd (*Coccinia indica*, family: Cucurbitaceae), rhizome of Turmeric (*Curcuma longa*, family: Zingiberaceae), fruit of Indian gooseberry (*Embelica officinalis*, family: Euphorbiaceae), leaves of Ram's horn (*Gymnema sylvestre*, family: Asclepiadaceae), fruit of Bitter gourd (*Momordica charantia*, family: Cucurbitaceae), whole plant of Sweet broom weed (*Scoparia dulcis*, family: Scrophulariaceae), seed of Jamun (*Syzigium cumini*, family: Myrtaceae), root of *Gulancha tinospora* (*Tinospora cardifolia*, family: Menispermacea) and seed of Fenugreek (*Trigonella foenum graecum*, family: Fabaceae). The antidiabetic effect of *Diasulin* has been investigated in alloxan-induced diabetic rats at graded oral doses of 50, 100 and 200 mg/kg/day for 30 days. Results showed that *Diasulin* lowered the fasting blood glucose and free insulin, significantly bringing their values to about normal levels, dose dependently [126]. *Diasulin* was also reported to possess significant free radical scavenging activity, in addition to significantly decreasing cholesterol, triglyceride, free fatty acids and phospholipids contents of the liver and kidney of the diabetic rats [126]. However, the antidiabetic and antihyperlipidaemic effects of *Diasulin* were proposed to be mediated by the active phytoprinciples in the constituent plants namely alkaloids and pectins from *Coccinia indica*, alkaloids from *Tinospora cordifolia*, *emlicanin A* and *emlicanin B* from *Emblica officinalis*, *trigonelline* and *scopoltin* from *Trigonella foenum graecum*, alkaloid (6-methoxybenzolinone) and terpenoids such as *scoparic acids A, B, C* and *scopadulcic acid A* and *B* from *Scoparia dulcis*, which may also account for the antioxidant and free radical scavenging activities of the polyherbal formulation [126, 127].

In a similar study, oral treatment of alloxan-induced diabetic rats with 200 mg/kg/day of Diasulin resulted in a significant reduction in blood glucose, glycosylated haemoglobin and an increase in plasma insulin and total haemoglobin and a significant improvement in oral glucose tolerance [127]. Diasulin caused a significant reduction in the activities of glucose-6-phosphatase and fructose-1,6- bisphosphatase in the liver while increasing hepatic hexokinase activity [128].

CONCLUSIONS

Based on the fact that the interest in and the use of herbal hypoglycaemic remedies have grown at an exponential proportion in the last two decades, it becomes very imperative that more definitive clinical evaluations (including the safety and standardization, identification of active ingredients and the definitive mechanism(s) of therapeutic action of the existing hypoglycaemic herbal alternatives) must be conducted. These will further strengthen and consolidate the preliminary results available on the therapeutic efficacies of some of these remedies.

ACKNOWLEDGEMENTS

The authors extend their thanks to the Editors and Bentham Science Publishers.

DECLARATION OF CONFLICT OF INTEREST

No conflict of interest was declared by the authors.

REFERENCES

[1]   Krall LP, Beaser RS. Joslin Diabetes Manual. 12th edition. Williams and Wilkins 1989; pp. viii.
[2]   Diabetes Control and Complication Trial Research Group. Report of the Expert Committee on the Diagnosis and Classification of Diabetes Mellitus. Diabetes Care 1997; 20: 1183-97.
[3]   World Health Organization. Diabetes Mellitus: Report of a WHO Study Group. The Technical Report Series 1985; 727.
[4]   Winter WE, Maclaren NK, Riley WJ, Clarke DW, Kappy S, Spillar RP. Maturity-onset diabetes of youth in black Americans. N Engl J Med1987; 316: 285-91.
[5]   Morrison EY. Diabetes mellitus–a third syndrome (phasic insulin dependence). International Diab Fed Bul 1981; 26: 6.
[6]   Wild S, Roglic G, Green A, Sicree R, King H. Global prevalence of Diabetes: Estimates for the year 2000 and projections for 2030. Diabetes Care 2004; 27(5): 1047-53.
[7]   American Diabetes Association. Report of the Expert Committee on the Diagnosis and Classification of Diabetes Mellitus. Diabetes Care 1997; 20: 1183-97.
[8]   Sobngwi E, Mauyais-Javis F, Vexiau P, Mbanya JC, Gautier JF. Diabetes in Africas, I: Epidemiology and clinical specificities. Diab Metab. 2001; 27: 628-34.
[9]   Amoah AGB, Owusu SK, Adjei S. Diabetes in Ghana: a community based prevalence study in Greater Accra. Diab Res Clin Pract 2002; 56: 197-205.
[10]   Motala AA, Omar MA, Pirie FJ. Diabetes in Africa: Epidemiology of type 1 and type 2 diabetes in Africa. J Card Risk 2003; 10: 77-83.
[11]   Enwere OO, Salako BL, Falade CO. Prescription and cost consideration at a diabetic clinic in Ibadan, Nigeria: A Report. An Iba Post Med 2006; 4(2): 35-39.
[12]   Rotimi CN, Cooper RS, Okosun IS, *et al.* Prevalence of diabetes and impaired glucose tolerance in Nigerians, Jamaicans and US blacks. Ethn Dis 1999; 9(2): 190-200.
[13]   Owoaje EE, Rotimi CN, Kaufman JS, Tracy J, Cooper RS. Prevalence of adult diabetes in Ibadan, Nigeria. E Afri Med J 1997; 74(5): 299-302.

[14] Olatunbosun ST, Ojo PO, Fineberg NS, Bella AF. Prevalence of diabetes mellitus and impaired glucose tolerance in a group of urban adults in Nigeria. J Nat Med Ass 1998; 90(5): 293-301.

[15] Bach JF. Insulin-dependent diabetes mellitus as an autoimmune disease. End Rev 1994; 15: 516-42.

[16] DeFronzo RA, Bonadonna RC, Ferrannini E. Pathogenesis of NIDDM: a balanced overview. Diabetes Care 1992; 15: 318-68.

[17] Neel JV. Diabetes mellitus – a thrifty genotype rendered detrimental by progress? A J Hum Gen 1962; 14: 353-62.

[18] Hartz AJ, Rupley DC Jnr, Kalkhoff R, Rimm AA. Relationship of obesity to diabetes: influence of obesity and body fat distribution. Prev Med 1983; 12: 351-7

[19] Drury TF, Powell AL. Prevalence of known diabetes among black Americans. In: Diabetes in America Harris MI, Hamman RF (Eds.). DHHS publ. no. (NIH) 1987; 87-1250.

[20] Cowie CC, Harris MI, Silverman RE, Johnson EW, Rust KF. Effect of multiple risk factors on differences between blacks and whites in the prevalence of non-insulin-dependent diabetes mellitus in the United States. A J Epid 1993; 137: 719-32.

[21] Zimmet PZ, Collins VR, Dowse GK, *et al.* The relation of physical activity to cardiovascular disease risk factors in Mauritians. A J Epid 1991; 134: 862-75.

[22] Sicree RA, Zimmet P, King H, Coventry JS. Plasma insulin response among Nauruans: Prediction of deterioration in glucose tolerance over 6 years. Diabetes 1984; 36: 179-86.

[23] Bogardus C, Lillioja S, Foley J, *et al.* Insulin resistance predicts the development of non-insulin dependent diabetes mellitus in Pima Indians. Diabetes 1987; 36(Suppl. 1): 47A.

[24] Cline GW, Magnusson I, Rothman DL, Petersen KF, Laurent D, Shulman GI. Mechanism of impaired insulin-stimulated muscle glucose metabolism in subjects with insulin-dependent diabetes mellitus. J Clin Invest 1997; 20: 1183-97.

[25] Harris MI. Impaired glucose tolerance in the U.S. population. Diabetes Care 1989; 12: 464-74.

[26] Larsen S, Hilsted J, Tronier B, Worning H. Metabolic control and B cell function in patients with insulin-dependent diabetes mellitus secondary to chronic pancreatitis. Metabolism 1987; 36: 964-7

[27] Adeneye AA, Agbaje EO, Amole OO, Elias SO, Izegbu MC. Antidiabetic and antilipidaemic activities of metformin-ascorbic acid combination on glucose-induced insulin resistance rat. W Afr J Pharm Dr Res 2007; 22 & 23: 10-15.

[28] Raskin I, Ribnicky DM, Komarnytsky S, *et al.* Plants and human health in the twenty-first century. Trends in Biotechnology 2002; 20: 522-31.

[29] Vijayakumar MV, Bhat MK. Effect of a novel dialysed Fenugreek seeds extract is sustainable and is mediated, in part, by activation of of hepatic enzymes. Phyt Res 2008; 22; 500-5.

[30] Soejarto DD. Biodiversity prospecting and benefit-sharing: perspective from the field. J Ethnopharmacol 1996; 51: 1-5.

[31] World Health Organization. WHO guidelines for the assessment of herbal medicine. WHO Expert Committee on specification for pharmaceutical preparation. Technical Report Series 1996; No. 863.

[32] Nwabuisi C. Prophylactic effect of multi-herbal extract 'Agbo-Iba' on malaria induced in mice. East Afr Med J 2002; 79(7): 343-346.

[33] Ernst E. Prevalence of Use of Complementary/Alternative Medicine: A systematic review. Bull Worl Heal Org 2000; 78(2): 252-7.

[34] Parek J, Chanda S. *In-vitro* Antimicrobial Activities of Extracts of *Launaea procumbens Roxb.* (Labiateae), *Vitis vinifera L.* (Vitaceae) and *Cyperus rotundus L.* (Cyperaceae). Afr J Biomed Res 2006; 9: 89-93.

[35] Venkatesh-Babu KC, Krishnakumari S. *Cardiospermum halicacabum* suppresses the production of TNF-alpha and nitric oxide by human peripheral blood mononuclear cells. Afr J Biomed Res 2006; 9: 95-99.

[36] Escot N. Fenugreek. ATOM (1994/95): 7-12.

[37] Al-Habori A, Raman A. Pharmacological Properties. In: Fenugreek the Genus *Trigonella.* Taylor and Francis 2002; pp. 163-82.

[38] Basch E, Ulbricht C, Kuo G, Szapary P, Smith M. Therapeutic applications of fenugreek. Alter Med Rev 2003; 8: 20-7.

[39] Ribes G, Sauvaire Y, Baccou JC, *et al.* Effects of Fenugreek seeds on endocrine pancreatic secretions in dogs. An Nutr Metabol 1984; 28: 37-43.

[40] Sharma RD, Raghuram TC, Rao NS. Effect of Fenugreek seeds on blood glucose and serum lipids in type 1 diabetics. Eur J Clin Nut 1990; 44: 301-6.

[41] Mada Z, Abel R, Samish S, Arad J. Glucose-lowering effect of Fenugreek in non-insulin dependent diabetics, Eur J Clin Nutr 1988; 42: 51-4.

[42] Petit PR, Sauvaire YD, Hillaire-Buys DM, *et al.* Steroid saponins from fenugreek seed: extraction, purification, and pharmacological investigation on feeding behaviour and plasma cholesterol. Steroids 1995; 60: 674-80.

[43] Ribes G, Sauvaire Y, Da Costa C, Baccou JC, Loubatieres-Mariani MM. Antidiabetic effects of subfraction from fenugreek seeds in diabetic dogs. Proceed Soc Exp Biol Med 1986; 182: 159-66.

[44] Sauvaire Y, Ribes G, Baccou JC, Loubatieres-Mariani MM. Implication of steroid saponins and sapogenins in the hypocholesterolaemic effect of fenugreek. Lipids 1991; 26: 191-7.

[45] Raju J, Gupta D, Rao AR, Yadava PK, Baquer NZ. *Trigonella foenum graecum* (fenugreek) seed powder improves glucose homeostasis in alloxan diabetic rat tissues by reversing the altered glycolytic, gluconeogenic and lipogenic enzymes. Mol Cell Biochem 2001; 224: 45-51.

[46] Handa T, Yamaguchi K, Sono Y, Yazawa K. Effect of fenugreek seed extract in obese mice fed a high-fat diet. Biosc Biotech Biochem 2005; 69(6): 1186-8.

[47] Blumenthal M, Goldberg A, Brinckman J. Fenugreek. In: Herbal Medicine: Expanded Commission E Monographs. Lippincott Williams and Wilkins 2000; pp. 130-133.

[48] Kuriyan R, Rajendran R, Bantwal G, Kurpad AV. Effect of supplementation of *Coccinia cordifolia* extract on newly detected diabetic patients. Diabetes Care 2007; 31(2): 216-20.

[49] Azad-Khan AK, Akhtar S, Mahtab H. *Coccinia indica* in the treatment of patients with diabetes mellitus. Bangladesh Medical Research Council Bulletin 1979; 5: 60-6.

[50] Kamble SM, Kamlakar PL, Vaidya S, Bambole VD. Influence of *Coccinia indica* on certain enzymes in glycolytic and lipolytic pathway in human diabetes. Ind J Med Sci 1998; 52: 143-6.

[51] Kamble SM, Jyotishi GS, Kamlakar PL, Vaidya SM. Efficacy of *Coccinia indica* W & A in diabetes mellitus. J Res Ayurv Sid 1996; XVII: 77-84.

[52] Sotaniemi EA, Haapakoski E, Rautio A. Ginseng therapy in non-insulin dependent diabetic patients: effect on psychophysical performance, glucose homeostasis, serum lipids, serum aminoterminalpropeptide concentration, and body weight. Diabetes Care 1995; 18: 1373-5.

[53] Vuksan V, Sievenpiper JL, Xu Z, *et al.* Konjac-mannan and American ginseng: emerging (*Panax quinquefolius*): emerging alternative therapies for type 2 diabetes mellitus. J Amer Col Nutr 2001; 20: 370S-80S.

[54] Shane-McWhorter L. Biological complementary therapies: a focus on botanical products in diabetes. Diabetes Spectrum 2001; 14: 199-208.

[55] Khanna P, Jain SC, Panagariya A, Dixit VP. Hypoglycaemic activity of *polypeptide-p* from a plant source. J Nat Prod 1981; 44: 648-55.

[56] Shibib BA, Khan IA, Rahman R. Hypoglycaemic activity of *Coccinia indica* and *Momordica charantia* in diabetic rats: depression of the hepatic gluconeogenic enzymes glucose-6-phosphatase and fructose-1, 6-biphosphatase and elevation of liver and red-cell shunt enzyme glucose-6-phosphate dehydrogenase. Biochem J 1993; 292: 267-70.

[57] Welihinda J, Karananayake EH, Sheriff MHR, Jayasinghe KSA. Effect of *Momordica charantia* on the glucose tolerance in maturity onset diabetes. J Ethnopharmacol 1986; 17(3): 277-82.

[58] Brinker F. Herb Contraindications and Drug Interactions. 3rd Edition. Eclectic Medical Publications. Sandy 2001; pp. 39.

[59] Tennekoon KH, Jeevathayaparan S, Angunawala P, Kurananayake EH, Jayasinghe KSA. Effect of *Momordica charantia* on key hepatic enzymes. J Ethnopharmacol 1994; 44(2): 93-7.

[60] Leung SO, Yeung HW, Leung KN. The immunosuppressive activities of two abortifacient proteins isolated from the seeds of bitter melon (*Momordica charantia*). Immunopharmacology 1987; 13(3):159-71.

[61] Bailey CJ, Day C. Traditional plant medicines as treatments for diabetes. Diabetes Care 1989; 12: 553-64.

[62] Ige SF, Salawu EO, Olaleye SB, Adeeyo OA, Badmus J, Adeleke AA, Onion (Allium cepa) extract prevents cadmium induced renal dysfunction. Ind J Nephrol 2009; 19: 140-4.

[63] Roman-Ramos R, Flores-Saenz JL, Alaricon-Aguilar FJ. Antihyperglycaemic effect of some edible plants. J Ethnopharmacol 1995; 48: 25-32.

[64] Kumari K, Mathew BC, Augusti KT. Antidiabetic and hypolipidaemic effects of S-methyl cysteine sulphoxide isolated from *Allium cepa* Linn. Ind J Biochem Biophysiol 1995; 32: 49-54.

[65] Mathew PT, Augusti KT. Hypoglycaemic effects of onion, *Allium cepa* Linn. on diabetes mellitus – a preliminary report. Ind J Physiol Pharmacol 1975; 19: 213-7.

[66] Augusti KT, Benaim ME. Effect of essential oil of onion on blood glucose, free fatty acid and insulin levels of normal subjects. Clin Chim Act 1975; 60: 121-123.

[67] Sheela CG, Augusti KT. Antidiabetic effects of S-allyl cysteine suphoxide isolated from garlic, *Allium sativum* Linn. Ind J Exp Biol 1992; 30: 532-6.

[68] Zacharia NT, Sebastian KL, Philip B, Augusti KT. Hypoglycaemic and hypolipidaemic effects of garlic in sucrose-fed rabbits. Ind J Physiol Pharmacol 1980; 24: 151-4.

[69] Augusti KT, Shella CG. Antiperoxide effect of S-allyl cysteine sulphoxide, an insulin secretagogue in diabetic rats. Experintia 1996; 52: 115-20.

[70] Jain RC, Vyas CR, Mahatma OP. Hypoglycemic action of onion and garlic. Lancet 1973; 2: 1491.

[71] Keisewetter H, Jung F, Pindur G, Jung EM, Mrowietz C, Wenzel E. Effect of garlic on thrombocyte aggregation, microcirculation, and other risk factors. Inter J Clin Pharmacol, Ther Toxicol 1991; 29: 151-5.

[72]   Chattopadhyay RR. Hypoglycemic effect of *Ocimum sanctum* leaf extract in normal and streptozotocin diabetic rats. Ind J Exp Biol 1993; 31: 891-3.

[73]   Agrawal P, Rai V, Singh RB, Azad Khan AK, Akhtar S, Mahtab H. Randomized placebo-controlled single-blind trial of holy basil leaves in patients with non-insulin-dependent diabetes mellitus. Int J Clin Pharmacol Ther 1996; 34: 406-9.

[74]   Al-Awadi FM, Gumaa KA. Studies on the activity of individual plants of an antidiabetic plant mixture. Act Diabetol 1987; 24: 215-20.

[75]   Ajabnoor MA. Effect of aloes on blood glucose levels in normal and alloxan diabetic mice. J Ethnopharmacol 1990; 28: 215-220.

[76]   Yongchaiyudha S, Rungpitarangsi V, Bunyapraphatsara N, Chokechaijaroenporn O. Antidiabetic activity of *Aloe vera* L. juice. I. Clinical trial of new cases of diabetes mellitus. Phytomedicine 1996; 3: 241-3.

[77]   Bunyapraphatsara N, Yongchaiyudha S, Rungpitarangsi V, Chokechaijaroenporn O. Antidiabetic activities of *Aloe vera* L. juice. II. Clinical trial in diabetes mellitus patients in combination with glibenclamide. Phytomedicine 1996; 3: 244- 5.

[78]   Ghannam N, Kingston M, Al-Meshaal IA, Tariq M, Parman NS, Woodhouse N. The antidiabetic activity of aloes: preliminary clinical and experimental observations. Horm Research 1986; 24: 288-94.

[79]   Chakrabarti S, Biswas TK, Rokeya B, *et al.* Advanced studies on the hypoglycaemic effect of *Caesalpinia bonducella* F. in type 1 and 2 diabetes in Long Evans rats. J Ethnopharmacol 2003; 84: 41-6.

[80]   Sharma SR, Dwivedi SK, Swarup D. Hypoglycaemic, antihyperglycaemic and hypolipidaemic activities of *Caesalpinia bonducella* seeds in rats. J Ethnopharmacol 1997; 58: 39-44.

[81]   Shapiro K, Gong WC. Natural products used for diabetes. J Amer Pharm Ass 2002; 42: 217-26.

[82]   Frati AC, Diaz NX, Altamirano P, Ariza P. Ariza R, Lopez-Ledesma R. The effect of two sequential doses of *Opuntia streptacantha* upon glycaemia. Arch Invest Med (Mexico) 1991; 22: 333-6.

[83]   Frati AC, Gordillo BE, Altamirano P, Ariza CR, Cortes-Franco R, Chavez-Negrete A. Acute hypoglycaemic effects of *Opuntia streptacantha* Lemiare in NIDDM (Letter). Diabetes Care 1990; 13: 455-6.

[84]   Adeneye AA, Ajagbonna OP, Ayodele OW. Hypoglycaemic and antidiabetic activities on the stem bark aqueous and ethanol extracts of *Musanga cecropioides* in normal and alloxan-induced diabetic rats. Fitoterapia 2007; 78: 502-5.

[85]   Gill LS. Enumeration of ethnomedical uses of plants in Nigeria. In: Ethnomedical uses of plants in Nigeria. Uniben Press 1992; pp. 72-5.

[86]   Adeneye AA. Methanol seed extract of *Citrus paradisi* Macfad lowers blood glucose, lipids and cardiovascular disease risk indices in normal Wistar rats. Nigerian Quarterly Journal of Hospital Medicine 2008; 18(1): 16-20.

[87]   Ramakrishnan PN, Murugesan R, Palanichamy S, Murugesh N. Oral hypoglycaemic effect of *Phyllanthus niruri* Linn. Ind J Pharm Sc 1982; 44(1): 10-12.

[88]   Nwajo HU. Studies on the effect of aqueous extract of *Phyllanthus niruri* leaf on plasma glucose level and some hepatospecific markers in diabetic Wistar rats. The Internet Journal of Laboratory Medicine 2007; 2(2). Available online at http//: www.ispub.com/ostia/index.php?xml/FilePath=journals/ijlm/vol2n2/niruri.xml

[89] Adeneye AA, Amole OO, Adeneye AK. Hypoglycaemic and hypocholesterolaemic activities of the aqueous leaf and seed extract of *Phyllanthus amarus* in mice. Fitoterapia 2006; 77: 511-4.

[90] Raphael KR, Sabu MC, Kuttan R. Hypoglycaemic effect of methanol extract of *Phyllanthus amarus* on alloxan induced diabetes mellitus in rats and its relation with antioxidant potential. Ind J Exp Biol 2002; 40: 905-9.

[91] Moshi MJ, Lutale JKJ, Rimoy GH, Abbas ZG, Josiah RM, Swai ABM. The effect of *Phyllanthus amarus* aqueous extract on blood glucose in non-insulin dependent diabetic patients. Phy Res 2001; 15: 577-80.

[92] Tuomilehto J, Hu G, Bidel S, Lindstrm J, Jousilahti P. Coffee consumption and risk of type 2 diabetes mellitus among middle-aged Finnish men and women. Journal of American Medical Association 2004; 291(10): 1213-19.

[93] Iso H, Date C, Wakai K, Fukui M, Tamakoshi A and the JACC Study Group. The relationship between green tea and total caffeine intake and risk for self-reported type 2 diabetes among Japanese adults. An Inter Med 2006; 144: 554-62.

[94] Salazar-Martinez E, Willett WC, Ascherio A, *et al.* Coffee consumption and risk for type 2 diabetes mellitus. Annals of Internal Medicine 2004; 140: 1-8.

[95] Van Dam RM, Willet WC, Manson JE, Hu FB. Coffee, caffeine, and risk of type 2 diabetes: A prospective cohort study in younger and middle-aged U.S. women. Diabetes Care 2006; 29: 398-403.

[96] Grover JK, Vats V, Rathi SS. Anti-hyperglycaemic effect of *Eugenia jambolana* and *Tinospora cordifolia* in experimental diabetes and their effects on key metabolic enzymes involved in carbohydrate metabolism. J Ethnopharmacol 2000; 73(3): 461-70.

[97] Achrekar S, Kakljil GS, Pote MS, Kelkar SM. Hypoglycaemic activity of *Eugenia jambolana* and *Ficus bengalensis*: mechanism of action. *In vivo* 1991; 5(2): 143-7.

[98] Sharma B, Balomajumder C, Roy P. Hypoglycaemic and hypolipidaemic effects of flavonoid rich extract from *Eugenia jambolana* seeds on streptozotocin induced diabetic rats. Food and Chemical Toxicology 2008; 46(7): 2376-83.

[99] Sharma SB, Nasir A, Prabhu KM, Murthy PS, Dev G. Hypoglycaemic and hypolipidaemic effect of ethanolic extract of seeds of *Eugenia jambolana* in alloxan-induced diabetic rabbits. J Ethnopharmacol 2003; 85(2-3): 201-6.

[100] Marco AJ, Sanz-Cervera JF, Ocete G, Carda M, Rodrìguez S, Vallès-Xirau J. New Germacranolides and Eudesmanolides from North Africa *Artemesia herba-alba*. J Nat Prod 1994; 57(7): 939-46.

[101] Al-Waili NSD. Treatment of diabetes mellitus by *Artemisia herba-alba* extract: preliminary study. Clin Exp Pharmacol Physiol 1986; 13(7): 569-74

[102] Shukla R, Gupta S, Gambhir JK, Prabhu KM, Murthy PS. Antioxidant effect of aqueous extract of the bark of *Ficus bengalensis* in hypercholesterolaemic rabbits. J Ethnopharmacol 2004; 92(1): 47-51.

[103] Cherian S, Kumar RV, Augusti KT, Kidwai JR. Antidiabetic effect of a glycoside of pelargonidin isolated from the bark of *Ficus bengalensis* Linn. Ind J Biochem Biophy 1992; 29(4): 380-2.

[104] Geetha BS, Mathew BC, Augusti KT. Hypoglycemic effects of leucodelphinidin derivative isolated from *Ficus bengalensis* (Linn). Ind J Physiol Pharmacol 1994; 38(3): 220-2.

[105] Augusti KT. Hypoglycaemic action of bengalenoside, a glucoside isolated from *Ficus bengalensis* Linn. in normal and alloxan diabetic rabbits. Ind J Physiol Pharmacol 1975; 19(4): 218-20.

[106] Scherian S, August KT. Antidiabetic effects of a glycoside of leucoperlagonidin isolated from *Ficus bengalensis* Linn. Ind J of Exp Biol 1993; 31(1): 26-29.

[107] Daniel RS, Mathew BC, Devi KS, Augusti KT. Antioxidant effect of two flavonoids from the bark of *Ficus bengalensis* Linn. in hyperlipidaemic rats. Ind J Exper Biol 36(9): 902-6.

[108] Panchabhai TS, Kulkarni UP, Rege NN. Validation of therapeutic claims of *Tinospora cordifolia*: A review. Phy Res 2008; 22: 425-441.

[109] Singh B, Sharma ML, Gupta DK, Atal CK, Arya RK. Protective effect of *Tinospora codifolia* Miers on carbon tetrachloride induced hepatoxicity. Ind J Pharmacol 1984; 16: 139-42.

[110] Gupta SS, Verma SCL, Garg VP, Rai M. Anti-diabetic effect of *T. cordifolia*. Part I. Effect on fasting blood sugar level, glucose tolerance and adrenaline induced hyperglycemia. Ind J Med Res 1967; 55: 733-45.

[111] Raghunathan K, Sharma PV. Madhumeha (Diabetes mellitus) – a backward glance. J Res Ind Med 1969; 3: 192-202.

[112] Stanely P, Prince M, Menon VP. Hypoglycemic and other related actions of *Tinospora cordifolia* roots in alloxan-induced diabetic rats. J Ethnopharmacol 2000; 70: 9-15.

[113] Prince PSM, Menon VP. Hypoglycaemic and hypolipidaemic action of alcohol extract of *Tinospora cordifolia* root in chemical induced diabetes in rats. Phy Res 2003; 17: 410-3.

[114] Kar A, Choudhary BK, Bandyopadhyay NG. Comparative evaluation of hypoglycaemic activity of some Indian medicinal plants in alloxan diabetic rats. J Ethnopharmacol 2003; 84: 105-8.

[115] Nadkarni AK (1992). Material medica; vol. 1, 3rd edition.

[116] Yajnik VH, Acharya HK, Vithlani MP, Yajnik NV. Efficacy and safety of Diabecon (D-400), a herbal formulation, in diabetic patients. The Indian Practitioner 1993; 46(12): 917-922.

[117] Dubey GP, Dixit SP, Singh A. Alloxan-induced diabetes in rabbits and effect of a herbal formulation D-400. Ind J Pharmacol 1994; 26: 225-6.

[118] Mohan AR, Chauhan BL, Mitra SK, Kulkarni RD. Safety, efficacy and tolerability of Diabecon (D-400), an Ayurdevic hypoglycaemic formulation, in healthy male medical students. Cur Med Pract 1993; 37: 245-55.

[119] Dubey GP, Agarwal A, Singh A. Evaluation of Diabecon (D-400), an indigenous herbal preparation, in diabetes mellitus. Ind J Inter Med 1993; 3(6): 183-6.

[120] Maji D, Singh AK. Effect of Diabecon (D-400), an ayurvedic herbal formulation on plasma insulin and C-peptide levels in NIDDM patients 1996; 49(1): 69-73.

[121] Pari L, Saravanan G. Antidiabetic effect of Cogent db, a herbal drug, in alloxan-induced diabetes mellitus. Comparative Biochemistry and Physiology Part C: Toxicol Pharmacol 2002; 131(1): 19-25.

[122] Pari L, Ramakrishnan R, Venkateswaran S. Antihyperglycaaemic effect of Diamed, a herbal formulation, in experimental diabetes in rats. J Pharm Pharmacol 2001; 53(8): 1139-43.

[123] Episulin (Active ingredient - Epicatechin). http://www.episulin.com

[124] Mutalik S, Chetam M, Sulochana B, Uma-Devi P, Udupa N. Effect of dianex, a herbal formulation on experimentally induced diabetes mellitus. Phyt Res 2005; 19(5): 409-15.

[125] Chang MS, Oh MS, Kim DR, *et al.* Effects of Okchun-San, a herbal formulation, on blood glucose levels and body weight in a model of type 2 diabetes. J Ethnopharmacol 2006; 103(3): 491-5.

[126] Saravanan R, Pari L. Antihyperlipidaemic and antiperoxidative effect of Diasulin, a polyherbal formulation in alloxan induced hyperglycaemic rats. BMC Comp Altern Med 2005; 5: 14-21.

[127] Pari L., Saravanan R. Role of Diasulin, an herbal formulation on antioxidant status in chemical induced diabetes. Int J Pharmacol 2006; 2(1): 110-115.

[128] Pari L., Saravanan R. Antidiabetic effect of diasulin, a herbal drug, on blood glucose, plasma insulin and hepatic enzymes of glucose metabolism in hyperglycaemic rats. Diab Obes Metabol 2004; 6(4): 286-292.

CHAPTER 5

Hypoglycemic Plants: Folklore to Modern Evidence Review

Mohamed Eddouks[*] and Naoufel Ali Zeggwagh

Moulay Ismail University, BP 21, Errachidia, 52000, Morocco

Abstract: The increasing worldwide incidence of diabetes mellitus in adults constitutes a global public health burden. It is predicted that by 2030, India, China and the United States will have the largest number of people with diabetes. By definition, diabetes mellitus is categorized as a metabolic disease characterized by hyperglycemia resulting from defects in insulin secretion, insulin action, or both. The vast majority of cases of diabetes fall into two broad etiopathogenetic categories. The first category, type 1 diabetes, is caused by an absolute deficiency of insulin secretion. While the second type is much a more prevalent category, called as type 2 diabetes, the cause is a combination of resistance to insulin action and an inadequate compensatory insulin-secretory response. Despite the great interest in the development of new drugs to prevent the burden of complications associated with this disease and the increased interest in the scientific community to evaluate either raw or isolated natural products in experimental studies, few of them were tested in humans. This chapter is a contribution to the understanding of ethnopharmacology of plants having hypoglycemic activity and its contribution to the elaboration of new treatment of diabetes mellitus.

Keywords: Diabetes, hypoglycemic activity, ethnopharmacology, type 1, type 2, glucose, insulin, secretory, mechanism of action, public health.

INTRODUCTION

Throughout the ages, humans have relied on Nature to cater for their basic needs-particularly for the treatment of a wide spectrum of diseases. Plants, in particular, have formed the basis of traditional medicine systems, with the earliest records, dating around 2900–2600 BC, documenting the uses of approximately 1000 plant-derived substances in Mesopotamia and the active transportation of medicinal plants and oils around what is now known as Southwest Asia. These include oils of *Cedrus* species (cedar) and *Cupressus sempervirens* (cypress), *Glycyrrhiza glabra* (liquorice), *Commiphora* species (myrrh) and *Papaver somniferum* (poppy juice), all of which are still used today for the treatment of ailments ranging from

*Address correspondence to Mohamed Eddouks: Moulay Ismail University, BP 21, 52000, Errachidia, Morocco; Tel: 00212535570024; Fax: 00212535573588; E-mail: mohamed.eddouks@laposte.net

Mohamed Eddouks and Debprasad Chattopadhyay (Eds)
All rights reserved-© 2012 Bentham Science Publishers

coughs and colds to parasitic infections and inflammation [1-3].

In addition to plants, around 120 mineral substances were also listed as "medicinal in nature" including arsenic sulfide, sulfur, lime, potassium permanganate and even rock salt. In most cases, the materials were delivered as infusions (teas), ointments, medicated wines and even by fumigation, methods still used in pharmaceutical delivery systems [4-7]. By approximately 700 BC, the concept of "contagion" was developed, though it would be millennia before the relationship of microbes to plagues, was formally established. Although what is interesting is a description of the use of "rotten grain" in treating wounds; it is tempting to speculate that this might have been a method of administering a crude antibiotic formulation to a patient [3, 8-11].

Much research on antidiabetic plants has been undertaken in academia. Indeed, the majority of the data described on crude extract or active components of these plants is from diverse source [4-6, 12]. This situation is likely to continue and, hopefully, increase in response to the growing prevalence of diabetes worldwide [2, 9, 11-14]. Academia has traditionally been more inclined to follow ethnobotanical leads, but much of the early research led to publications rather than patents. A greater awareness of intellectual property issues coupled with greater synergy with the pharmaceutical industry may well lead to the development of new drugs from this route [6, 7, 12, 15-20].

ETHNOPHARMACOLOGY

It is hard to define ethnopharmacology, for example, in Google the word ethnobotany shows approximately 3,000 listings featuring a variety of descriptions about how plants were used in primitive cultures. Within the definitions will be words like indigenous, rain forest, ancient, pharmaceuticals, folklore, hallucinogens, and endangered. However, if you try to look up ethnobotany in the latest edition of Webster's New World College Dictionary you will not find an entry [1, 2, 16, 17, 21].

Ask an archeologist to explain ethnobotany and you may receive a scholarly lecture on Hawthorne seeds found among the bones of a Delaware Indian ossuary. While a chemist will describe ethnobotany about the pharmaceutical benefits of

Digitalis (foxglove) as a treatment for heart disease [5, 6, 12, 13, 22, 23]. Visit a Navajo sweat lodge and experience ethnobotany yourself when a brew of water, cedar, and pinon needles is poured over searing red rocks to release spiritual and physical healing vapors. So, what is ethnobotany? It is all of these things. Ethnobotany is a subject that fills volumes of historical and biological texts yet is a subject largely ignored in modern texts [2, 8, 9, 17, 24, 25]. It is an ancient way of life and a relatively new and thriving scientific field. Perhaps the simplest definition of ethnobotany is provided by the word itself: *ethno* (people) and *botany* (science of plants). In essence, it is a study of how people of particular cultures and regions make use of the plants in their local environments. These uses can include as food, medicine, fuel, shelter, and in many cultures, in religious ceremonies [4, 13, 20, 23].

TRADITIONAL *VERSUS* MODERN MEDICINE

Much of the knowledge is actually quite new, but it has a social meaning and legal character, entirely unlike the knowledge indigenous peoples acquire from settlers and industrialized societies.' The use of the term 'traditional medicine' to describe ethnomedicine in this volume should be understood to denote merely the historical and cultural context of the origin of the healing systems [1, 3, 16, 19, 24-26].

Ethnomedicine covers a very wide spectrum, which may be classified into two types, the *personalistic* systems, where supernatural causes ascribed to angry deities, ghosts, ancestors and witches predominate, and the *naturalistic* systems, where illness is explained in impersonal, systemic terms [5, 7, 8, 11, 23, 25, 27]. The personalistic system appears to predominate (although not to the exclusion of the naturalistic explanations) in the traditional medical systems of native America, parts of China, South Asia, Latin America and most of the communities in Africa [1, 15, 17, 20, 27, 28]. Naturalistic explanations (also not to the exclusion of personalistic causation) predominate in *Ayurveda, Unani, Khampo* (Japan) and traditional Chinese medicine. In the later types, part of the belief is that intrusion of heat or cold into, or their loss from, the body upsets its basic equilibrium; that is, the balance of humors, or of the *dosha* of *Ayurveda,* or the *yin* and *yang* of Chinese medicine, and these must be restored if the patient is to recover. In the personalistic system, as exemplified by the traditional African system of medicine, healing is concerned with the utilization of human energy, the environment, and the cosmic balance of natural forces as tools in healing. In the African world, the natural environment is a living entity, whose components, the land, sea, atmosphere, and the faunas and floras, are bound to man in an intrinsic manner. Plants therefore play a participatory role in healing [22, 26]. A healer's power is not determined by the number of efficacious herbs they know, but by the magnitude of their understanding of the natural laws. The ability of the healer to utilize these natural laws for the benefit of his patient and the whole community is the ultimate measure of his success. Treatment therefore is not limited to the sterile use of different leaves, roots, fruits, barks, grasses and various objects like minerals, dead insects bones, feathers, shells, eggs, powders, and the smoke from different burning objects for the cure and prevention of diseases. If a sick person is given a leaf infusion to drink, they drink it believing not only in the organic properties of the plant but also in the magical or spiritual force imbibed by nature in all living things and also the role of his ancestors, spirits and gods in the healing processes [15, 16, 21, 29]. The patient also believes in the powers of the incantation recited by the healer and assists them in the designation of the ingredients of the remedies given. The patient is also an active participant in the art of healing, not a passive subject of therapy. According to the World Health Organization, a large segment of human population still depends on traditional medicine, or the so-called alternative medicine, as the preferred form of healthcare, even with improved access to modern medicine [17, 18, 24, 25].

DEFINITION OF DIABETES

Diabetes mellitus, long considered a disease of minor significance to world health, is now taking its place as one of the main threats to human health in the 21st century. The past two decades have seen an explosive increase in the number of people diagnosed with diabetes worldwide. Pronounced changes in the human environment, and in human behaviour and lifestyle, have accompanied globalization, and these have resulted in escalating rates of both obesity and diabetes [30-33]. Recently, the term of *diabesity* have been suggested by several epidemiological reports [30, 31, 34].

There are two main forms of diabetes. Type 1 diabetes is due primarily to autoimmune-mediated destruction of pancreatic β-cell islets, resulting in absolute insulin deficiency [35-40]. People with type 1 diabetes must take exogenous insulin for survival to prevent the development of ketoacidosis. Its frequency is low relative to type 2 diabetes, which accounts for over 90% of cases globally. Type 2 diabetes is characterized by insulin resistance and/or abnormal insulin secretion, either of which may predominate [41-45]. People with type 2 diabetes are not dependent on exogenous insulin, but may require it for control of blood glucose levels if this is not achieved with diet alone or with oral hypoglycaemic agents [46, 47].

The diabetes epidemic relates particularly to type 2 diabetes, and is taking place both in developed and developing nations [48-50]. Paradoxically, part of the problem relates to the achievements in public health during the 20th century, with people living longer owing to elimination of many of the communicable diseases [51-55]. Non-communicable diseases (NCD) such as diabetes and cardiovascular disease (CVD) have now become the main public health challenge for the 21st century, as a result of their impact on personal and national health and the premature morbidity and mortality associated with the NCDs [56-61].

TRADITIONAL MEDICINE OF DIABETES MELLITUS

Survey of Plants Used in the Treatment of Diabetes in the World

The *Ebers Papyrus* written in approximately 1550 B.C. provides the earliest documentation about the use of plants in the treatment of conditions associated with diabetes. In India, the early Ayurvedic texts such as the *Sushruta Samhita* and the *Charaka Samhita* written in the 4th to 5th century B.C. describe the use of about 760 and 500 species of medicinal plants, respectively, including those prescribed for conditions such as glycosuria, polyphagia, and polyuria associated with diabetes. In China, Ben Jing, written in about 104 B.C., contains detailed descriptions of 252 species with reference to those used to treat diabetes. It is easier to track the traditional and modern uses of species in the treatment of diabetes in cultures with strong written documentations like those in India, China, and the Middle East than in South America and Africa, where much less documentation is available [62-64].

Despite their long tradition of use in most parts of the world, very few of these species have been exposed to modern, large-scale, clinical trials to test their efficacy. Some species used in the ancient civilizations of India and China have been used for hundreds of years and some people would suggest that they are effective. However, it is clear that more research needs to be undertaken on these species because, in most cases, the active compounds and their mode of action still remain unclear. For example, hundreds of species are used in Chinese medicine for treating diabetes, but only seven multiple-species antidiabetic products have been approved for clinical use in China [65-70].

Currently, many countries face large increases in the number of people suffering from diabetes. The World Health Organization estimated that about 30 million people suffered from diabetes in 1985 and the number increased to more than 171 million in 2000 [71, 72]. Researchers estimate the number will increase to over 366 million by 2030 largely in developing countries, especially in people aged between 45 and 64 years [73-75]. This is in contrast to the developed world in which most people diagnosed with diabetes are over 64 years. Despite the lack of robust scientific data to support the efficacy of many species of plants, they remain the main source of medication for patients with diabetes in many parts of the world and are sometimes taken in preference to other treatments [76-79]. Plants thought to play a role in the treatment of diabetes are taken as food or as medication. Some studies provided an overview of the species of plants reported to be used to treat diabetes [80, 81]. Their review remains a classic reference work for those using ethnobotanical data to study the potential of plants in the treatment of diabetes. It was based on a search of information about antidiabetic plants up to the year 1994, available in the database NAPRALERT at the College of Pharmacy, University of Illinois, Chicago. In their review, they identified about 1200 species of plants from 725 genera representing 183 families [82, 83]. Another review by Perez *et al.,* identified about 800 species. In the 10 years since Marles and Farnsworth completed their review, knowledge about the potential uses and chemistry of the plants that they listed has increased. Most natural product and pharmacology groups still tend to search for new actives in poorly studied species instead of undertaking further research on species with proven activity. This could be due in part to researchers finding it difficult to find funds to support work on plants with proven activity and commercial companies not wanting to invest funds into developing a product in which they will not be able to protect the intellectual property. These reasons are justified, but more research needs to be undertaken on species containing compounds with proven activity in order to turn a "potential" into an "actual" lead [84, 85]. Very few examples of plant-based leads, such as metformin, a biguanide derived from two linked guanidine units (guanidine derivatives are reported to be the active constituents of *Galega officinalis* (Fabaceae), are currently prescribed in mainstream Western medicine. The challenge will be to see whether any of these species or their active compounds progress through the validation system. In the last 5 years, the species that received the most citations for their antidiabetic activity include species of *Panax*, *Phyllanthus*, *Momordica charantia*, *Allium cepa*, and *A. sativum*. A growing body of evidence indicates that the traditional uses of these species can be supported by scientific evidence [86-89]. Many of the active compounds in these species have been identified, but more research is needed if products are going to be developed from these species [90, 91]. Currently, *Panax ginseng* is included in some of the products currently prescribed in China for treating diabetes and the same is true in India for the use of products containing *Momordica charantia* [92-94].

Knowledge about the toxicity of the species is an important criterion of hypoglycemic plants. For example, species of plants used as vegetables and have hypoglycemic activity could be of high priority. Onion and garlic meet this criterion; they have been well studied and contain compounds that modulate biochemical processes involved in diabetes. Allicin and S-allylcysteine sulfoxide, from *Allium sativum* bulbs, are reported to be the active constituents associated with prevention of diabetics related cardiovascular complications. Administration of S-methylcysteine sulfoxide and S-allylcysteine sulfoxide, from *Allium* species, to alloxan-diabetic rats ameliorated glucose intolerance, weight loss, and depletion of liver glycogen; however, they were not as effective as glibenclamide and insulin in relation to glucose utilization [95-98]. To dismiss a plant because it contains toxic compounds could result in dropping species with potent antidiabetic leads, such as the *vinca* alkaloids. The alkaloids vindoline, vindolinine, and leurosine, isolated from the leaves of *Catharanthus roseus* are reported to be antidiabetic [99-102]. Conophylline, a vinca alkaloid from *Ervatamia microphylla* leaves, induced insulin expression in pancreatic cells *in vitro* and induced differentiation of pancreatic precursor cells. However, because neuropathy is associated with the use of *vinca* alkaloids, their clinical potential in the management of diabetes is limited. Another group of alkaloids, the polyhydroxylated piperidines, pyrrolidines indolizidines, pyrrolizidines, and nortropanes have potential in the management of a range of different diseases including diabetes [103-106]. These compounds are found in species used to treat diabetes, such as 1-deoxynojirimycin (DNJ). DNJ is a piperidine alkaloid (also known as moranoline) from roots of *Morus alba* that inhibits α-glucosidase activity *in vitro*; however, its efficacy *in vivo* has not been as promising. Other polyhydroxy alkaloids have been isolated from species known to be toxic. For example, the 7-O-β-D-glucoside of the piperidine alkaloid α-homonojirimycin from *Aglaonema treubii* and *Hyacinthus orientalis* bulbs has been investigated as a potential antidiabetic drug [107-109].

Several nitrogen-containing compounds isolated from *Xanthocercis zambesiaca* root and leaves have been evaluated for potential antihyperglycemic effects *in vivo*. An aqueous methanol extract and the isolated compounds fagomine, 4-O-β-D-glucopyranosylfagomine, (2R,5R)-dihydroxymethyl-(3R,4R) dihydroxypyrrolidine (DMDP), and castanospermine reduced blood glucose level in streptozotocin diabetic mice; while fagomine was also shown to increase the plasma insulin level. Isolated compounds 2, 5-imino-1, 2, 5-trideoxy- L-glucitol, β-homofuconojirimycin, and 2, 5-dideoxy-2, 5-imino-D-fucitol from the pods and bark of *Angylocalyx pynaertii*, were identified as specific inhibitors of α-L-fucosidase [110, 111].

Toxicity is a relative term and will vary on the part of the plant being extracted or eaten and the amounts taken. However, it is critical that the crude extract and individual compounds are tested for toxicity, although most of the currently used tests only measure acute toxicity. These tests do not provide information about adverse responses that might result from long-term exposure to the species. Knowledge about whether compounds taken in low amounts over time could result in the accumulation of a toxic dose is important because diabetes is a chronic condition and a patient might need to take a daily supply of a medication over a long period [112-114]. Thus, it is very important to gather data on the profile of compounds in a proposed antidiabetic plant to see whether they have been shown to cause any adverse responses. For example, ephedrine, from

Ephedra species, is reported to suppress hyperglycemia in diabetic mice (induced by streptozotocin) and to promote the regeneration of pancreas islets following atrophy induced by streptozotocin. Ephedrine is also reported to improve microcirculation in the diabetic europathic foot [115-118]. However, in view of the adverse effects associated with administration of ephedrine, such as hypertension, it should be used with caution in those with cardiovascular disease and diabetes [119-121].

Publicizing the medicinal properties of a species is always a concern because this may result in overharvesting unless the species is already commercially produced. Thus, as part of a research project on a species with relatively restricted geographical distribution, procedures need to be considered at an early stage to establish their sustainable production [122-125].

Overall, researchers facing many challenges are interested in further understanding of the value of plants in the control of diabetes. These include not only the criteria used to select the plants, the selection of appropriate bioassays, and the isolation of the active compounds but also the issues associated with ownership of the plant material being studied. The implementation of the Convention on Biodiversity (CBD) (www.biodiv.org) by different countries has resulted in a complex array of procedures that need to be in place to enable scientists to gain access to plant material. All scientists involved in plant-based research, especially those involved in research that might result in the discovery of a lead molecule, need to keep copies of the appropriate paperwork to enable them to trace the source of their plant material and any knowledge they used to assist their research. Readers are referred to the CBD Website to obtain information about how different countries implement the CBD and which authorities need to be contacted in these countries to obtain "prior informed consent" before collecting genetic resources [126-128].

Hypoglycemic Plants and Biodiversity

Molecular data have enabled significant advances to be made in understanding of the phylogenetic relationships among different plant families. Species used to treat diabetes can be found distributed throughout the plant kingdom. However, some trends justify further study [11, 43, 57].

Of the 656 species of flowering plants identified a high proportion of 437 genera, representing 111 families, come from the rosids and asteroids. However, there are representatives with potent activity in the magnoliids and monocots. Within the Ranunculales, alkaloids with potential antidiabetic activity have been isolated from the Berberidaceae, Menispermaceae, Papaveraceae, and Ranunculaceae. The best studied example is berberine from rhizomes of *Coptis chinensis* (Ranunculaceae). It is reported to be hypoglycemic in normal and in diabetic mice. Treating impaired glucose tolerance rats with berberine resulted in a reduction in levels of fasting blood glucose, triglycerides, and total cholesterol. Berberine also aided insulin secretion of HIT-TI5 cells and murine pancreatic islets in a dose-dependent manner *in vitro*. It has been shown that oral administration of berberine to hypercholesterolemic patients reduced serum cholesterol, triglycerides, and low-density lipoprotein (LDL) cholesterol *in vitro*, berberine elevated LDL receptor expression through a post-transcriptional mechanism that stabilizes mRNA [14, 24, 89, 98].

Other studies suggest that berberine may mediate antihyperglycemic effects by inhibiting α-glucosidase and decreasing glucose transport through the intestinal epithelium. Some *in vitro* studies suggest that berberine exerts a glucose-lowering effect in hepatocytes that is insulin independent and similar to the action of metformin, but has no effect on insulin secretion. Other alkaloids with potential use in the treatment of diabetes from this group of plants include dehydrocorydaline from *Corydalis turtschaninovii* (Papaveraceae) tuber and tetrandrine from *Stephania tetrandra* (Menispermaceae) root. Polysaccharides from this group of plants also justify further study including aconitans A, B, C, and D from the roots of *Aconitum carmichaelii* (Ranunculaceae), which lower blood glucose in normal and diabetic mice [4, 65, 112].

The diversity of active compounds increases within the rosids, including examples of alkaloids, flavonoids, and terpenoids. The legume family (Fabaceae) contains a large number of species, of which 81 are identified as having hypoglycemic activity. For example, (–)-multiflorine was isolated from seeds of *Lupinus* species (Fabaceae). It produced a hypoglycemic effect when administered to mice with streptozotocin-induced diabetes; in addition, synthetic compounds also containing the quinolizidin-2-one ring system were active *in vivo*. Some other quinolozidine alkaloids, lupanine, 13-α-hydroxylupanine, and 17-oxolupanine isolated from *Lupinus* species, enhance insulin secretion *in vitro*, an effect that could be explained by blocking β -cell KATP -sensitive channels [92, 100].

Flavonoids that ameliorate the condition of patients with diabetes occur in many plant families and have been well studied in members of the Fabales. Quercetin dose dependently decreased the plasma glucose level in streptozotocin-induced diabetic rats, which may be related to an increase in the number of pancreatic islets. Quercetin may also be of value in diabetic nephropathy because treatment of diabetic rats with quercetin attenuated renal dysfunction and oxidative stress. Diabetic neuropathy may also be attenuated by treatment with quercetin because antinociceptive activity has been associated with quercetin in a mouse model of diabetic neuropathic pain. Quercetin-3-O-methyl ether may have some potential in treating diabetic complications [3, 127, 128].

Isorhamnetin-3,7-di-O-β-D-glucopyranoside isolated from *Brassica juncea* (Brassicaceae) leaf appears to be metabolized to isorhamnetin *in vivo*, and intraperitoneal (*i.p*) administration of isorhamnetin reduced serum glucose in diabetic rats. Kaempferitrin isolated from *Bauhinia forficata* (Fabaceae) leaves lowered blood glucose in diabetic rats. Administration of naringin to hyperglycemic rats dose dependently decreased the blood glucose level, increased insulin level, and increased the total antioxidant status [18, 33].

The possible mechanisms to explain the hypoglycemic effect of brazilin from *Caesalpinia sappan* (Fabaceae) wood have been investigated and some studies suggest an association with insulin action. It has been shown that brazilin increases the rate of glucose oxidation and lipogenesis in the presence of insulin and that it may regulate the enzymatic processes involved in glucose metabolism. The hypoglycemic effect of brazilin may be associated with enhancement of insulin receptor function by a decrease in serine phosphorylation. Other studies show that brazilin stimulates glucose transport *in vitro* and decreases gluconeogenesis in hepatocytes isolated from diabetic rats. Brazilin is also reported to inhibit aldose reductase activity [3, 17].

Hypoglycemic and hypolipidemic effects were observed when streptozotocin-induced diabetic rats were treated with tectorigenin, an isoflavone isolated from the flowers of *Pueraria thunbergiana* (Fabaceae); these effects were proposed to be associated with the antioxidant effects of tectorigenin. Oral administration of tectorigenin, an aldose reductase inhibitor isolated from *Belamcanda chinensis* (Iridaceae) rhizomes, to streptozotocin-induced diabetic rats caused a significant inhibition of sorbitol accumulation in tissues such as lens, sciatic nerves, and red blood cells, thus indicating the potential of tectorigenin in the prevention or treatment of some diabetic complications. It has been proposed that 6″-O-xylosyltectoridin and tectoridin, isolated from the flowers of *Pueraria thu*nbergiana act as pro-drugs because they are metabolized to tectorigenin by human intestinal bacteria; tectorigenin showed more potent hypoglycemic activity than 6″-O-xylosyltectoridin and tectoridin [3, 7].

Puerarin isolated from the roots of *Pueraria lobata* increased glucose utilization and lowered plasma glucose in diabetic rats lacking insulin. Daidzein is reported to inhibit the activities of α-amylase and α-glucosidase. Daidzein and genistein occur in many species of legumes and they have been associated with a reduction in glucose toxicity-induced cardiac mechanical dysfunction and thus may be beneficial against diabetes-associated cardiac defects. Long-term (6 months) oral administration of genistein to streptozotocin-induced diabetic rats inhibited retinal vascular leakage, which may have some clinical relevance [18, 128].

An oleanane triterpenoid, kaikasaponin III (KS III), isolated from the flowers of *Pueraria thunbergiana*, also showed hypoglycemic and hypolipidemic effects when given to streptozotocin induced diabetic rats. These effects were proposed to be associated with the antioxidant effect of KS III. More recent studies show that KS-III may exhibit its hypoglycemic and hypolipidemic effects by up-regulating or down-regulating antioxidant mechanisms *via* the changes in phase I and II enzyme (*e.g.,* superoxide dismutase [SOD], glutathione peroxidase and catalase) activities [21, 46, 129-132].

Other taxonomic clade that contains many active species is euasterid I. This clade contains families with numerous species that, in traditional practices of medicine, have been reputed to possess antidiabetic activity. Many of these species contain oleanolic and ursolic acids, which have been isolated from the dried stem of *Bouvardia ternifolia* (Rubiaceae) and have lowered blood sugar levels in normal and alloxan-diabetic mice [115, 123].

Another study identified oleanolic acid as an anti-β-amylase compound from *Olea europaea* leaves; it inhibited postprandial hyperglycemia in diabetic rats. The mechanism of action of oleanolic acid glycosides and some other triterpenoids has been investigated. It has been proposed that oral administration of oleanolic acid 3-O -glucuronide, momordin Ic, escins Ia and IIa, and E, Z -senegin II do not initiate insulin-like activity or promote insulin release; however, they may exert their hypoglycemic activity by suppressing the transfer of glucose from the stomach to the small intestine and by inhibiting glucose transport at the brush border of the small intestine. In contrast, an *in vitro* study has suggested that oleanolic acid may act *via* a different mechanism [23, 51]. Using an INS-1 cell assay, oleanolic acid and oleanolic aldehyde isolated from grape skin were shown to stimulate insulin production dose dependently. Oleanolic acid is also reported to inhibit α-glucosidase. Some oleanolic acid monodesmosides (oleanolic acid 3-O-glucuronide, momordin Ic, momordin I and 28-O-deglucosyl-chikusetsusaponins IV and V) have been associated with inhibition of gastric emptying in mice, but oleanolic acid 3, and 28-O-bisdesmosides (momordin IIc, chikusetsusaponins IV and V, oleanolic acid 28-O-monodesmoside) and their aglycone oleanolic acid were not associated with this activity [31]. It has been proposed that the 3-O-monodesmoside structure and 28-carboxyl group were important for such activity, and that the 28-ester glucoside moiety and 2′-O-β-D-glucopyranoside moiety reduced the activity [31].

Luteolin-7-O-β-glucoside and luteolin-4′-O-β-glucoside were identified as anti-α -amylase compounds from *Olea europaea* (Oleaceae) leaves, and luteolin inhibited postprandial hyperglycemia in diabetic rats. Luteolin, amentoflavone, and luteolin-7-O -glucoside are reported to inhibit the activities of α -amylase and α -glucosidase. However, other studies indicate that, when administered orally to rats treated with maltose or sucrose, luteolin does not suppress the glucose production from carbohydrates through the inhibition of α -glucosidase action in the gut [2, 84].

When ethnobotanical information about the uses of plants in diabetes is superimposed onto a phylogeny of the angiosperms, it is clear that clusters of related species of plants are reported to have activity. Within the asterids, the clades that contain the Lamiales, Solanales, and Gentianales have 134 species of plants used traditionally to treat diabetes. This represents 20% of the species covered in this review. Whether the activity could be explained by a similar group of compounds seems highly unlikely because the families in these orders contain a high diversity of compounds many with a diverse range of biological properties [75].

METHODOLOGY FOR THE EVALUATION OF THE HYPOGLYCEMIC ACTIVITY OF PLANTS IN ANIMAL MODELS

Background

Animal models have been used extensively to investigate the *in vivo* efficacy, mode of action and side effects of antidiabetic plants and their active principles. Due to the heterogeneity of diabetic conditions in man, no single animal model is entirely representative of a particular type of human diabetes. Thus, many different animal models have been used, each displaying a different selection of features seen in human diabetic states [9, 10]. Normal nondiabetic animals and animals with impaired glucose tolerance and insulin resistance (but not overt diabetes) have also been used to demonstrate hypoglycemic activity and to investigate the mode of action of antidiabetic plant materials [10, 99].

For initial efficacy testing of antidiabetic activity, it is advisable to replicate the traditional method of preparation of the plant closely because activity may be altered by minor deviations. Most traditional antidiabetic plant materials are taken orally, so initial tests with unrefined plant materials or plant extracts usually involve oral administration in the diet. Oral gavage may be necessary if the smell or taste of the plant creates an aversion to feeding or drinking. Monitoring of feeding, drinking, general behavior, and standard parameters of glucose homeostasis (detailed later) in as much detail as possible is recommended. Isolation of active hypoglycemic fractions and principles and their effects in animal models of diabetes are reviewed in detail in other chapters of this volume. It is generally inappropriate to administer a crude plant extract by a parenteral route due to the risk of a local adverse reaction or more disseminated toxicity from a high concentration of the antidiabetic principle or other components of the extract. Even highly purified extracts may have adverse effects if administered intravenously, but adverse effects may not occur after oral administration. Thus, the enteral route of administration provides a natural barrier against unnecessary toxicity and facilitates initial dose-ranging studies. Some plant extracts may be modified chemically as they pass along the alimentary tract; thus, enteral and parenteral administration may give rise to a different profile of effects [2, 9].

With this caution in mind, it can still be useful to compare the pharmacodynamic effects of purified extracts administered by different routes. For example, comparing the effects of enteral *vs.* parenteral administration in the fed and fasted state might indicate the importance of the intestine as a site of action of an isolated principle to inhibit intestinal digestion and/or nutrient absorption. Comparing different intravenous administration sites, such as peripheral *vs.* hepatic portal injection, could indicate the relative importance of the liver as a site of action [25, 26].

The efficacy of antidiabetic plant materials can vary with time; this is customarily investigated through a sequence of acute, subchronic, and chronic studies. The typical measures of glucose homeostasis to be undertaken usually include basal (fasting) or random blood/plasma glucose and insulin concentrations and oral (or intravenous or intraperitoneal) glucose tolerance tests. Although experimental protocols to investigate mode of action are beyond the scope of this chapter, it is relevant to note that measures of β-cell function (*e.g.*, insulin secretion in response to a range of secretagogues), insulin action (*e.g.*, whole-body glucose disposal), glucose handling by key glucoregulatory tissues (*e.g.*, muscle and liver), and intestinal glucose absorption are likely to yield valuable information [28, 40].

An appreciation of the mode of action of an antidiabetic plant material indicates the types of diabetes against which the material is most likely to be effective. For example, plant materials that slow intestinal glucose absorption are most effective in the prandial and early postprandial periods and can be used as dietary adjuncts to all types of diabetes. Knowledge of the mode of action also indicates the risk of "over-lowering" blood glucose. Substances that stimulate insulin secretion at low glucose concentrations strongly inhibit hepatic glucose output, or block counter-regulatory mechanisms to raise blood glucose can induce overt hypoglycemia and are often referred to as "hypoglycemic". Substances that enhance or partially mimic insulin action or reduce intestinal glucose absorption are not likely to lower glucose to the extent of hypoglycemia and are considered to be "antihyperglycemic". Indicators of long-term glycemic control such as glycated hemoglobin and fructosamine have received relatively little use during chronic studies in animal models. Most studies of antidiabetic plants have preceded the availability of these assays for small sample volumes, and further standardization of the assays may be required for application to blood samples from animals [15, 25].

Extraction and Fractionation of Hypoglycemic Plant Extract

Plant preparations include powdered plant material, extract, tincture, and fatty or essential oils. They may be produced by extraction, fractionation, purification, concentration, or other physical or biological procedure. The herbal materials or herbal preparations are considered to be active ingredients of herbal medicines. Therapeutic activity refers to any beneficial alteration or regulation of the physical and mental status of the body, yet safety and efficacy of herbal medicine with a well-documented history of traditional use should be evaluated. If constituents with therapeutic activities are known, the preparation should be standardized to contain a defined amount of the active ingredients. Markers are chemically defined constituents of an herbal medicine [15, 26]. There is a need to approach scientific proof and clinical validation with chemical standardization, biological assays, animal models, and clinical trials. However, standardization of herbal extract to create a uniform product for clinical trial is a crucial subject under discussion since, according to herbalist's perspective, quality and effectiveness of traditional medicines could be compromised. In the case of active constituent extract, the high degree of concentration may cause a partial representation of all normally occurring constituents thus limiting the broad range of traditionally known properties. Some constituents could be lost that are even more effective than the presumed active compounds. In the case of chemical marker compounds, their use encourages the misconception of herbs as a substitute for drugs. Different standardization procedures may produce different finished products; furthermore, manufacture sometimes involves the use of toxic solvents. Another important consideration concerns the amount of herb necessary to obtain the active extract or the single biochemical constituent: herbalists do not foster harvesting of wild herbs, yet wild herbs are considered to be superior to cultivated herbs [25, 68].

IN VITRO ASSESSMENT OF HYPOGLYCEMIC PLANTS

Antidiabetic effects of plants can be assessed clinically in humans, *in vivo* using animal models or *in vitro* using a variety of test systems. Each level of testing has its advantages and limitations. Human studies are ultimately necessary because the product is tested by the intended route in the eventual beneficiary of an effective treatment. However, in many cases it is neither feasible nor ethical to conduct initial trials in humans because little is known about the safety or efficacy of the herb or even of a suitable dose or method of preparation. It is therefore appropriate to conduct studies in animals prior to administering the herb to humans [16, 78].

Preliminary testing of a herb in an animal model can give valuable information on the type of extract to be made, a suitable dose, likely toxic effects, and, of course, efficacy. This information can then be translated to human studies, although species differences and ethical considerations may be limiting factors. Animal and human studies are essential to determine the ultimate safety and efficacy of a herb or its components when used clinically. However, they provide limited information on the mechanism of action of a particular therapeutic agent [41, 88].

In vitro tests can play an important role in the evaluation of antidiabetic or other medicinal plants, as initial screening tools or as follow-up to human or animal studies. Biological material used in these includes, in increasing order of simplicity, perfused whole organs, isolated tissues, cells in primary or immortal culture, subcellular membranes or purified receptors, and enzymes. *In vitro* assays are typically based on a specific biological process relevant to the disease and its treatment. The advantages of *in vitro* assays in ethnobotanical research and general drug discovery programs are as follows:

Mechanism of action; *in vitro* models are based on a fairly specific process, *e.g.*, activity of a particular enzyme, binding to a particular receptor, or effects on a particular metabolic reaction within a given cell type or organ. They are of considerable value in identifying the mechanism of action of a therapeutic agent [100].

- Amount of material needed; *in vitro* tests require far less test material than clinical and animal studies do. This is of particular relevance to natural products, which may be hard to obtain for reasons of conservation or low abundance:

- Lower cost; in the vast majority of cases, *in vitro* assays are more economical (per sample tested) than tests using animals or humans as subjects.

- Reduced use of animals; *in vitro* tests provide an alternative to animal testing for many aspects of an investigation. Organs or tissues derived from one or a few animals can be used to test many replicates or many samples, whereas for *in vivo* studies, several individual animals would be required per sample or dose. Immortalized cell lines, although originally derived from animals or humans, do away completely with the repeated need for animal tissue in assays.

- Reduced variability; cells from a single cell line or tissues derived from one animal have the advantage of genetic homogeneity, resulting in minimum inherent variability. Thus, comparison of data between treatments or with control conditions is less complex than using animal or human subjects in which genotypic or phenotypic variations between individuals can complicate the interpretation of results and increase the number of replicates required. Automation and fast throughput *in vitro* assays can be adapted to rapid or high throughput formats using automation for liquid handling and end-point measurements. This makes them essential to high-throughput screening programs such as those employed by drug discovery programs in the pharmaceutical industry and academia.

- Bioassay-guided fractionation of plant extracts; there is a dearth of information on the active components of many plant materials known to be useful for diabetes. This is largely due to practical difficulties and high cost of coupling the fractionation of an active extract to biological testing using an animal model often the first model in which activity was seen. *In vitro* assays, by virtue of their more rapid output, lower cost, and need for less material, are an ideal means of following the active components during a fractionation process. The end result is one or more components with defined biological activity. These components may then be isolated in larger quantities and tested *in vivo* to confirm their effects [78].

A range of *in vitro* models are available to study potential antidiabetic activity in plant extracts. They are based on the primary need to control hyperglycemia in diabetes and the various means of achieving this goal. *In vitro* models may be used to screen randomly or ethnobotanically selected materials for a specific activity that would result in the lowering of blood glucose levels. Alternatively, the models may be used to determine the mechanism of action of a plant extract with traditional use and/or human or *in vivo* data to support an antidiabetic effect [18].

It is relevant, in the context of *in vitro* tests for antidiabetic activity, to examine the source and fate of glucose in the body in the normal and diabetic states. Glucose is derived primarily from the digestion of dietary carbohydrates in the gastrointestinal tract, from which it is absorbed into the blood by passive and active mechanisms. In the fed state, a rise in blood glucose normally stimulates insulin secretion from the pancreas. This hormone initiates glucose uptake into specific target tissues, primarily liver, muscle, and fat cells (adipocytes). It promotes glucose oxidation and glycogen deposition in liver and muscle and the incorporation of glucose (as glycerol) into triglycerides in adipocytes. These combined activities have the effect of lowering elevated plasma glucose resulting from the intake of a meal. In the fasted state, glucose and insulin levels decrease. Glucose is then mobilized from glycogen stores in the liver (glycogenolysis) [82, 117].

Another important source of glucose in the fasted state is gluconeogenesis - the *de novo* formation of glucose from smaller, non-sugar, precursor molecules. This occurs in the liver and, to a lesser extent, kidneys and is under the control of glucagon, a counter-hormone whose levels rise as those of insulin fall, and *vice versa*. When glucagon levels are high and those of insulin are low, gluconeogenesis and glycogenolysis are stimulated and glucose enters the bloodstream. In diabetes, insulin is absent, (type I diabetes), or insufficient, (type II diabetes) [56, 131]. In type II diabetes, insulin target tissues are generally less responsive to insulin (insulin resistant) than normal. The fine balance between glucose uptake into target organs and release of hepatic glucose is impaired, resulting in abnormally high fasting glucose levels as well as poor glucose tolerance following a meal. From the foregoing, the following mechanisms have been proposed for an agent that would lower or control plasma glucose levels:

- Inhibition of carbohydrate-digesting enzymes, reducing the amount or rate of glucose release from the diet.

- Impairment of glucose uptake from the small intestine.

- Stimulation of insulin secretion from β-cells of the pancreas [43, 57].

- Insulinomimetic or insulin-sensitizing activity at insulin target tissues, *i.e.*, liver, skeletal muscle, or adipocytes [85, 117].

- Antagonism of glucagon activity [85].

In vitro tests offer a number of significant advantages for research on antidiabetic plants. A wide range of tests is available based on various mechanisms that would alleviate hyperglycemia in diabetes. The use of specific tests is recommended when screening natural products or other samples for a particular mode of action. However, if the mechanism by which a plant material is acting is to be elucidated, a full range of tests should be used. Multiple mechanisms and active components are possible in antidiabetic plants. In conducting the tests, attention should be paid to potential interferents in the plant extracts [121].

CONCLUSIONS

The NAPRALERT database has over 1200 plant species used worldwide for their antidiabetic activity. Many of these have yet to be extensively investigated. Of the most popular ones growing in Asia and Africa, *Gymnema sylvestre* and *Momordica* species have been found in various studies to be of benefit when used as adjunct therapy in non-insulin-dependent DM. Of particular interest in this review are the hypoglycemic potential of edible plants and their role in controlling DM. In most cases, these plants are cheap and easily accessible and should be promoted as part of the global strategy to combat DM once additional data supporting their use are available. Their safety profile appears to be unquestionable. These foods could become an important source for nutraceutical products.

The most common modes of action of several antidiabetic plants include inhibition of glucose digestion absorption, stimulation of insulin secretion, and stimulation of peripheral glucose utilization. However, the actual cellular/molecular targets remain elusive. We have also seen that several factors may influence the outcome of scientific research on antidiabetic plants. Of importance, we note that seasonal and geographical variations can affect the activity of the plant material. Also, the choice of animal model can affect the experimental outcome. In this regard, chemically induced animal models, widely used because they are economical and well characterized, mimic type I diabetes, although type II is the most prominent form in human populations. Therefore, these models are not the most appropriate to assess beneficial effects on insulin resistance.

Bioassays using isolated cells or tissues are only beginning to be applied in research on antidiabetic plants and they offer much promise to elucidate the modes of action of active principles. Of all the plants described here, fenugreek, *momordica*, onion, and garlic appear to be the safest and have the most scientific evidence supporting their antidiabetic potential. Patients should nonetheless advise their physicians of their use of these plants in light of potential interaction with commonly prescribed drugs, particularly oral hypoglycemic agents.

ACKNOWLEDGEMENTS

The authors extend their thanks to Bentham Science Publishers.

DECLARATION OF CONFLICT OF INTEREST

No conflict of interest was declared by the authors.

REFERENCES

[1]   Phillipson JD and Anderson, LA. Ethnopharmacology and Western medicine. J Ethnopharmacol 1989; 25: 61-72.
[2]   Soejarto DD, Fong HH, Tan GT, Zhang HJ, Ma CY, Franzblau SG, *et al.* Ethnobotany/ethnopharmacology and mass bioprospecting: issues on intellectual property and benefit-sharing. J Ethnopharmacol 2005; 100: 15-22.
[3]   Patwardhan B. Ethnopharmacology and drug discovery. J Ethnopharmacol 2005; 100: 50-2.
[4]   Lewis K, and Ausubel FM. Prospects for plant-derived antibacterials. Nat Biotechnol 2006; 24: 1504-7.
[5]   Elisabetsky E, Shanley P. Ethnopharmacology in the Brazilian Amazon. Pharmacol Ther 1994; 64: 201-14.
[6]   Bernard P, Scior T, Didier B, Hibert M, Berthon JY. Ethnopharmacology and bioinformatic combination for leads discovery: application to phospholipase A(2) inhibitors. Phytochemistry 2001; 58: 865-74.

[7]   Phillipson JD. Phytochemistry and pharmacognosy. Phytochemistry 2007; 68: 2960-72.

[8]   Uprety Y, Asselin H, Boon EK, Yadav S, Shrestha KK. Indigenous use and bio-efficacy of medicinal plants in the Rasuwa District, Central Nepal. J Ethnobiol Ethnomed 2010; 6: 3.

[9]   Soh PN, Benoit-Vical F. Are West African plants a source of future antimalarial drugs? J Ethnopharmacol 2007; 114: 130-40.

[10]   Subash-Babu P, Ignacimuthu S, Agastian P, Varghese B. Partial regeneration of beta-cells in the islets of Langerhans by Nymphayol a sterol isolated from Nymphaea stellata (Willd.) flowers. Bioorg Med Chem 2009; 17: 2864-70.

[11]   Chattopadhyay D, Khan MT. Ethnomedicines and ethnomedicinal phytophores against herpes viruses. Biotechnol Annu Rev. 2008; 14: 297-348.

[12]   Heinrich M, Gibbons S. Ethnopharmacology in drug discovery: an analysis of its role and potential contribution. J Pharm Pharmacol 2001; 53: 425-32.

[13]   Mans DR, da Rocha AB, Schwartsmann G. Anti-cancer drug discovery and development in Brazil: targeted plant collection as a rational strategy to acquire candidate anti-cancer compounds. Oncologist 2000; 5: 185-98.

[14]   Farnsworth NR. Ethnopharmacology and drug development. Ciba Found Symp 1994; 185: 42-51.

[15]   Samy RP, Gopalakrishnakone P. Therapeutic Potential of Plants as Anti-microbials for Drug Discovery. Evid Based Complement Alternat Med 2008; 5: 107–13.

[16]   Muthaura CN, Keriko JM, Derese S, Yenesew A. Rukunga GM. Investigation of some medicinal plants traditionally used for treatment of malaria in Kenya as potential sources of antimalarial drugs. Exp Parasitol. In Press.

[17]   Patwardhan B, Vaidya AD. Natural products drug discovery: accelerating the clinical candidate development using reverse pharmacology approaches. Indian J Exp Biol 2010; 48: 220-7.

[18]   Nanyingi MO, Mbaria JM, Lanyasunya AL, Wagate CG, Koros KB, Kaburia HF, Munenge RW, Ogara WO. Ethnopharmacological survey of Samburu district, Kenya. J Ethnobiol Ethnomed 2008; 4: 14.

[19]   Gertsch J. How scientific is the science in ethnopharmacology? Historical perspectives and epistemological problems. J Ethnopharmacol 2009; 122: 177-83.

[20]   Fernandes P. Antibacterial discovery and development--the failure of success? Nat Biotechnol 2006; 24: 1497-503.

[21]   Burns WR. East meets West: how China almost cured malaria. Endeavour 2008; 32: 101-6.

[22]   Svetaz L, Zuljan F, Derita M, Petenatti E, Tamayo G, Caceres A, Cechinel Filho V, Gimenez A, Pinzon R, Zacchino SA, Gupta M. Value of the ethnomedical information for the discovery of plants with antifungal properties. A survey among seven Latin American countries. J Ethnopharmacol 2010; 127: 137-58.

[23]   Wang ZD, Huang C, Li ZF, Yang J, Li BH, Liang RR, Dai ZJ, Liu ZW. Chrysanthemum indicum ethanolic extract inhibits invasion of hepatocellular carcinoma *via* regulation of MMP/TIMP balance as therapeutic target. Oncol Rep 2010; 23: 413-21.

[24]   Houghton PJ. The role of plants in traditional medicine and current therapy. J Altern Complement Med 1995; 1: 131-43.

[25]   Rollinger JM, Haupt S, Stuppner H, Langer T. Combining ethnopharmacology and virtual screening for lead structure discovery: COX-inhibitors as application example. J Chem Inf Comput 2004; 44: 480-8.

[26] Robert S, Baccelli C, Devel P, Dogne JM, Quetin-Leclercq J. Effects of leaf extracts from Croton zambesicus Muell. Arg. on hemostasis. J Ethnopharmacol 2010; 128: 641-8.

[27] Elisabetsky E. Sociopolitical, economical and ethical issues in medicinal plant research. J Ethnopharmacol 1991; 32: 235-9.

[28] Raza M. A role for physicians in ethnopharmacology and drug discovery. J Ethnopharmacol 2006; 104: 297-301.

[29] Hegde HV, Hegde GR, Kholkute SD. Herbal care for reproductive health: ethno medicobotany from Uttara Kannada district in Karnataka India. Complement Ther Clin Pract 2007, 13: 38-45.

[30] Szalat A, Fraenkel M, Doviner V, Salmon A, Gross DJ. Malignant pheochromocytoma: predictive factors of malignancy and clinical course in 16 patients at a single tertiary medical center. Endocrine, In Press.

[31] Sun W, Bi Y, Liang H, Cai M, Chen X, Zhu Y, *et al*. Inhibition of obesity-induced hepatic ER stress by early insulin therapy in obese diabetic rats. Endocrine, In Press.

[32] Liu XH, Qin C, Du JQ, Xu Y, Sun N, Tang JS, Li Q, Foreman RD. Diabetic rats show reduced cardiac-somatic reflex evoked by intrapericardial capsaicin. Eur J Pharmacol 2011; 651: 83-8.

[33] Ohsawa M, Aasato M, Hayashi SS, J. Kamei J. RhoA/Rho kinase pathway contributes to the pathogenesis of thermal hyperalgesia in diabetic mice. Pain 2011; 152: 114-22.

[34] Cumaoglu A, Ozansoy G, Irat AM, Aricioglu A, Karasu C, Ari N. Effect of long term, non cholesterol lowering dose of fluvastatin treatment on oxidative stress in brain and peripheral tissues of streptozotocin-diabetic rats. Eur J Pharmacol 2011; 654(1): 80-5.

[35] Dogrul A, Gul H, Yesilyurt O, Ulas UH, O. Yildiz O. Systemic and spinal administration of etanercept, a tumor necrosis factor alpha inhibitor, blocks tactile allodynia in diabetic mice. Acta Diabetol, In Press.

[36] Kim HJ, Koo SY, Ahn BH, Park O, Park DH, Seo DO, *et al*. NecroX as a novel class of mitochondrial reactive oxygen species and ONOO scavenger. Arch Pharm Res 2010; 33; 1813-23.

[37] Smolock AR, Mishra G, Eguchi K, Eguchi S, Scalia R. Protein Kinase C Upregulates Intercellular Adhesion Molecule-1 and Leukocyte-Endothelium Interactions in Hyperglycemia *via* Activation of Endothelial Expressed Calpain. Arterioscler Thromb Vasc Biol; 2010; 19: 2894-900.

[38] Ghaboura N, Tamareille S, Ducluzeau PH, Grimaud L, Loufrani L, Croue A, Tourmen Y, Henrion D, Furber A, Prunier F. Diabetes mellitus abrogates erythropoietin-induced cardioprotection against ischemic-reperfusion injury by alteration of the RISK/GSK-3beta signaling. Basic Res Cardiol 2010; 106: 147-162.

[39] Satake M, Ikarashi N, Kagami M, Ogiue N, Toda T, Kobayashi Y, Ochiai W, Sugiyama K. Increases in the expression levels of aquaporin-2 and aquaporin-3 in the renal collecting tubules alleviate dehydration associated with polyuria in diabetes mellitus. Biol Pharm Bull 2010; 33: 1965-70.

[40] Rawat P, Kumar M, Rahuja N, Srivastava DS, Srivastava AK, Maurya R. Synthesis and antihyperglycemic activity of phenolic C-glycosides. Bioorg Med Chem Lett 2011; 21: 228-33.

[41] H.R. Madkor HR, S.W. Mansour SW and G. Ramadan G. Modulatory effects of garlic, ginger, turmeric and their mixture on hyperglycaemia, dyslipidaemia and oxidative stress in streptozotocin-nicotinamide diabetic rats. Br J Nutr 2010; 1-8.

[42]   Shobana S, Harsha MR, Platel K, Srinivasan K, Malleshi NG. Amelioration of hyperglycaemia and its associated complications by finger millet (Eleusine coracana L.) seed coat matter in streptozotocin-induced diabetic rats. Br J Nutr; 2010: 104: 1787-95.

[43]   Boku A, Sugimura M, Morimoto Y, Hanamoto H, Niwa H. Hemodynamic and autonomic response to acute hemorrhage in streptozotocin-induced diabetic rats. Cardiovasc Diabetol 2010; 9: 78.

[44]   Kim KC, Kim JS, Kang KA, Kim JM, Won Hyun J. Cytoprotective effects of catechin 7-O-beta-D glucopyranoside against mitochondrial dysfunction damaged by streptozotocin in RINm5F cells. Cell Biochem Funct 2010; 28: 651-60.

[45]   Luo C, Zhang W, Sheng C, Zheng C, Yao J, Miao Z. Chemical composition and antidiabetic activity of opuntia milpa alta extracts. Chem Biodivers 2010; 7: 2869-79.

[46]   Pisarev VB, Snigur GL, Spasov AA, Samokhina MP, Bulanov AE. Mechanisms of toxic effect of streptozotocin on beta-cells in the islets of langerhans. Bull Exp Biol Med 2009; 148: 937-9.

[47]   Iwamoto J, Seki A, Sato Y, Matsumoto H, Takeda T, Yeh JK. Vitamin K(2) Prevents Hyperglycemia and Cancellous Osteopenia in Rats with Streptozotocin-Induced Type 1 Diabetes. Calcif Tissue Int, In Press.

[48]   do Carmo JM, Junior RF, Salgado HC, Fazan VP. Methods for exploring the morpho-functional relations of the aortic depressor nerve in experimental diabetes. J Neurosci Methods 2010; 30; 195(1):30-5.

[49]   Qiu X, Lin H, Wang Y, Yu W, Chen Y, Wang R, Dai Y. Intracavernous Transplantation of Bone Marrow-Derived Mesenchymal Stem Cells Restores Erectile Function of Streptozocin-Induced Diabetic Rats. J Sex Med 2010; 7: 314–26.

[50]   Kamboj SS, Sandhir R. Protective effect of N-acetylcysteine supplementation on mitochondrial oxidative stress and mitochondrial enzymes in cerebral cortex of streptozotocin-treated diabetic rats. Mitochondrion 2011; 11: 214-22.

[51]   Wang H, Zheng Z, Gong Y, Zhu B, Xu X. U83836E Inhibits Retinal Neurodegeneration in Early-Stage Streptozotocin-Induced Diabetic Rats. Ophthalmic Res 2010; 46: 19-24.

[52]   Yu R, Zhang H, Huang L, Liu X, Chen J. Anti-hyperglycemic, antioxidant and anti-inflammatory effects of VIP and a VPAC1 agonist on streptozotocin-induced diabetic mice. Peptides 2011; 32(2): 216-22.

[53]   Gupta LH, Badole SL, Bodhankar, Sabharwal SG. Antidiabetic potential of alpha-amylase inhibitor from the seeds of Macrotyloma uniflorum in streptozotocin-nicotinamide-induced diabetic mice. Pharm Biol 2011; 49(2): 182-9.

[54]   Juang JH, Kuo CH. Effects of cyclooxygenase-2 inhibitor and adenosine triphosphate-sensitive potassium channel opener in syngeneic mouse islet transplantation. Transplant Proc 2010; 42: 4221-4.

[55]   Kim J, Kim CS, Sohn E, Jeong IH, Kim H, Kim JS. Involvement of advanced glycation end products, oxidative stress and nuclear factor-kappaB in the development of diabetic keratopathy. Graefes Arch Clin Exp Ophthalmol 2010; 229: 254-257.

[56]   Alfarano C, Suffredini S, Fantappie O, Mugelli A, Cerbai E, Manni ME, Raimondi L. The effect of losartan treatment on the response of diabetic cardiomyocytes to ATP depletion. Pharmacol Res; In Press.

[57]   Bu T, Liu M, Zheng L, Guo Y, Lin X. alpha-Glucosidase inhibition and the *in vivo* hypoglycemic effect of butyl-isobutyl-phthalate derived from the Laminaria japonica rhizoid. Phytother Res 2010; 24: 1588-91.

[58] Kane MA, Folias AE, Pingitore A, Perri M, Obrochta KM, Krois CR, Cione E, Ryu JY, Napoli JL. Identification of 9-cis-retinoic acid as a pancreas-specific autacoid that attenuates glucose-stimulated insulin secretion. Proc Natl Acad Sci 2010; 107(50): 21884-9.

[59] Yang Y, Gurung B, Wu T, Wang H, Stoffers DA, Hua X. Reversal of preexisting hyperglycemia in diabetic mice by acute deletion of the Men1 gene. Proc Natl Acad Sci 2010; 107: 20358-63.

[60] Solomon M, Flodstrom-Tullberg M, Sarvetnick N. Beta-cell specific expression of suppressor of cytokine signaling-1 (SOCS-1) delays islet allograft rejection by down-regulating Interferon Regulatory Factor-1 (IRF-1) signaling. Transpl Immunol, In Press.

[61] Kopelman PG. Obesity as a medical problem. Nature 2000; 404: 635-43.

[62] Wang TH, Lin TF. Monascus rice products. Adv Food Nutr Res 2007; 53: 123-59.

[63] Kiefer D, Pantuso T. Panax ginseng. Am Fam Physician 2003; 68: 1539-42.

[64] Xie JT, McHendale S, Yuan CS. Ginseng and diabetes. Am J Chin Med 2005; 33: 397-404.

[65] Kim JJ, Xiao H, Tan Y, Wang ZZ, J. Paul J, Seale J, Qu X. The effects and mechanism of saponins of Panax notoginseng on glucose metabolism in 3T3-L1 cells. Am J Chin Med 2009; 37: 1179-89.

[66] Albutt EC, Chance GW. Fasting plasma cholesteryl esters in diabetic children consuming corn oil. Am J Clin Nutr 1969; 22: 1552-4.

[67] Wadhwa PS, Young EA, Schmidt K, Elson CE, Pringle DJ. Metabolic consequences of feeding frequency in man. Am J Clin Nutr 1973; 26: 823-30.

[68] Reaven GM. Effects of differences in amount and kind of dietary carbohydrate on plasma glucose and insulin responses in man. Am J Clin Nutr 1979; 32: 2568-78.

[69] Crapo PA,. Kolterman OG, Waldeck N, Reaven GM, Olefsky JM. Postprandial hormonal responses to different types of complex carbohydrate in individuals with impaired glucose tolerance. Am J Clin Nutr 1980; 33: 1723-8.

[70] Jenkins DI, Wolever TM, Taylor RH, Griffiths C, Krzeminska K, Lawrie JA, Bennett CM, Goff DV, Sarson DL, Bloom SR. Slow release dietary carbohydrate improves second meal tolerance. Am J Clin Nutr 1982: 35: 1339-46.

[71] Shutler SM, Bircher GM, Tredger JA, Morgan LM, Walker AF, Low AG. The effect of daily baked bean (Phaseolus vulgaris) consumption on the plasma lipid levels of young, normo-cholesterolaemic men. Br J Nutr 1989; 61: 257-65.

[72] Rasmussen O, Gregersen S, Hermansen K. Influence of the amount of starch on the glycaemic index to rice in non-insulin-dependent diabetic subjects. Br J Nutr 1992; 67: 371-7.

[73] Hannan JM, Ali L, Khaleque J, Akhter M, Flatt PR, Abdel-Wahab YH. Aqueous extracts of husks of Plantago ovata reduce hyperglycaemia in type 1 and type 2 diabetes by inhibition of intestinal glucose absorption. Br J Nutr 2006; 96: 131-7.

[74] Lutsey PL, Jacobs DRJ, Kori S, Mayer-Davis E, Shea S, Steffen LM, Szklo M, Tracy R. Whole grain intake and its cross-sectional association with obesity, insulin resistance, inflammation, diabetes and subclinical CVD: The MESA Study. Br J Nutr 2007; 98: 397-405.

[75] Sridhar MG, Vinayagamoorthi R, Arul Suyambunathan V, Bobby Z, Selvaraj N. Bitter gourd (Momordica charantia) improves insulin sensitivity by increasing skeletal muscle insulin-stimulated IRS-1 tyrosine phosphorylation in high-fat-fed rats. Br J Nutr 2008; 99: 806-12.

[76]   Lo HC, Wang YH, Chiou HY, Lai SH, Yang Y. Relative efficacy of casein or soya protein combined with palm or safflower-seed oil on hyperuricaemia in rats. Br J Nutr 2010; 104: 67-75.

[77]   Chung MJ, Cho SY, Bhuiyan MJ, Kim KH, Lee SJ. Anti-diabetic effects of lemon balm (Melissa officinalis) essential oil on glucose- and lipid-regulating enzymes in type 2 diabetic mice. Br J Nutr 2010; 104: 180-8.

[78]   Muthusamy VS, Saravanababu C, Ramanathan M, Bharathi Raja R, Sudhagar S, Anand S, Lakshmi BS. Inhibition of protein tyrosine phosphatase 1B and regulation of insulin signalling markers by caffeoyl derivatives of chicory (Cichorium intybus) salad leaves. Br J Nutr 2010; 104: 813-23.

[79]   Latha M,Pari L. Effect of an aqueous extract of Scoparia dulcis on blood glucose, plasma insulin and some polyol pathway enzymes in experimental rat diabetes. Braz J Med Biol Res. 2004; 37: 577-86.

[80]   Marles R, Durst T, Kobaisy M, Soucy-Breau C, Abou-Zaid M, Arnason JT, Kacew S, Kanjanapothi D, Rujjanawate C, Meckes M. Pharmacokinetics, metabolism and toxicity of the plant-derived photoxin alpha-terthienyl. Pharmacol Toxicol 1995; 77: 164-8.

[81]   Jordan SA, Cunningham DG, Marles RJ. Assessment of herbal medicinal products: challenges, and opportunities to increase the knowledge base for safety assessment. Toxicol Appl Pharmacol 2010; 243: 198-216.

[82]   Attama AA, Nwabunze, OJ. Mucuna gum microspheres for oral delivery of glibenclamide: In vitro evaluation. Acta Pharm 2007; 57: 161-71.

[83]   Yang XB, Huang ZM, Cao WB, Zheng M, Chen HY, Zhang JZ. Antidiabetic effect of Oenanthe javanica flavone. Acta Pharmacol Sin 2000; 21: 239-42.

[84]   Svetina A, Jerkovic I, Vrabac L, Curic S. Thyroid function, metabolic indices and growth performance in pigs fed 00-rapeseed meal. Acta Vet Hung 2003; 51: 283-95.

[85]   Bedekar A, Shah K, Koffas M. Natural products for type II diabetes treatment. Adv Appl Microbiol 2010; 71: 21-73.

[86]   Xie JT, Wang CZ, Wang AB, Wu J, Basila D, Yuan CS. Antihyperglycemic effects of total ginsenosides from leaves and stem of Panax ginseng. Acta Pharmacol Sin 2005; 26: 1104-10.

[87]   Chen CF, Chiou WF and Zhang JT. Comparison of the pharmacological effects of Panax ginseng and Panax quinquefolium. Acta Pharmacol Sin 2008; 29: 1103-8.

[88]   Malviya N, Jain S, Malviya S. Antidiabetic potential of medicinal plants. Acta Pol Pharm 2010; 67: 113-8.

[89]   Holmberg MB, Jansson, B. Experiences from an out-patient department for drug addicts in Goteborg. Acta Psychiatr Scand 1968; 44: 172-89.

[90]   Liljeberg HG, Akerberg AK, Bjorck IM. Effect of the glycemic index and content of indigestible carbohydrates of cereal-based breakfast meals on glucose tolerance at lunch in healthy subjects. Am J Clin Nutr 1999; 69: 647-55.

[91]   Lang V, Bornet FR, Vaugelade P, van Ypersele de Strihou M, Luo J, Pacher N, Rossi F, La Droitte P, Duee PH, Slama G. Euglycemic hyperinsulinemic clamp to assess posthepatic glucose appearance after carbohydrate loading. 2. Evaluation of corn and mung bean starches in healthy men. Am J Clin Nutr 1999; 1183-8.

[92]   McKeown NM, Meigs JB, Liu S, Wilson PW, Jacques PF. Whole-grain intake is favorably associated with metabolic risk factors for type 2 diabetes and cardiovascular disease in the Framingham Offspring Study. Am J Clin Nutr 2002; 76: 390-8.

[93]   Juntunen KS, Laaksonen DE, Poutanen KS, Niskanen LK, Mykkanen HM. High-fiber rye bread and insulin secretion and sensitivity in healthy postmenopausal women. Am J Clin Nutr 2003; 77: 385-91.

[94]   Schafer G, Schenk U, Ritzel U, Ramadori G, Leonhardt U. Comparison of the effects of dried peas with those of potatoes in mixed meals on postprandial glucose and insulin concentrations in patients with type 2 diabetes. Am J Clin Nutr 2003; 78: 99-103.

[95]   Grassi D, Lippi C, Necozione S, Desideri G, Ferri C. Short-term administration of dark chocolate is followed by a significant increase in insulin sensitivity and a decrease in blood pressure in healthy persons. Am J Clin Nutr 2005; 81: 611-4.

[96]   Laaksonen DE, Toppinen LK, Juntunen KS, Autio K, Liukkonen KH, Poutanen KS, L. Niskanen L, Mykkanen HM. Dietary carbohydrate modification enhances insulin secretion in persons with the metabolic syndrome. Am J Clin Nutr 2005; 82: 1218-27.

[97]   Ahuja KD, Robertson IK, Geraghty DP, Ball MJ. Effects of chili consumption on postprandial glucose, insulin, and energy metabolism. Am J Clin Nutr 2006; 84: 63-9.

[98]   Hatonen KA, Simila ME, Virtamo JR, Eriksson JG, Hannila ML, Sinkko HK, Sundvall JE, Mykkanen HM, Valsta LM. Methodologic considerations in the measurement of glycemic index: glycemic response to rye bread, oatmeal porridge, and mashed potato. Am J Clin Nutr 2006; 84: 1055-61.

[99]   Stanhope KL, Griffen SC, Bair BR, Swarbrick MM, Keim NL, Havel PJ. Twenty-four-hour endocrine and metabolic profiles following consumption of high-fructose corn syrup-, sucrose-, fructose-, and glucose-sweetened beverages with meals. Am J Clin Nutr 2008; 87: 1194-203.

[100]   Moisey LL, Kacker S, Bickerton AC, Robinson LE, Graham TE. Caffeinated coffee consumption impairs blood glucose homeostasis in response to high and low glycemic index meals in healthy men. Am J Clin Nutr 2008; 87: 1254-61.

[101]   Kallio P, Kolehmainen M, Laaksonen DE, Pulkkinen L, Atalay M, Mykkanen H, Uusitupa M, Poutanen K, Niskanen L. Inflammation markers are modulated by responses to diets differing in postprandial insulin responses in individuals with the metabolic syndrome. Am J Clin Nutr 2008; 87: 1497-503.

[102]   Berry SE, Tydeman EA, Lewis HB, Phalora R, Rosborough J, Picout DR, Ellis PR. Manipulation of lipid bioaccessibility of almond seeds influences postprandial lipemia in healthy human subjects. Am J Clin Nutr 2008; 88: 922-9.

[103]   Chase CK, McQueen CE. Cinnamon in diabetes mellitus. Am J Health Syst Pharm 2007; 64: 1033-5.

[104]   Roca B. Rhabdomyolysis and hemolysis after use of Coutarea latiflora. Am J Med 2003; 115: 601-688.

[105]   Wolf G, Haberstroh U, Neilson EG. Angiotensin II stimulates the proliferation and biosynthesis of type I collagen in cultured murine mesangial cells. Am J Pathol 1992; 140: 95-107.

[106]   Livingston JN, Purvis BJ. Effects of wheat germ agglutinin on insulin binding and insulin sensitivity of fat cells. Am J Physiol 1980; 238: E267-75.

[107]   Kakade ML, Liener IE. Determination of available lysine in proteins. Anal Biochem 1969; 27: 273-80.

[108]   Palecek E, Pechan Z. Estimation of nanogram quantities of proteins by pulse-polarographic technique. Anal Biochem 1971; 42: 59-71.

[109] Salinas M, Fando JL, Grisolia S. A sensitive and specific method for quantitative estimation of carbamylation in proteins. Anal Biochem 1974; 62: 166-72.

[110] Guruvayoorappan C, Sudha G. Phytopharmacological evaluation of Byesukar for hypoglycaemic activity and its effect on lipid profile and hepatic enzymes of glucose metabolism in diabetic rats. Ann Hepatol 2008; 7: 358-63.

[111] Galvano F, La Fauci L, Vitaglione P, Fogliano V, Vanella L, Felgines C. Bioavailability, antioxidant and biological properties of the natural free-radical scavengers cyanidin and related glycosides. Ann Ist Super Sanita 2007; 43: 382-93.

[112] Kim HK, Kim MJ, Shin DH. Improvement of lipid profile by amaranth (Amaranthus esculantus) supplementation in streptozotocin-induced diabetic rats. Ann Nutr Metab 2006; 50: 277-81.

[113] Islam MS, Choi H, Loots T.Effects of dietary onion (*Allium cepa* L.) in a high-fat diet streptozotocin-induced diabetes rodent model. Ann Nutr Metab 2008; 53: 6-12.

[114] Cheng HH, Huang HY, Chen YY, Huang CL, Chang CJ, Chen HL, Lai MH. Ameliorative effects of stabilized rice bran on type 2 diabetes patients. Ann Nutr Metab 2010; 56: 45-51.

[115] Sobieraj DM, Freyer CW. Probable hypoglycemic adverse drug reaction associated with prickly pear cactus, glipizide, and metformin in a patient with type 2 diabetes mellitus. Ann Pharmacother 2010; 44: 1334-7.

[116] Bueno L, Weekes TE, Ruckebusch Y. Effects of diet on the motility of the small intestine and plasma insulin levels in sheep. Ann Rech Vet 1977; 8: 95-104.

[117] Altraif I, Dafalla M. Murrah, Sunn M. Herbs induced liver failure. Ann Saudi Med 2010; 30: 165-7.

[118] Nagasawa H, Fujii Y, Kageyama Y, Segawa T, Ben-Amotz A. Suppression by beta-carotene-rich algae Dunaliella bardawil of the progression, but not the development, of spontaneous mammary tumours in SHN virgin mice. Anticancer Res 1991; 11: 713-7.

[119] Ong KC, Khoo HE. Insulinomimetic effects of myricetin on lipogenesis and glucose transport in rat adipocytes but not glucose transport translocation. Biochem Pharmacol 1996; 51: 423-9.

[120] Desikan R, Hancock JT, Neill SJ, Coffey MJ, Jones OT. Elicitor-induced generation of active oxygen in suspension cultures of Arabidopsis thaliana. Biochem Soc Trans 1996; 24: 199S.

[121] Bogacheva AM, Rudenskaya GN, Preusser A, Tchikileva IO, Dunaevsky YE, Golovkin BN, Stepanov VM. A new subtilisin-like proteinase from roots of the dandelion Taraxacum officinale Webb S. L. Biochemistry (Mosc) 1999; 64: 1030-7.

[122] Hanada K, Hirano H. Interaction of a 43-kDa receptor-like protein with a 4-kDa hormone-like peptide in soybean. Biochemistry 2004; 43: 12105-12.

[123] Sim L, Jayakanthan K, Mohan S, Nasi R, Johnston BD, Pinto BM, Rose DR. New glucosidase inhibitors from an ayurvedic herbal treatment for type 2 diabetes: structures and inhibition of human intestinal maltase-glucoamylase with compounds from Salacia reticulata. Biochemistry 2010; 49: 443-51.

[124] Kozlovskaya EP, Elyakova LA. Purification and properties of trypsin-like enzymes from the starfish Lysastrosoma anthosticta. Biochim Biophys Acta 1974; 371: 63-70.

[125] Schobert B, Tschesche H. Unusual solution properties of proline and its interaction with proteins. Biochim Biophys Acta 1978; 541: 270-7.

[126] Kwon DY, Jang JS, Lee JE, Kim YS, Shin DH, Park S. The isoflavonoid aglycone-rich fractions of Chungkookjang, fermented unsalted soybeans, enhance insulin signaling and

peroxisome proliferator-activated receptor-gamma activity *in vitro*. Biofactors 2006, 26: 245-58.

[127] Parmar HS, Kar A. Antidiabetic potential of Citrus sinensis and Punica granatum peel extracts in alloxan treated male mice. Biofactors. 2007; 31: 17-24.

[128] Parmar HS, Kar A. Possible amelioration of atherogenic diet induced dyslipidemia, hypothyroidism and hyperglycemia by the peel extracts of Mangifera indica, Cucumis melo and Citrullus vulgaris fruits in rats. Biofactors 2008; 33: 13-24.

[129] Nagata M, Hidaka M, Sekiya H, Kawano Y, Yamasaki K, Okumura M, Arimori K. Effects of pomegranate juice on human cytochrome P450 2C9 and tolbutamide pharmacokinetics in rats. Drug Metab Dispos 2007; 35: 302-5.

[130] Rao AV, Gurfinkel DM. The bioactivity of saponins: triterpenoid and steroidal glycosides. Drug Metabol Drug Interact. 2000; 17: 211-35.

[131] Abdel-Barry JA, Abdel-Hassan IA, Jawad AM, Al-Hakiem MH. Hypoglycaemic effect of aqueous extract of the leaves of Trigonella foenum-graecum in healthy volunteers. East Mediterr Health J 2000; 83-8.

[132] Gaedeke N, Klein M, Kolukisaoglu U, Forestier C, Muller A, Ansorge M, *et al.* The Arabidopsis thaliana ABC transporter AtMRP5 controls root development and stomata movement. EMBO J 2001; 20: 1875-87.

Send Orders of Reprints at reprints@benthamscience.org

Phytotherapy in the Management of Diabetes and Hypertension, 2012, 193-233 193

CHAPTER 6

Phytotherapy of Hypertension in Morocco

Mohamed Eddouks[*] and Naoufel Ali Zeggwagh

Moulay Ismail University, BP 21, Errachidia, 52000, Morocco

Abstract: There is an increasing interest in the health and wellness benefits of herbs and *botanical*s. The reason behind this interest is the fact that herbs and *botanical*s might offer a natural safeguard against the development of certain pathological conditions and are used in several cultures as a putative treatment for some diseases. One such area may be the lowering of blood pressure activity. Ethnopharmacological surveys in Morocco demonstrated the use of 21 plant species belonging to different families in the treatment of ailments related to high blood pressure. Our bibliographic review establishes the fact that most plants used in the traditional treatment of hypertension effectively reduce blood pressure when used with different extraction procedures and protocols. In most cases, the hypotensive effect is accompanied by a diuretic activity or a vasorelaxant effect. This study confirms the richness of our traditional medicine and supports the use of plants in the treatment of hypertension in Morocco.

Keywords: Hypertension, medicinal plants, diuretic activity, vasorelaxation, hypotensive, ethnopharmacology, traditional, blood, pressure, Morocco.

INTRODUCTION

Since the dawn of human civilization, plant materials have played an important role in the treatment of diseases. In many regions of the world, herbal remedies continue to be more accessible and affordable than conventional drugs and represent the first line of the treatment of common ailments or diseases [1, 2]. Concurrently, societies with well-developed modern health care systems have a growing demand for nature-based remedies that can complement the prescribed modern therapies for many diseases [3-5].

Hypertension is a disease of worldwide significance and increasing prevalence [6-10]. In many countries, several studies have demonstrated the effective richness of local traditional knowledge in the treatment of hypertension [11-13]. These

*Address correspondence to Mohamed Eddouks: Moulay Ismail University, BP 21, 52000, Errachidia, Morocco; Tel: 00212535570024; Fax: 00212535573588; E-mail: mohamed.eddouks@laposte.net

Mohamed Eddouks and Debprasad Chattopadhyay (Eds)
All rights reserved-© 2012 Bentham Science Publishers

studies have provided an exhaustive list of plant species used as herbal remedies to treat hypertension. Pharmacological studies using different *in vivo* and *in vitro* tools have confirmed the effective hypotensive effect of many plants and plant derived natural products [14-18].

In Morocco, plants and natural products are the privileged sources of remedies in both rural and urban populations [19, 20]. Ethnopharmacological surveys in different Moroccan regions demonstrated that more than 231 plant species are used in the traditional medicine to cure different infectious and metabolic pathologies [19, 21-24]. Concerning hypertension, studies demonstrated that the Moroccan population uses an average of 72 plant species in the treatment of hypertension. Among these plants, only 19 are popularly used and highly recommended by traditional healers [22, 24].

The present work aims at giving a literature review of the major plants used in the treatment of hypertension in Morocco with the description of the major experimental studies related to their hypotensive activity and the underlying mode of action of each plant. The aim of this work is also to contribute to a better understanding of the major Moroccan hypotensive plants activity and the scientific relevance of the use of plants in the treatment of hypertension.

HYPERTENSION

Hypertension is one of the major risk factors for coronary heart disease (CHD), myocardial infarction (MI), cerebrovascular accidents (CVA), chronic renal failure (CRF), and congestive heart failure (CHF) in the United States of America and in industrialized countries around the world [25-28]. In industrialized countries, the risk of becoming hypertensive (blood pressure >140/90 mm Hg) over a lifetime is more than 90%. CHD is the leading cause of death in the United States, accounting for more than 800 000 deaths per year (more than one death per minute), and CVA is the fourth leading cause of death in the US. The annual expenditure on CHD is over 200 billion dollars [29-31]. Hypertension is defined as an increase in BP of unknown cause with an increased risk for cardiovascular (CV) diseases such as cerebral, cardiac, large artery, and renal events [25, 30, 32]. However, subclinical vascular target organ damage (TOD) occurs very early in the course of hypertension and can be identified with noninvasive testing [31, 33-36]. These CV diseases include left ventricular hypertrophy (LVH), diastolic dysfunction, microalbuminuria, abnormal vascular compliance, and abnormal cognitive dysfunction or vascular dementia [28].

Hypertension is part of a heterogeneous condition best described as an atherosclerotic syndrome or hypertension syndrome with genetic and acquired structural and metabolic disorders including the following:

1. Dyslipidemia or hyperlipidemia.

2. Insulin resistance, impaired glucose tolerance, and diabetes mellitus (DM).

3. Central obesity (android or portal obesity).

4. Endocrine and neurohormonal changes (sympathetic nervous system [SNS], Renin-Angiotensin-Aldosterone System [RAAS]).

5. Renal function abnormalities (sodium, water, uric acid, protein load excretion, and microalbuminuria).

Abnormalities of vascular and cardiac smooth muscle structure and function, such as arterial compliance abnormalities with loss of arterial elasticity, diastolic dysfunction and LVH.

1. Membranopathy and abnormal cellular cation transport (Ca^{++}, Mg^{++}, Na^+ and K^+).

2. Abnormalities of coagulation (prothrombotic).

3. Endothelial dysfunction.

4. Vascular inflammation (high sensitivity C-reactive protein (HS-CRP))

5. Aging.

6. Accelerated atherogenesis.

FREQUENCY AND CLINICAL IMPORTANCE

According to the World Health Organization, it has been estimated that approximately 24% of adults in Western or industrialized nations have high blood pressure. In many developing nations, there has been a rapid development of a 'second wave' epidemic of hypertension so serious that death and disability from coronary heart disease and cerebrovascular disease will rank first and fourth, respectively, as causes of the global burden of disease by the year 2020 [28, 36, 37].

The prevalence of high blood pressure increases with age, affecting approximately 65% of the population aged between 65 and 74 years in developed nations [28]. The systolic pressure rises throughout life, while the diastolic pressure rises until the age of 55–60 and then declines later [38-40]. This age-related phenomenon leads to a widened pulse pressure, which is predominantly due to a rise in the stiffness of the large arteries [28]. Hypertension is more common in men than in women until about the age of 50. After that time, it is more common in women [41-44]. In most industrialized societies, non-Hispanic black people have a slightly higher prevalence of hypertension, and definitely have a more severe form of the disease [28].

TRADITIONAL TREATMENT OF HYPERTENSION IN THE WORLD

Nutritionally speaking, it is well-known that vegetables and many natural products may reduce the risk of cardiovascular disease generally and especially hypertension [45-47]. In addition, when used as traditional medicine, plants demonstrate an effective role in the reduction of arterial blood pressure [48-51]. Plants used in the treatment of hypertension belong to different families such as Alliaceae, Verbenaceae, Rosaceae and Lauraceae [52-56]. Populations belonging to different cultural environments use these plants in different preparations such as aqueous and alcoholic extracts with single or mixed preparations [2, 4, 57-59]. The hypotensive mechanisms elucidated in advanced pharmacological studies seem to be very large and vary from an increasing renal water excretion to the inhibition of RAS [15, 60-69]. In addition, many studies have revealed the association between the observed *in vivo* hypotensive activity and the *in vitro* vasorelaxation [17, 18, 70-72]. However, the observed hypotensive effect seems to be lasting in most of the studies [52, 73-79]. As an important part in the control of blood pressure, many studies have demonstrated that the central nervous system may be implicated in the hypotensive effect of some medicinal plants [80-84]. Other studies attributed the hypotensive activity of some plants to the diuretic activity, and the use of different animal models of hypertension gives the evidence that plants may reduce blood pressure by inhibiting angiotensin, converting enzyme or increasing endothelial nitric oxide synthesis [81, 85-90].

TRADITIONAL TREATMENT OF HYPERTENSION IN MOROCCO

Taking philosophies and idioms from the ancestral Arabic medicine, Moroccan pharmacopeia uses plants and different natural products to treat different pathologies [4, 5, 19]. In most cases, traditional healers prescribe aqueous extract as the main part of treatment with different posologies and doses [22, 91]. However, the prescription of plant mixtures seems to be rare in Moroccan ethnopharmacology [19, 21]. Concerning hypertension, ethnopharmacological surveys in different Moroccan regions show that 72 plant species are used in the treatment of hypertension [22, 24, 92], but only 19 plants are popularly used in Morocco.

APIACEAE FAMILY

Carum Carvi L.

Botanical Description

Caraway (*Carum carvi*) also known as Meridian Fennel, or Persian Cumin, is a biennial plant in the family Apiaceae, native to western Asia, Europe and Northern Africa.

The plant is similar in appearance to a carrot plant, with finely divided feathery leaves containing thread-like divisions, growing on 20–30 cm of stems. The main floral part is 40–60 cm tall, with small white or pink flowers in umbels. Caraway fruits (erroneously called seeds) are crescent-shaped achenes, around 2 mm long, with five pale ridges. The plant prefers warm, sunny locations and well-drained soil.

Ethnobotany

The fruits, usually used completely, have a pungent [93-98], anise-like flavor and aroma of essential oils, mostly carvone and limonene [99-101]. They are used as a spice in breads, especially rye bread [94]. Seeded rye bread is denser partly because the limonene from the caraway fruits has yeast-killing properties [93-98].

Caraway is also used in liquors, casseroles, curry and other foods, and is more commonly found in European cuisine. It is also used to add flavor to cheeses such as havarti. Akvavit and several liqueurs are made with caraway [97, 102, 103]. A carminative or a tea (tisane) made from the seeds is used as a remedy for colic, loss of appetite and digestive disorders and to dispel worms. Caraway seed oil is also used as a fragrance component in soaps, lotions, and perfumes [23, 104-106].

Hypotensive Activity

Oral administration of ripe fruits of *Carum carvi* L. at a dose of 100 mg/kg produces a significant increase of renal excretion of water, sodium and potassium in a pattern similar to furosemide [97]. However, the effect of *Carum carvi* L. in arterial blood pressure is not identified.

Foeniculum vulgare L.

Botanical Description

Foeniculum vulagre is a plant species in the genus Foeniculum (treated as the sole species in the genus by most botanists). It is a member of the family Apiaceae (formerly the Umbelliferae). It is a hardy, perennial, umbelliferous herb, with yellow flowers and feathery leaves. It is generally considered indigenous to the shores of the Mediterranean, but has become widely naturalized elsewhere and may now be found growing wild in many parts of the world, especially in dry soils near the seacoast and on riverbanks.

It is a highly aromatic and flavorful herb with culinary and medicinal uses, and is one of the primary ingredients of absinthe.

Ethnobotany

Foeniculum dulce is widely used in the treatment of gastrointestinal disorders [107, 108] in addition to its traditional uses as an antibacterial [109] and anti-inflammatory agent [110-113].

Hypotensive Activity

After an intravenous injection to normal rats, *Foeniculum vulgare* produced a significant dose dependent reduction in arterial blood pressure. A single intravenous injection of *Foeniculum vulgare* extract seems to act *via* a histamine antagonism action [114]. Furthermore, oral administration of *Foeniculum vulgare* aqueous extract produced a significant reduction of the rat's blood pressure with a significant increase in diuresis and renal electrolytes excretion [115].

ASTERACEA FAMILY

Artemisia absinthium A

Botanical Description

It is a herbaceous perennial plant, with a hard, woody rhizome. The straight growing silvery-green stems are 0.8-1.2 m (rarely 1.5 m) tall, grooved and branched. The leaves are spirally arranged, greenish-grey above and white below, covered with silky silvery-white trichomes, and bear minute oil-producing glands; the basal leaves are up to 25 cm long, bipinnate to tripinnate with long petioles, and small, less divided cauline leaves (those on the stem), 5-10 cm long, with short petioles. The uppermost leaves can be both simple and sessile (without a petiole). Flowers are pale yellow, tubular, and clustered in spherical bent-down heads (capitula), which are in turn clustered in leafy and branched panicles. Flowering occurs from early summer to early autumn; pollination is anemophilous. The fruit is a small achene, and seed dispersal is by gravity.

Ethnobotany

The leaves and flowering tops are collected when the plant is in full bloom, and dried naturally or with artificial heat. Its active substances include silica, two bitter elements (absinthine and anabsinthine), thujone, tannin and resinous substances, malic acid and succinic acid [118-120]. It is known to act as a remedy of indigestion and gastric pain, antiseptic, and as a febrifuge. Medicinally, the herb is used to make a tea for helping pregnant women during labor pain. A dried encapsulated form of the plant is used as an anthelmintic [116, 117], and the oil of the plant can be used as a cardiac stimulant to improve blood circulation [118-122].

Hypotensive Activity

No experimental study has demonstrated the hypotensive activity of this plant.

Artemisia herba alba A

Botanical Description

Artemisia herba alba is a perennial herb, oblong with a tapering base. It grows up to 20-30 cm in height. The stems are rigid and erect. The grey leaves of sterile shoots are petiolate, ovate to orbicular in outline whereas the leaves of the flowering stems are much smaller. The flowering heads are sessile, oblong and tapering at the base and flowering happens from September to December. This plant is commonly found on the steps of the Middle East and North Africa and sometimes stands forming [123, 124].

Ethnobotany

Artemisia herba-alba is used in the Middle East against a variety of ailments including enteritis and intestinal disturbance [125-127]. In a study aimed at a rational use of this plant, the essential oil of *A. herba-alba* was tested against various bacteria which have been reported to cause intestinal problems as well as for antispasmodic activity on the rabbit jejunum. The essential oil of *A. herba-alba* showed antibacterial activity for example towards *Escherichia coli*, *Shigella sonnei* or *Salmonella typhosa* at 1-2 mg/ml. Oral administration of an aqueous extract (0.39 g plant material/kg body weight) of *Herba-alba* for 2-4 weeks in rabbits produced a significant hypoglycaemic activity [128]. The extract caused a pronounced fall in plasma glucose level. The maximal effect on plasma glucose concentration (reduction of 22% when compared to untreated diabetic animals) was observed 6 h after the treatment [128, 129]. Oral administration of the aqueous *Herba alba* extract to rabbits also protected the animals from body weight loss compared to untreated control diabetic animals [127].

Hypotensive Activity

The aqueous extract of *Artemisia herba alba* produced a significant reduction in arterial blood pressure after intravenous injection in normal rats. In addition, oral administration of the extract to spontaneous hypertensive rats produced a significant reduction of systolic blood pressure accompanied with diuretic activity [130].

BRASSICACEA FAMILY

Lepidium sativum

Botanical Description

Garden cress (*Lepidium sativum*) is a fast-growing, edible herb, *botanical*ly related to watercress and mustard, sharing their peppery, tangy flavor and aroma. In some regions, garden cress is known as garden pepper cress, pepper grass, pepperwort or poor man's pepper.

This annual plant can reach a height of 60 cm with many branches on the upper part. The white to pinkish flowers are only 2 mm ($1/12^{th}$ of an inch) across, clustered in branched racemes.

Ethnobotany

Garden Cress is added to soups, sandwiches and salads for its tangy flavor. It is also eaten as sprouts, and the fresh or dried seedpods can be used as a peppery seasoning [131-134]. Garden cress is also known to be used as a medicine in the Ayurveda system of medicine in India to prevent postnatal complications. In Morocco, cress may be given to pet birds such as budgerigars for a healthy and fresh treat [108, 135], and is used in the traditional treatment of diabetes [136].

Hypotensive Effect

Oral administration of a *Lepidium sativum* aqueous extract produced a significant reduction in systolic blood pressure with an increasing diuresis [136].

CAPPARACEAE FAMILY

Capparis *spinosa* L.

Botanical Description

Caper (*Capparis spinosa* L.) is a perennial spiny bush that bears rounded, fleshy leaves while the flower is big, white to pinkish-white in colour. The pickled bud of this plant is also called Caper. The bush is native to the Mediterranean region, growing wild on walls or in rocky coastal areas. The plant is best known for the edible bud and fruit (caper berry) which are usually consumed as pickle. Other species of *Capparis* are also picked along with C. *spinosa* for their buds or fruits.

Ethnobotany

In Greek popular medicine, a herbal tea made of caper root and young shoots is considered to be beneficial against rheumatism [137]. The bioflavonoid rutin, isolated from this plant is a powerful antioxidant [138-142] and has no known toxicity. The plant is also used as a dietary supplement for capillary fragility. Studies also showed that Capers contain more quercetin per weight than any other plant [143-145]. Ethnobotanical survey in Morocco demonstrated the use of this plant as a treatment for diabetes mellitus [94, 146].

Hypotensive Activity

An intravenous injection of *Capparis spinosa* produced a hypotensive and diuretic effect in normal rats. In addition, oral administration to hypertensive rats produced significant reduction in arterial blood pressure (data not shown).

CUCURBITACEAE FAMILY

Citrullus colocynthis L.

Botanical Description

The stems are herbaceous and beset with rough hairs; the leaves stand alternately on long petioles. They are triangular, many cleft, variously sinuated, obtuse, hairy, a fine green on the upper surface, rough and pale under. Yellow flowers appear singly at the axils of leaves. The fruit is globular. It is the size of an orange, yellow and smooth. The ripe fruit contains a hard coriaceous rind within, a white spongy pulp enclosing numerous ovate compressed white or brownish seeds.

The colocynth, also known as bitter apple, bitter cucumber, egusi, or vine of Sodom, is a viny plant native to the Mediterranean Basin and Asia, especially Turkey (regions such as İzmir), Nubia, and Trieste. The plant was originally named *Colocynthis citrullus*, but is now classified as *Citrullus colocynthis*.

Ethnobotany

The characteristic small seed of the colocynth has been found in several early archeological sites in northern Africa and the Near East, specifically at Neolithic Armant, Nagada (dated 3650-2850 BC), and Hierakonopolis (3500-3300 BC) in Egypt dated back from 3800 BC to Roman times in Libya.

Desert Bedouins are said to make a type of bread from the ground seeds. There is some confusion between this species and the closely-related watermelon, whose seeds may be used in the same way. In particular, the name "*egusi*" may refer to either or both plants (or more generically to other cucurbits) as seed crops, or to a soup made from these seeds and popular in West Africa. A traditional food plant in Africa, this little-known vegetable has the potential to improve nutrition, boost food security, and foster rural development and support sustainable land care. Experimental studies demonstrated a large variety of pharmacological activity such as hypoglycaemic and hypolipidaemic activity [147, 148], antibacterial activity [149-151] and anticancer activity [152].

Hypotensive Activity

The active principle present in the pulp of *Citrullus colocynthis,* which exhibits a cathartic abortifacient activity, is not well established yet. The cardiovascular and smooth musculature contraction activities of a recently identified glycoside alpha-elaterin-2-D-glucopyranoside (coloside A) failed to stimulate the uterus, but exhibited purgative properties. Additionally, it demonstrated an antihistaminic and anti-acetylcholine-like activity on the intestinal musculature and exhibited a negative chronotropic and negative inotropic activity in isolated mammalian and amphibian heart [153].

FUMARIACEAE FAMILY

Fumaria officinalis L.

Botanical Description

The herb is small and slender, with weak, straggling, or climbing stems, de-compound leaves, and clusters or spikes of small flowers of a pinkish hue, topped with purple, or more rarely white. The leaves have no odor, but taste bitter and saline. The plant flowers almost throughout the summer in fields, gardens, and on banks, and in ditches, spreading with great rapidity. At Mudgee, in New South Wales, it was reported to have smothered a wheat crop. Shakespeare makes several references to the herb. An interesting peculiarity is that it is very seldom visited by insects.

Ethnobotany

The plant has been demonstrated to have many activities: slightly diaphoretic, diuretic, and aperient; valuable in all visceral obstructions, particularly those of the liver, in scorbutic affections, and in troublesome eruptive diseases, even those of the leprous disorder [154-157]. A decoction makes a curative lotion for milk-crust on the scalp of an infant. Physicians and writers from Dioscorides to Chaucer and from the fourteenth century to Cullen to modern times value its purifying power [158, 159]. The Japanese make a tonic from it. Cows and sheep eat it, and the latter are said to derive great benefit from it. The leaves, in decoction or extract, may be used in almost any doses. The inspissated juice has also been employed, also a syrup, powder, cataplasm, distilled water, and several tinctures [160, 161].

Hypotensive Activity

The hypotensive activity is still unknown.

LAMIACEAE FAMILY

Ajuga iva L.

Botanical Description

It is a short and small growing plant usually found as individual specimen or in few numbers as tufts (growing very close to each other). Their roots live all year round and make the plant to be described as perennial.

The herbaceous stem (with a woody base) is covered with long, fine, white hairs (villous) and forms opposite leaves. The leaves are linear-lanceaolate to linear-oblong and vary in either being entire, or with 2, 4 or 6 opposite teeth-like lobes. The mature leaves measure around 24 mm long and 6 mm wide. They have a pleasant, lemon-like aromatic smell.

Ethnobotany

The plant is used in the treatment of diabetes and hypertension in Morocco [162-166]. In addition, some studies have reported its use in gastrointestinal disorders and demonstrated that the plant possesses anti-inflammatory, anticancer and antiulcer activities [167, 168].

Hypotensive Activity

Pharmacological studies using both *in vivo* and *in vitro* investigations have demonstrated that the aqueous extract of this plant does not exert hypotensive activity after oral administration in normal rats. However, in isolated aortic rings, it exerts a vasorelaxant activity probably mediated *via* nitric oxide depending pathway [164].

Marrubium vulgare L.

Botanical Description

It is a gray-leaved herbaceous perennial plant, somewhat resembling mint in appearance, which grows to 25-45 cm tall. The leaves are 2-5 cm long with a densely crinkled surface, and are covered in downy hairs. The flowers are white, borne in clusters on the upper part of the main stem.

Ethnobotany

Preparations of horehound are still largely used as expectorants and tonics [169, 170]. It may, indeed, be considered one of the most popular pectoral remedies, being given with benefit for chronic cough, asthma, and some cases of consumption [171-173]. For children's cough and croup, it is given to advantage in the form of syrup. It is also useful as a tonic and a corrective of the stomach [169, 174]. Hypoglycemic activity of *Marrubium vulgare* has been demonstrated by several studies [169, 174].

Hypotensive Activity

Marrubium vulgare demonstrated a hypotensive effect in both normal and hypertensive rats with a nitric oxide independent mechanism [175]. Phytochemical investigation allowed the isolation of a diterpenoid: marrubenol which demonstrated an *in vitro* vasorelaxant activity with a calcium dependent mechanism [16, 65].

Rosmarinus officinalis L.

Botanical Description

Rosemary (*Rosmarinus officinalis*) is a woody, perennial herb with fragrant evergreen needle-like leaves. It is native of the Mediterranean region. It is a member of the mint family Lamiaceae which also includes many other herbs.

Ethnobotany

Rosemary has a very old reputation for improving memory, and has been used as a symbol for remembrance (during weddings, war commemorations and funerals) in Europe and Australia [176-179]. The results of a study suggest that carnosic acid, found in rosemary, may shield the brain from free radicals, lowering the risk of strokes and neurodegenerative diseases like Alzheimer's and Lou Gehrig's [180-182]. Rosemary contains a number of potentially bioactive compounds, including antioxidants such as carnosic acid and rosmarinic acid, camphor (up to 20% in dry leaves), caffeic acid, ursolic acid, betulinic acid, rosmaridiphenol, and rosmanol [183-186].

Hypotensive Activity

The aqueous extract of *Rosmarinus officinalis* possesses a potent diuretic activity in normal rats after seven days of oral administration [66]. However, the effect of the aqueous extract on arterial blood pressure has not been assessed.

Thymus serpyllum L.

Botanical Description

Thymus is a perennial low aromatic shrub with much-branched woody stems forming dense tufts from which arise tiny, paired opposite leaves on short stalks, each with two minutes leaflets at the base. The leaves are 6-8mm long, the underside covered with fine hairs. The flowers are arranged in whorls in the axils of the upper leaves, and are of a typical labiate appearance, pink to lilac in color. The plant is indigenous to Mediterranean regions and southern Europe, but is widely cultivated throughout the world, where it thrives in temperate climates, particularly on waste ground.

Ethnobotany

The volatile oil of Thymus exerts a calming influence on smooth muscles. It is a useful carminative in dyspepsia, and the high tannin content helps to relieve diarrhea [187]. Thymol is twenty times more antiseptic than phenol, but does not have an irritant effect on the mucosa and may safely be taken internally. It is active against a variety of intestinal infections and infestations, particularly hookworm and ascarids, and can significantly alter the bacterial populations of the gut, actions which are enhanced by the poor absorption of thymol into the bloodstream [188, 189]. Rosmarinic acid has an anti-inflammatory activity [185, 190-192]. Thymus' bitter component stimulates the appetite, aids a sluggish digestion and improves liver function [193, 194].

The small proportion of thymol that is absorbed into the bloodstream carries the antiseptic effect to the lungs and kidneys where it is excreted from the body in the urine and on the breath [190, 195-197]. Thymus is therefore used in the treatment of bronchial, pulmonary and urinary infections. It has an expectorant action, increasing the production of fluid mucus to ensure a productive cough [187, 191, 198]. The carvacrol stimulates the mucous membranes into secretory activity, while the saponins are reflex-stimulating expectorants [188, 199-201]. Thymus has a specific use in asthma and coughs with a nervous component, and thyme oil may be added to oil and used as a rub for chest infections, or included in a steam inhalation for asthma [202-204].

Hypotensive Activity

The effect of *Thymus serpyllum* on arterial blood pressure has never been studied.

LILIACEAE FAMILY

Allium cepa L.

Botanical Description

Onion is a term used for many plants in the genus *Allium*. They are known by the common name "onion" but, used without qualifiers, it usually refers to *Allium cepa* which is also known as the "garden onion" or "bulb" onion. It is grown underground by the plant as a vertical shoot that is used for food storage, leading to the possibility of confusion with a tuber.

Ethnobotany

Onions, one of the oldest vegetables, are found in a large number of recipes and preparations spanning almost the totality of the world's cultures [205, 206]. They are now available in fresh, frozen, canned, caramelized, pickled, powdered, chopped, and dehydrated forms. Onions can be used, usually chopped or sliced, in almost every type of food, including cooked foods and fresh salads and as a spicy garnish [178, 207-211]. They are rarely eaten on their own, but usually act as accompaniment to the main course. Depending on the variety, an onion can be sharp, spicy, tangy and pungent or mild and sweet [212, 213].

Hypotensive Activity

Allium cepa has been studied for its hypotensive activity both in animal and clinical studies. The results showed that the plant possesses hypotensive activity in SHR and a renovascular model of hypertension, the underlying mechanism seems to be dependent on nitric oxide synthesis [214-216]. In clinical studies, Quercetin isolated from *Allium cepa* seems to reduce arterial blood pressure in hypertensive patients [216].

Allium sativum

Botanical Description

Allium sativum, commonly known as garlic, is a species of the onion family Alliaceae. Its close relatives include the onion, shallot, leek, and chive. Garlic has been used throughout recorded history for both culinary and medicinal purposes. It has a characteristic pungent, spicy flavor that mellows and sweetens considerably with cooking. A bulb of garlic, the most commonly used part of the plant, is divided into numerous fleshy sections called cloves. Single clove garlic (also called Pearl garlic or Solo garlic) also exists. It originated from the Yunnan province of China. The cloves are used as seed, for consumption (raw or cooked), and for medicinal purposes. The leaves, stems (scape), and flowers (bulbils) on the head (spathe) are also edible and are most often consumed while immature and still tender. The papery, protective layers of "skin" over various parts of the plant and the roots attached to the bulb are the only parts not considered palatable.

Ethnobotany

In test tube studies, garlic has been found to have antibacterial, antiviral, and antifungal activities. However, these actions are less clear in humans [217-221]. Garlic is also known to prevent heart disease (including atherosclerosis, high cholesterol and high blood pressure) and cancer. Animal studies, and some early studies in humans, have suggested possible cardiovascular benefits of garlic. A Czech study found that garlic supplementation reduces accumulation of cholesterol on the vascular walls of animals [222-226]. Another study had similar results, with garlic supplementation significantly reducing aortic plaque deposits of cholesterol-fed rabbits [227-230]. Another study showed that supplementation with garlic extract inhibits vascular calcification in human patients with high blood cholesterol [231-235].

Hypotensive Effect

The known vasodilatory effect of garlic is possibly caused by catabolism of garlic-derived polysulfides to hydrogen sulfide in red blood cells, a reaction that depends on reduced thiol in or on the RBC membrane, and hydrogen sulfide is an endogenous cardioprotective vascular cell-signaling molecule [219, 224, 228, 230, 236, 237].

MYRTACEAE FAMILY

Myrtus communis L.

Botanical Description

Myrtle often grows as a rounded bush, with large specimens reaching 3-5 m. The small, pointed, oval leaves are in pairs or spirally arranged along a stem and when crushed are pleasantly aromatic. A profusion of fragrant flowers is borne from

May to July. Each flower is solitary arising from leaf axils and consists of four white petals and numerous conspicuous anthers. Pollination is done by bees and the dark purple fruits are fragrant.

Ethnobotany

The plant has long been considered to be an aphrodisiac. In the past, many Mediterranean brides carried bouquets that incorporated Myrtle sprigs, a tradition still seen in Palestine today [238, 239]. Leaves contain various aromatic oils, malic acid, citric acid and tannins as well as vitamin C [240-242]. Its leaf oils and related aroma have made myrtle a popular ingredient of traditional Mediterranean cosmetics, and extracts have been used both as astringents and antiseptics [243-248]. The berries have long been used to treat indigestion and stimulate the digestive system and for hypoglycemic activity [243, 244, 249, 250].

Hypotensive Activity

The hypotensive activity of *Myrtus communis* is still to be known.

OLEACEAE FAMILY

Fraxinus excelsior L.

Botanical Description

The Common Ash (*Fraxinus excelsior*, L.), a tall, handsome tree, common in Britain, is readily distinguished by its light-grey bark (smooth in younger trees, rough and scaly in older specimens), and by its large compound leaves, divided into four to eight pairs of lance-shaped leaflets, tipped by a single one, an arrangement which imparts a light feathery arrangement to the foliage.

Ethnobotany

Fraxinus excelsior L. has been employed as a bitter tonic and astringent, and is said to be valuable as an antiperiodic [115, 251]. Because of its astringency, it has been used, in decoction, extensively in the treatment of intermittent fever and ague, as a substitute for Peruvian bark. The decoction is odorless, though its taste is fairly bitter. It has been considered useful to remove obstructions of the liver and spleen, and in rheumatism of an arthritic nature [252-254]. The leaves have diuretic, diaphoretic and purgative properties, and are employed in modern herbal medicine for their laxative action, especially in the treatment of gouty and rheumatic complaints, proving a useful substitute for Senna and having a less griping effect [115, 255]. The distilled water of the leaves, taken every morning, is considered good for dropsy and obesity [255-257].

Hypotensive Activity

The aqueous extract of *Fraxinus excelsior* has demonstrated a potent diuretic activity with a hypotensive effect in both normal and hypertensive rats [255].

Olea europea L.

Botanical Description

The olive (*Olea europaea*) is a species of a small tree in the family Oleaceae, native to the coastal areas of the eastern Mediterranean Basin (the adjoining coastal areas of southeastern Europe, western Asia and northern Africa) as well as northern Iran at the south end of the Caspian Sea. Its fruit, also called the olive, is of major agricultural importance in the Mediterranean region as the source of olive oil. The tree and its fruit give their name to the plant family, which also includes species such as lilacs, jasmine, Forsythia and the true ash trees (*Fraxinus*). The word 'oil' in many languages ultimately derives from the name of the tree and its fruit.

Ethnobotany

While olive oil is well known for its flavor and health benefits, the leaf has been used medicinally in various times and places. Natural olive leaf and olive leaf extracts (OLE) are now marketed as anti-aging, immunostimulators, and even antibiotics [149, 258-261]. Clinical evidence has proven the blood pressure lowering effects of carefully extracted olive leaf extracts [262, 263]. Bioassays support its antibacterial, antifungal, and anti-inflammatory effects at a laboratory level [23, 24, 259, 264-269].

Hypotensive Activity

Olive oil possesses a beneficial effect on the cardiovascular system. Leaf plant seems to produce a potent hypotensive activity *via* an action in calcium channels [24, 263].

PLANTAGINACEAE FAMILY

Globularia alypum L.

Botanical Description

Globularia is a genus of about 22 species of flowering plants in the family Plantaginaceae, native of central and southern Europe, Macaronesia, northwest Africa and southwest Asia. They are dense low evergreen mat-forming herbs or subshrubs, with leathery oval leaves 1–10 cm long. The flowers are produced in dense inflorescences (capitula) held above the plant on a 1–30 cm tall stem; the capitula is 1–3 cm in diameter, with numerous tightly packed purple, violet, pink or white flowers.

Ethnobotany

Globularia alypum is largely used in the treatment of several infectious diseases [270, 271] and diabetes [24, 272].

Hypotensive Activity

No study has demonstrated the effect of this plant on arterial blood pressure.

RANUNCULACEAE FAMILY

Nigella sativa L.

Botanical Description

The plant has a stiff, erect, branching stem, bears deeply-cut greyish-green leaves and terminal greyish-blue flowers, followed by odd, toothed seed vessels, filled with small compressed seeds, usually three-cornered, with two sides flat and one convex, black or brown externally, white and oleaginous within, of a strong, agreeable aromatic odour, like nutmegs, and a spicy, pungent taste.

Ethnobotany

Nigella sativa has been used for medicinal purposes for centuries, both as a herb and as pressed oil, in Asia, the Middle East and Africa [273-275]. It has been traditionally used for a variety of conditions and treatments related to respiratory health, stomach and intestinal health, kidney and liver function, circulatory and immune system support, as analgesic, anti-inflammatory, anti-allergic, antioxidants, anticancer, antiviral and for general well-being [276-281].

Hypotensive Activity

Experimental studies have demonstrated that *Nigella sativa* possesses a hypotensive activity associated with a diuretic activity in hypertensive rats [72]. In addition, volatile oil of the plant seems to reduce arterial blood pressure *via* muscarinic mechanism [2282-284].

URTICACEAE FAMILY

Urtica dioica L.

Botanical Description

The stinging nettle is a dioecious and herbaceous perennial herb, 1 to 2 m tall in the summer and dying down to the ground in winter. It has widely spreading rhizomes and stolons, which are bright yellow roots. The soft green leaves are 3 to 15 cm (1 to 6 in) long and are borne oppositely on an erect wiry green stem. The leaves have a strongly serrated margin, a cordate base and an acuminate tip with a terminal leaf tooth longer than adjacent laterals. It bears small greenish or brownish 4-merous flowers in dense axillary inflorescences. The leaves and stems are very hairy with non-stinging hairs and also bear many stinging hairs (trichomes), whose tips come off when touched, transforming the hair into a needle that will inject several chemicals: acetylcholine, histamine, 5-HT or serotonin, and possibly formic acid. This mixture of chemical compounds causes a sting or paresthesia from which the species derives its common name, as well as the colloquial names: burn nettle, burn weed, burn hazel. The pain and itching from a nettle sting can last from only a few minutes to as long as a week.

Ethnobotany

The nettle is one of the nine plants invoked in the pagan Anglo-Saxon Nine Herbs Charm, recorded in the 10th century. It is believed to be a galactagogue, and a clinical trial has shown that its juice is diuretic in patients with congestive heart failure [285, 286]. Urtication, or flogging with nettles, is the process of deliberately applying stinging nettles to the skin in order to provoke inflammation. An agent thus used is known as a rubefacient [287-291]. It is used as a folk remedy for rheumatism, providing temporary relief from pain. The counter-irritant action to which this is often attributed can be preserved by the preparation of an alcoholic tincture which can be applied as part of a topical preparation, but not as an infusion, which drastically reduces the irritant action. Extracts are also used to treat arthritis, anemia, hay fever, kidney problems, and pain [292-294].

Hypotensive Activity

The aqueous extract has demonstrated a hypotensive activity after intravenous injection in normal rats, and it also induces a strong bradycardia through non-cholinergic and non-adrenergic pathways which might compensate for its vascular effect and account for the hypotensive action of *Urtica dioica* L described *in vivo* [83]. In addition, the aqueous extract has demonstrated an acute diuretic and natriuretic effect in normal rats [89].

ZYGOPHYLLACEAE FAMILY

Peganum harmala L.

Botanical Description

Harmal (*Peganum harmala*) is a plant of the family Nitrariaceae, native of the eastern Mediterranean region east to India. Its trade name, "*Syrian Rue*," refers to its resemblance to plants of the rue (*Ruta*, Rutaceae) family.

It is a perennial plant which can grow to about 0.8 m tall, but normally it is about 0.3 m tall. The roots of the plant can reach a depth of up to 6.1 m. It blossoms between June and August in the Northern Hemisphere. The flowers are white and are about 2.5–3.8 cm in diameter. The round seed capsules measure about 1–1.5 cm in diameter and have three chambers and carry more than 50 seeds.

Ethnobotany

Peganum harmala is used as an analgesic and anti-inflammatory agent. In Yemen, it has been used to treat depression, and it has been established in the laboratory that harmaline, an active ingredient in *Peganum harmala*, is a central nervous system stimulant and a "reversible inhibitor of MAO-A (RIMA)", a category of antidepressant. Smoke from the seeds kills algae, bacteria, intestinal parasites and molds [295-297]. The root is applied to kill lice and when burned, the seeds kill insects. It also inhibits the reproduction of the *Tribolium castaneum* beetle. It is also used as an anthelmintic (to expel parasitic worms) [298-305]. The ancient

Greeks used powdered *Peganum harmala* seeds to get rid of tapeworms and to treat recurring fevers (possibly malaria). *Peganum harmala* is an abortifacient, and, in large quantities, it can reduce spermatogenesis and male fertility in rats [23, 306-310].

Hypotensive Activity

Alkaloids isolated from *Peganum harmala* have demonstrated a potent vasorelaxant activity in isolated aortic rings [311, 312]. However, the *in vivo* hypotensive effect of these two compounds is still unknown.

DISCUSSION AND CONCLUSION

From the 1994 WHO data, it appears that 90% of the world's population use medicinal plants for curing several ailments and diseases, and 81% have no access to synthetic drugs. Although this is unfortunate for the less developed countries in Africa, Asia and South-America, these data show that in many parts of the world, drugs from plants are an important therapeutic source [5, 52, 57, 58]. The present paper aims at reviewing most plants used in the treatment of hypertension in Morocco. The traditionally used plants and herbs belong to different families and experimental studies effectively confirm the hypotensive activity of most plants. The experimental studies used different protocols and animal models of hypertension to evaluate the hypotensive activity of medicinal plants. Plant extracts were administrated intravenously or orally and the arterial blood pressure was measured throughout invasive or non-invasive methods. Globally, the experimental studies demonstrated that Moroccan plants effectively reduce arterial blood pressure in different manners. Some plants like *Urtica dioica*, *Marrubium vulgare* and *Artemisia herba alba* produce a rapid and short lasting reduction in arterial blood pressure. This rapid effect seems to be due to an action of the central nervous system [9, 29]. Other groups of plants like *Fraxinus excelsior*, *Carum carvi*, *Rosmarinus officinalis* demonstrated a diuretic activity but unfortunately in the case of *Rosmarinus officinalis* no information is available concerning the effect on arterial blood pressure and this is also the same for *Globularia alypum*. *Allium cepa*, *Allium sativa* and *Nigella sativa*, which are the most studied plants for their hypotensive effect. Studies have reported the potent hypotensive effect of these plants, and the mechanism of action seems to be more potent and long lasting than any other plants used in the treatment of hypertension. It is noteworthy that increasing diuresis is the common point of most Moroccan hypotensive plants. Mechanistic studies related to the hypotensive effect of plants have clearly demonstrated the similarity between plant hypotensive and mechanisms of action [282, 283]: for example *Allium sativum* reduces blood pressure more effectively than Angiotensine converting enzyme inhibitors [224, 230, 313, 314]. The use of aortic rings allowed the evaluation of most vasorelaxant activity of hypotensive plants. In this context, *Artemisia herba alba* and *Ajuga iva* are good examples of the link between hypotensive activity and vasorelaxant effect. However, for unknown reasons, hypotensive plants: *Carum carvi* and *Foeniculum vulgare* are still not studied when the vasorelaxant activity is concerned. In all experimental studies, the hypotensive effect is not accompanied with deep and longer remodeling of the cardiovascular system.

In spite of the observed and interesting hypotensive activity, the phytochemistry of Moroccan hypotensive plants is not totally explored.

Taken in all, most plants used in the traditional treatment of hypertension have demonstrated effective hypotensive activity *in vivo* and/or *in vitro* investigations. However, toxicological studies are extremely needed for a safe popular use of plants.

ACKNOWLEDGEMENTS

The authors extend their thanks to the Editors and Bentham Science Publishers.

DECLARATION OF CONFLICT OF INTEREST

No conflict of interest was declared by the authors.

REFERENCES

[1]   Balunas MJ, Kinghorn AD. Drug discovery from medicinal plants. Life Sciences 2005; 78(5): 431-41.
[2]   Borris RP. Natural products research: perspectives from a major pharmaceutical company. J Ethnopharmacol 1996; 51(1-3): 29-38.
[3]   Brower V. Back to nature: extinction of medicinal plants threatens drug discovery. J Natl Cancer Inst 2008; 100(12): 838-9.
[4]   Cordell GA, Colvard MD. Some thoughts on the future of ethnopharmacology. J Ethnopharmacol 2005; 100(1-2): 5-14.

[5]   Cragg GM, Newman DJ, Snader KM. Natural Products in Drug Discovery and Development. J Nat Pr 1997; 60 (1): 52-60.

[6]   Allen W, Cowley R. Long-term control of arterial blood pressure. Physiol Rev 1992; 72(1): 231-99.

[7]   Asmar R. Préssion artérielle. Régulation et épidemiologie: Mesures et valeurs normales. Néphrologie & Thérapeutique 2007; 3(4): 163-84.

[8]   Bakris GL, Mensah GA. Pathogenesis and clinical physiology of hypertension. Cur Prob Cardiol 2003; 28(2): 137-55.

[9]   Bohr D, Dominiczak AF. Experimental hypertension. Hypertension 1991; 17(Sup I): 39-44.

[10]   Guyton AC. Hypertension. A neural disease? Archives of neurology 1988; 45(2): 178-9.

[11]   Heinrich M. Ethnobotany and its role in drug development. Phytother Res 2000; 14(7): 479-88.

[12]   Houghton PJ, Howes MJ, Lee CC, Steventon G. Uses and abuses of *in vitro* tests in ethnopharmacology: Visualizing an elephant. J Ethnopharmacol 2007; 110(3): 391-400.

[13]   Joubert E, Gelderblom WCA, Louw A, de Beer D. South African herbal teas: Aspalathus linearis, Cyclopia spp. and Athrixia phylicoides - a review. Journal of Ethnopharmacology; In Press.

[14]   Al-Qattan KK, Khan I, Alnaqeeb MA, Ali M. Mechanism of garlic (*Allium sativum*) induced reduction of hypertension in 2K-1C rats: a possible mediation of Na/H exchanger isoform-1. Prostaglandins Leukot Essent Fatty Acids 2003; 69(4): 217-22.

[15]   Eddouks M, Maghrani M, Zeggwagh NA, Haloui M, Michel JB. Fraxinus excelsior L. evokes a hypotensive action in normal and spontaneously hypertensive rats. J Ethnopharmacol 2005; 99(1): 49-54.

[16]   El Bardai S, Morel N, Wibo M, Fabre N, Llabres G, Lyoussi B, Quetin-Leclercq J. The vasorelaxant activity of marrubenol and marrubiin from Marrubium vulgare. Planta Med 2003; 69(1): 75-7.

[17]   Kalus U, Pindur G, Jung F, Mayer B, Radtke H, Bachmann K, Mrowietz C, Koscielny J, Kiesewetter H. Influence of the onion as an essential ingredient of the Mediterranean diet on arterial blood pressure and blood fluidity. Arzneimittelforschung 2000; 50(9): 795-801.

[18]   Khayyal MT, el-Ghazaly MA, Abdallah DM, Nassar NN, Okpanyi SN, Kreuter MH. Blood pressure lowering effect of an olive leaf extract (Olea europaea) in L-NAME induced hypertension in rats. Arzneimittelforschung 2002; 52(11): 797-802.

[19]   Bellakhdar J, Claisse R, Fleurentin J, Younos C. Repertory of standard herbal drugs in the Moroccan pharmacopoea. J Ethnopharmacol 1991; 35(2): 123-43.

[20]   Bellakhdar J, Passannanti S, Paternostro MP, Piozzi F. Constituents of Origanum compactum. Planta Med 1988; 54(1): 94-9.

[21]   Bellakhdar J. A new look at traditional medicine in Morocco. World Health Forum 1989; 10(2): 193-9.

[22]   Eddouks M, Maghrani M, Lemhadri A, Ouahidi ML, Jouad H. Ethnopharmacological survey of medicinal plants used for the treatment of diabetes mellitus, hypertension and cardiac diseases in the south-east region of Morocco (Tafilalet). J Ethnopharmacol 2002; 82(2-3): 97-103.

[23]   Tahraoui A, El-Hilaly J, Israili ZH, Lyoussi B. Ethnopharmacological survey of plants used in the traditional treatment of hypertension and diabetes in south-eastern Morocco (Errachidia province). J Ethnopharmacol 2007; 110(1): 105-17.

[24]   Ziyyat A, Legssyer A, Mekhfi H, Dassouli A, Serhrouchni M, Benjelloun W. Phytotherapy of hypertension and diabetes in oriental Morocco. J Ethnopharmacol 1997; 58(1): 45-54.

[25]   Elliott WJ. Systemic Hypertension. Current Problems in Cardiology 2007; 32(4): 201-59.

[26]   Guidlines subcommittee WHO, International society of hypertension Guidlines for the management of hypertension. J Hyper 1999; 17: 151-83.

[27]   Kurtz TW, Griffin KA, Bidani AK, Davisson RL, Hall JE. Recommendations for blood pressure measurement in humans and experimental animals. Part 2: Blood pressure measurement in experimental animals: a statement for professionals from the subcommittee of professional and public education of the American Heart Association council on high blood pressure research. Hypertension 2005; 45(2): 299-310.

[28]   Oparil S, Zaman MA, Calhoun DA. Pathogenesis of Hypertension. Ann Intern Med 2003, 2003; 139(9): 761-76.

[29]   Blaustein MP, Zhang J, Chen L, Hamilton BP. How does salt retention raise blood pressure? Am J Physiol Regul Integr Comp Physiol 2006; 290(3): R514-23.

[30]   Del Colle S, Morello F, Rabbia F, Milan A, Naso D, Puglisi E, Mulatero P, Veglio F. Antihypertensive drugs and the sympathetic nervous system. J Cardiovasc Pharmacol 2007; 50(5): 487-96.

[31]   Gradman A, Vivas Y. New drugs for hypertension: what do they offer? Curr Hypertens Rep 2006; 8(5): 425-32.

[32]   Folkow B. Physiological aspects of primary hypertension. Physiol Rev 1982; 62: 3 47-504.

[33]   Geoffrey AH. The sympathetic nervous system in hypertension: assessment by blood pressure variability and ganglionic blockade. J Hypert 2003; 21: 1619-21.

[34]   Hall JE. The kidney, hypertension, and obesity. Hypertension 2003; 41: 625-33.

[35]   Joyner M, Charkoudian N, GunnarWallin B. A sympathetic view of the sympathetic nervous system and human blood pressure regulation. Exp Physiol 2008; 93(6): 715-24.

[36]   Lerman LO, Chade AR, Sica V, Napoli C. Animal models of hypertension: An overview. J Lab Clin Med 2005; 146(3): 160-73.

[37]   Michel JB, De Roux N, Plissonnier D, Anidjar S, Salzmann JL, Levy B. Pathophysiological role of the vascular smooth muscle cell. J Card Pharmacol 1990; 16 (Suppl 1): 4-11.

[38]   Pinto YM, Paul M, Ganten D. Lessons from rat models of hypertension: from Goldblatt to genetic engineering. Cardr Res 1998; 39(1): 77-88.

[39]   Pleuvry BJ. Drugs affecting the autonomic nervous system. Anaesth Intens Care Med 2008; 9(2): 84-7.

[40]   Rapp JP. Genetic Analysis of Inherited Hypertension in the Rat. Physiol Rev 2000, 2000; 80(1): 135-72.

[41]   Sharifi AM, Akbarloo N, Darabi R, Larijani B. Study of correlation between elevation of blood pressure and tissue ACE activity during development of hypertension in 1K1C rats. Vasc Pharmacol 2004; 41(1): 15-20.

[42]   Takahashi N, Smithies O. Human genetics, animal models and computer simulations for studying hypertension. Trends in Genet 2004; 20(3): 136-45.

[43]   Webb RC. Smooth muscle contraction and relaxation. Advan Physiol Edu 2003; 27(4): 201-6.

[44]   Woodrum DA, Brophy CM. The paradox of smooth muscle physiology. Mol Cel Endocrinol 2001; 177(1-2): 135-43.

[45]   Dauchet L. Dietary patterns and blood pressure change over 5-y follow-up in the SU.VI.MAX cohort. Am J Clin Nutr 2007; 85: 1650-6.

[46] Dauchet L, Amouyel P, Dallongeville J. Fruit and vegetable consumption and risk of stroke: a meta-analysis of cohort studies. Neurology 2005; 65: 1193-7.

[47] Dauchet L, Amouyel P, Hercberg S, Dallongeville J. Fruit and vegetable consumption and risk of coronary heart disease: a meta-analysis of cohort studies. J Nutr 2006; 136: 2588-93.

[48] Chang P, Koh YK, Geh SL, Soepadmo E, Goh SH, Wong AK. Cardiovascular effects in the rat of dihydrocorynantheine isolated from Uncaria callophylla. J Ethnopharmacol 1989; 25(2): 213-5.

[49] Landry Y, Gies JP. Drugs and their molecular targets: an updated overview. Fund Clin Pharmacol 2008; 22: 1-18.

[50] Newman DJ, Cragg GM. Natural products as sources of new drugs over the last 25 years. J Nat Prod 2007; 70(3): 461-77.

[51] Wang HX, Ng TB. Natural products with hypoglycemic, hypotensive, hypocholesterolemic, antiatherosclerotic and antithrombotic activities. Life Sci 1999; 65(25): 2663-77.

[52] Chen HB, Islam MW, Radhakrishnan R, Wahab SA, Naji MA. Influence of aqueous extract from Neurada procumbens L. on blood pressure of rats. J Ethnopharmacol 2004; 90 (2-3): 191-4.

[53] Fatehi M, Rashidabady T, Fatehi-Hassanabad Z. Effects of Crocus sativus petals' extract on rat blood pressure and on responses induced by electrical field stimulation in the rat isolated vas deferens and guinea-pig ileum. J Ethnopharmacol 2003; 84(2-3): 199-203.

[54] Guang-Wei L, Katsuyuki M, Tokihito Y, Kenjiro Y. Effects of extract from Clerodendron trichotomum on blood pressure and renal function in rats and dogs. J Ethnopharmacol 1994; 42(2): 77-82.

[55] Mackraj I, Ramesar S, Singh M, Govender T, Baijnath H, Singh R, Gathiram P. The *in vivo* effects of Tulbhagia violacea on blood pressure in a salt-sensitive rat model. J Ethnopharmacol 2008; 117(2): 263-9.

[56] Salazar MJ, El Hafidi M, Pastelin G, Ramírez-Ortega MC, Sánchez-Mendoza MA. Effect of an avocado oil-rich diet over an angiotensin II-induced blood pressure response. J Ethnopharmacol 2005; 98(3): 335-8.

[57] Boulos L. Medicinal plants of North Africa. Algonac, Mich.: Reference Publications, Inc.; 1983.

[58] Gilani AH, Atta ur R. Trends in ethnopharmacology. J Ethnopharmacol 2005; 100(1-2): 43-9.

[59] Gurib-Fakim A. Medicinal plants: Traditions of yesterday and drugs of tomorrow. Molecular Aspects of Medicine 2006; 27(1): 1-93.

[60] Afkir S, Nguelefack TB, Aziz M, Zoheir J, Cuisinaud G, Bnouham M, Mekhfi H, Legssyer A, Lahlou S, Ziyyat A. Arbutus unedo prevents cardiovascular and morphological alterations in L-NAME-induced hypertensive rats: Part I: Cardiovascular and renal hemodynamic effects of Arbutus unedo in L-NAME-induced hypertensive rats. J Ethnopharmacol 2008; 116(2): 288-95.

[61] Dehkordi FR, Kamkhah AF. Antihypertensive effect of Nigella sativa seed extract in patients with mild hypertension. Fund Clin Pharmacol 2008; 22(4): 447-52.

[62] Dimo T, Azay J, Tan PV, Pellecuer J, Cros G, Bopelet M, Serrano JJ. Effects of the aqueous and methylene chloride extracts of Bidens pilosa leaf on fructose-hypertensive rats. J Ethnopharmacol 2001; 76(3): 215-21.

[63]   Dimo T, Rakotonirina SV, Tan PV, Azay J, Dongo E, Cros G. Leaf methanol extract of Bidens pilosa prevents and attenuates the hypertension induced by high-fructose diet in Wistar rats. J Ethnopharmacol 2002; 83(3): 183-91.

[64]   El Bardai S, Lyoussi B, Wibo M, Morel N. Comparative study of the antihypertensive activity of Marrubium vulgare and of the dihydropyridine calcium antagonist amlodipine in spontaneously hypertensive rat. Clin Exp Hypertens 2004; 26(6): 465-74.

[65]   El-Bardai S, Wibo M, Hamaide MC, Lyoussi B, Quetin-Leclercq J, Morel N. Characterisation of marrubenol, a diterpene extracted from Marrubium vulgare, as an L-type calcium channel blocker. Br J Pharmacol 2003; 140(7): 1211-6.

[66]   Haloui M, Louedec L, Michel JB, Lyoussi B. Experimental diuretic effects of Rosmarinus officinalis and Centaurium erythraea. J Ethnopharmacol 2000; 71(3): 465-72.

[67]   Kubota Y, Tanaka N, Kagota S, Nakamura K, Kunitomo M, Umegaki K, Shinozuka K. Effects of Ginkgo biloba extract on blood pressure and vascular endothelial response by acetylcholine in spontaneously hypertensive rats. J Pharm Pharmacol 2006; 58(2): 243-9.

[68]   Lahlou S, Leylliane F, Leal I, Josè H, Leal-Cardoso G, Pinto D. Antihypertensive effects of the essential oil of Alpinia zerumbet and its main constituent, terpinen-4-ol, in DOCA-salt hypertensive conscious rats. Fund Clin Pharmacol 2003; 17(3): 323-30.

[69]   McMahon FG, Vargas R. Can garlic lower blood pressure? A pilot study. Pharmacotherapy 1993; 13(4): 406-7.

[70]   Haji Faraji M, Haji Tarkhani AH. The effect of sour tea (Hibiscus sabdariffa) on essential hypertension. J Ethnopharmacol 1999; 65(3): 231-6.

[71]   Ibarrola DA, Ibarrola MH, Vera C, Montalbetti Y, Ferro EA. Hypotensive effect of crude root extract of Solanum sisymbriifolium (Solanaceae) in normo- and hypertensive rats. J Ethnopharmacol 1996; 54(1): 7-12.

[72]   Zaoui A, Cherrah Y, Lacaille-Dubois MA, Settaf A, Amarouch H, Hassar M. [Diuretic and hypotensive effects of Nigella sativa in the spontaneously hypertensive rat]. Therapie 2000; 55(3): 379-82.

[73]   Aydin Y, Kutlay O, Ari S, Duman S, Uzuner K, Aydin S. Hypotensive effects of carvacrol on the blood pressure of normotensive rats. Planta Med 2007; 73(13): 1365-71.

[74]   Chen SJ, Wu BN, Yeh JL, Lo YC, Chen IS, Chen IJ. C-fiber-evoked autonomic cardiovascular effects after injection of Piper betle inflorescence extracts. J Ethnopharmacol 1995; 45(3): 183-8.

[75]   Corallo A, Foungbé S, Davy M, Cohen Y. Cardiovascular pharmacology of aqueous extract of the leaves of Bridelia atroviridis Muell. Arg. (Euphorbiaceae) in the rat. J Ethnopharmacol 1997; 57(3): 189-96.

[76]   Dwivedi S. Terminalia arjuna Wight & Arn.--A useful drug for cardiovascular disorders. J Ethnopharmacol 2007; 114(2): 114-29.

[77]   Gibbons S, Oriowo MA. Antihypertensive effect of an aqueous extract of Zygophyllum coccineum L. in rats. Phytother Res 2001; 15(5): 452-5.

[78]   Gilani AH, Aftab K. Hypotensive and spasmolytic activities of ethanolic extract of Capparis cartilaginea. Phytother Res 1995; 8(3): 145-8.

[79]   Gilani AH, Ghayur MN, Khalid A, Zaheer ul H, Choudhary M, Atta-ur R. Presence of Antispasmodic, Antidiarrheal, Antisecretory, Calcium Antagonist and Acetylcholinesterase Inhibitory Steroidal Alkaloids in Sarcococca saligna. Planta Med 2005; 2: 120-5.

[80]   Kamata K, Noguchi M, Nagai M. Hypotensive effects of lithospermic acid B isolated from the extract of Salviae miltiorrhizae Radix in the rat. Gen Pharmacol 1994; 25(1): 69-73.

[81]   Lahlou S, Magalhaes PJ, Carneiro-Leao RF, Leal-Cardoso JH. Involvement of nitric oxide in the mediation of the hypotensive action of the essential oil of Mentha x villosa in normotensive conscious rats. Planta Med 2002; 68(8): 694-9.

[82] Lahlou S, Magalhaes PJ, de Siqueira RJ, Figueiredo AF, Interaminense LF, Maia JG, Sousa PJ. Cardiovascular effects of the essential oil of Aniba canelilla bark in normotensive rats. J Cardiovasc Pharmacol 2005; 46(4): 412-21.

[83] Legssyer A, Ziyyat A, Mekhfi H, Bnouham M, Tahri A, Serrhouchni M, Hoerter J, Fischmeister R. Cardiovascular effects of Urtica dioica L. in isolated rat heart and aorta. Phytother Res 2002; 16(6): 503-7.

[84] Lima-Landman MT, Borges AC, Cysneiros RM, De Lima TC, Souccar C, Lapa AJ. Antihypertensive effect of a standardized aqueous extract of Cecropia glaziovii Sneth in rats: an *in vivo* approach to the hypotensive mechanism. Phytomedicine 2007; 14(5): 314-20.

[85] Abdul-Ghani AS, Amin R. The vascular action of aqueous extracts of Foeniculum vulgare leaves. J Ethnopharmacol 1988; 24(2-3): 213-8.

[86] Menezes IAC, Moreira ÍJA, Carvalho AA, Antoniolli AR, Santos MRV. Cardiovascular effects of the aqueous extract from Caesalpinia ferrea: Involvement of ATP-sensitive potassium channels. Vasc Pharmacol 2007; 47(1): 41-7.

[87] Ribeiro Rde A, de Barros F, de Melo MM, Muniz C, Chieia S, Wanderley MdG, Gomes C, Trolin G. Acute diuretic effects in conscious rats produced by some medicinal plants used in the state of Sao Paulo, Brasil. J Ethnopharmacol 1988; 24(1): 19-29.

[88] Santos MRV, Carvalho AA, Medeiros IA, Alves PB, Marchioro M, Antoniolli AR. Cardiovascular effects of Hyptis fruticosa essential oil in rats. Fitoterapia 2007; 7 8(3): 186-91.

[89] Tahri A, Yamani S, Legssyer A, Aziz M, Mekhfi H, Bnouham M, Ziyyat A. Acute diuretic, natriuretic and hypotensive effects of a continuous perfusion of aqueous extract of Urtica dioica in the rat. J Ethnopharmacol 2000; 73(1-2): 95-100.

[90] Tanida M, Niijima A, Fukuda Y, Sawai H, Tsuruoka N, Shen J, Yamada S, Kiso Y, Nagai K. Dose-dependent effects of L-carnosine on the renal sympathetic nerve and blood pressure in urethane-anesthetized rats. Am J Physiol Regul Integr Comp Physiol 2005; 288(2): R447-55.

[91] Bellakhdar A, Abi F, Khalidi A, Fadil A, Sibai M, Bouzidi A. A case of post-traumatic intrapericardial hernia in a child. Chir Pediatr 1988; 29(1): 47-9.

[92] Jouad H, Haloui M, Rhiouani H, El Hilaly J, Eddouks M. Ethnobotanical survey of medicinal plants used for the treatment of diabetes, cardiac and renal diseases in the North centre region of Morocco (Fez-Boulemane). J Ethnopharmacol 2001; 77(2-3): 175-82.

[93] Chaiyasit D, Choochote W, Rattanachanpichai E, Chaithong U, Chaiwong P, Jitpakdi A, Tippawangkosol P, Riyong D, Pitasawat B. Essential oils as potential adulticides against two populations of Aedes aegypti, the laboratory and natural field strains, in Chiang Mai province, northern Thailand. Parasitol Res 2006; 99(6): 715-21.

[94] Eddouks M, Lemhadri A, Michel JB. Caraway and caper: potential anti-hyperglycaemic plants in diabetic rats. J Ethnopharmacol 2004; 94(1): 143-8.

[95] Iacobellis NS, Lo Cantore P, Capasso F, Senatore F. Antibacterial activity of Cuminum cyminum L. and Carum carvi L. essential oils. J Agric Food Chem 2005; 53(1): 57-61.

[96] Lado C, Hajdu M, Farkas E, Then M, Taba G, Szentmihalyi K. Study on the transfer of components of Aetheroleum carvi and Aetheroleum foeniculi oils. Fitoterapia 2005; 76(2): 166-72.

[97] Lahlou S, Tahraoui A, Israili Z, Lyoussi B. Diuretic activity of the aqueous extracts of Carum carvi and Tanacetum vulgare in normal rats. J Ethnopharmacol 2007; 110(3): 458-63.

[98]   Luczaj L, Szymanski WM. Wild vascular plants gathered for consumption in the Polish countryside: a review. J Ethnobiol Ethnomed 2007; 3: 17-22.

[99]   Matsumura T, Ishikawa T, Kitajima J. Water-soluble constituents of caraway: aromatic compound, aromatic compound glucoside and glucides. Phytochemistry 2002; 61(4): 455-9.

[100] Naderi-Kalali B, Allameh A, Rasaee MJ, Bach HJ, Behechti A, Doods K, Kettrup A, Schramm KW. Suppressive effects of caraway (Carum carvi) extracts on 2, 3, 7, 8-tetrachloro-dibenzo-p-dioxin-dependent gene expression of cytochrome P450 1A1 in the rat H4IIE cells. Toxicol *In Vitro* 2005; 19(3): 373-7.

[101] Oka Y, Nacar S, Putievsky E, Ravid U, Yaniv Z, Spiegel Y. Nematicidal activity of essential oils and their components against the root-knot nematode. Phytopathology 2000; 90(7): 710-5.

[102] Lemhadri A, Hajji L, Michel JB, Eddouks M. Cholesterol and triglycerides lowering activities of caraway fruits in normal and streptozotocin diabetic rats. J Ethnopharmacol 2006; 106(3): 321-6.

[103] Nakano Y, Matsunaga H, Saita T, Mori M, Katano M, Okabe H. Antiproliferative constituents in Umbelliferae plants II. Screening for polyacetylenes in some Umbelliferae plants, and isolation of panaxynol and falcarindiol from the root of Heracleum moellendorffii. Biol Pharm Bull 1998; 21(3): 257-61.

[104] Park IK, Kim JN, Lee YS, Lee SG, Ahn YJ, Shin SC. Toxicity of plant essential oils and their components against Lycoriella ingenua (Diptera: Sciaridae). J Econ Entomol 2008; 101(1): 139-44.

[105] Pitasawat B, Champakaew D, Choochote W, Jitpakdi A, Chaithong U, Kanjanapothi D, Rattanachanpichai E, Tippawangkosol P, Riyong D, Tuetun B, Chaiyasit D. Aromatic plant-derived essential oil: an alternative larvicide for mosquito control. Fitoterapia 2007; 78(3): 205-10.

[106] Zare M, Shams-Ghahfarokhi M, Ranjbar-Bahadori S, Allameh A, Razzaghi-Abyaneh M. Comparative study of the major Iranian cereal cultivars and some selected spices in relation to support Aspergillus parasiticus growth and aflatoxin production. Iran Biomed J 2008; 12(4): 229-36.

[107] Ali-Shtayeh MS, Jamous RM, Al-Shafie JH, Elgharabah WA, Kherfan FA, Qarariah KH, Khdair IS, Soos IM, Musleh AA, Isa BA, Herzallah HM, Khlaif RB, Aiash SM, Swaiti GM, Abuzahra MA, Haj-Ali MM, Saifi NA, Azem HK, Nasrallah HA. Traditional knowledge of wild edible plants used in Palestine (Northern West Bank): a comparative study. J Ethnobiol Ethnomed 2008; 4: 13-17.

[108] Andrade-Cetto A. Ethnobotanical study of the medicinal plants from Tlanchinol, Hidalgo, Mexico. J Ethnopharmacol 2009; 122(1): 163-71.

[109] Aridogan BC, Baydar H, Kaya S, Demirci M, Ozbasar D, Mumcu E. Antimicrobial activity and chemical composition of some essential oils. Arch Pharm Res 2002; 25(6): 860-4.

[110] Boskabady MH, Khatami A, Nazari A. Possible mechanism(s) for relaxant effects of Foeniculum vulgare on guinea pig tracheal chains. Pharmazie 2004; 59(7): 561-4.

[111] Camacho-Corona Mdel R, Ramirez-Cabrera MA, Santiago OG, Garza-Gonzalez E, Palacios Ide P, Luna-Herrera J. Activity against drug resistant-tuberculosis strains of plants used in Mexican traditional medicine to treat tuberculosis and other respiratory diseases. Phytother Res 2008; 22(1): 82-5.

[112] Choi EM, Hwang JK. Antiinflammatory, analgesic and antioxidant activities of the fruit of Foeniculum vulgare. Fitoterapia 2004; 75(6): 557-65.

[113] Conforti F, Statti G, Uzunov D, Menichini F. Comparative chemical composition and antioxidant activities of wild and cultivated Laurus nobilis L. leaves and Foeniculum vulgare subsp. piperitum (Ucria) coutinho seeds. Biol Pharm Bull 2006; 29(10): 2056-64.

[114] Abdul-Ghani AS, Amin R. The vascular action of aqueous extracts of Foeniculum vulgare leaves. J Ethnopharmacol 1988; 24(2-3): 213-8.

[115] Wright CI, Van-Buren L, Kroner CI, Koning MM. Herbal medicines as diuretics: a review of the scientific evidence. J Ethnopharmacol 2007; 114(1): 1-31.

[116] Baker DD, Alvi KA. Small-molecule natural products: new structures, new activities. Current Opinion in Biotechnology 2004; 15(6):5 76-83.

[117] Balunas MJ, Kinghorn AD. Drug discovery from medicinal plants. Life Sci 2005; 78(5): 431-41.

[118] Baumann IC, Glatzel H, Muth HW. Studies on the effects of wormwood (Artemisia absinthium L.) on bile and pancreatic juice secretion in man. Z Allgemeinmed 1975; 51(17): 784-91.

[119] da Silva JB, Rocha AB. Chemical varieties of Artemisia absinthium L., compositae. Rev Farm Bioquim Univ Sao Paulo 1971; 9(1):101-6.

[120] Juteau F, Jerkovic I, Masotti V, Milos M, Mastelic J, Bessiere JM, Viano J. Composition and antimicrobial activity of the essential oil of Artemisia absinthium from Croatia and France. Planta Med 2003; 69(2): 158-61.

[121] Muto T, Watanabe T, Okamura M, Moto M, Kashida Y, Mitsumori K. Thirteen-week repeated dose toxicity study of wormwood (Artemisia absinthium) extract in rats. J Toxicol Sci 2003; 28(5): 471-8.

[122] Omer B, Krebs S, Omer H, Noor TO. Steroid-sparing effect of wormwood (Artemisia absinthium) in Crohn's disease: a double-blind placebo-controlled study. Phytomedicine 2007; 14(2-3): 87-95.

[123] Abid ZB, Feki M, Hedhili A, Hamdaoui MH. Artemisia herba-alba Asso (Asteraceae) has equivalent effects to green and black tea decoctions on antioxidant processes and some metabolic parameters in rats. Ann Nutr Metab 2007; 51(3): 216-22.

[124] Fenardji F, Klur M, Fourlon C, Ferrando R. White artemisia (Artemisia herba alba L.). Rev Elev Med Vet Pays Trop 1974; 27(2): 203-6.

[125] Hatimi S, Boudouma M, Bichichi M, Chaib N, Idrissi NG. *In vitro* evaluation of antileishmania activity of Artemisia herba alba Asso. Bull Soc Pathol Exot 2001; 94(1): 29-31.

[126] Marrif HI, Ali BH, Hassan KM. Some pharmacological studies on Artemisia herba-alba (Asso.) in rabbits and mice. J Ethnopharmacol 1995; 49(1): 51-5.

[127] Al-Waili NS. Treatment of diabetes mellitus by Artemisia herba-alba extract: preliminary study. Clin Exp Pharmacol Physiol 1986; 13(7): 569-73.

[128] al-Shamaony L, al-Khazraji SM, Twaij HA. Hypoglycaemic effect of Artemisia herba alba. II. Effect of a valuable extract on some blood parameters in diabetic animals. J Ethnopharmacol 1994; 43(3): 167-71.

[129] Twaij HA, Al-Badr AA. Hypoglycemic activity of Artemisia herba alba. J Ethnopharmacol 1988; 24(2-3): 123-6.

[130] Zeggwagh NA, Farid O, Michel JB, Eddouks M. Cardiovascular effect of Artemisia herba alba aqueous extract in spontaneously hypertensive rats. Methods Find Exp Clin Pharmacol 2008; 30(5): 375-81.

[131] Mimica-Dukic N, Kujundzic S, Sokovic M, Couladis M. Essential oil composition and antifungal activity of Foeniculum vulgare Mill obtained by different distillation conditions. Phytother Res 2003; 17(4): 368-71.

[132] Hawrelak JA, Cattley T, Myers SP. Essential oils in the treatment of intestinal dysbiosis: A preliminary *in vitro* study. Altern Med Rev 2009; 14(4): 380-4.

[133] Giosafatto CV, Mariniello L, Ring S. Extraction and characterization of Foeniculum vulgare pectins and their use for preparing biopolymer films in the presence of phaseolin protein. J Agric Food Chem 2007; 55(4): 1237-40.

[134] Fang L, Qi M, Li T, Shao Q, Fu R. Headspace solvent microextraction-gas chromatography-mass spectrometry for the analysis of volatile compounds from Foeniculum vulgare Mill. J Pharm Biomed Anal 2006; 41(3): 791-7.

[135] Alexandrovich I, Rakovitskaya O, Kolmo E, Sidorova T, Shushunov S. The effect of fennel (Foeniculum Vulgare) seed oil emulsion in infantile colic: a randomized, placebo-controlled study. Altern Ther Health Med 2003; 9(4): 58-61.

[136] Maghrani M, Zeggwagh NA, Michel JB, Eddouks M. Antihypertensive effect of Lepidium sativum L. in spontaneously hypertensive rats. J Ethnopharmacol 2005; 100(1-2): 193-7.

[137] Yang T, Liu YQ, Wang CH, Wang ZT. Advances on investigation of chemical constituents, pharmacological activities and clinical applications of Capparis spinosa. Zhongguo Zhong Yao Za Zhi 2008; 33(21): 2453-8.

[138] Tesoriere L, Butera D, Gentile C, Livrea MA. Bioactive components of caper (Capparis spinosa L.) from Sicily and antioxidant effects in a red meat simulated gastric digestion. J Agric Food Chem 2007; 55(21): 8465-71.

[139] Sharaf M, el-Ansari MA, Saleh NA. Quercetin triglycoside from Capparis spinosa. Fitoterapia 2000; 71(1): 46-9.

[140] Ramezani Z, Aghel N, Keyghobadi H. Rutin from different parts of Capparis spinosa growing wild in Khuzestan/Iran. Pak J Biol Sci 2008; 11(5): 768-72.

[141] Perez Pulido R, Omar NB, Lucas R, Abriouel H, Martinez Canamero M, Galvez A. Resistance to antimicrobial agents in lactobacilli isolated from caper fermentations. Antonie Van Leeuwenhoek 2005; 88(3-4): 277-81.

[142] Panico AM, Cardile V, Garufi F, Puglia C, Bonina F, Ronsisvalle G. Protective effect of Capparis spinosa on chondrocytes. Life Sci 2005; 77(20): 2479-88.

[143] Ozcan MM. Investigation on the mineral contents of capers (Capparis spp.) seed oils growing wild in Turkey. J Med Food 2008; 11(3): 596-9.

[144] Matthaus B, Ozcan M. Glucosinolates and fatty acid, sterol, and tocopherol composition of seed oils from Capparis spinosa Var. spinosa and Capparis ovata Desf. Var. canescens (Coss.) Heywood. J Agric Food Chem 2005; 53(18): 7136-41.

[145] Matthaus B, Ozcan M. Glucosinolate composition of young shoots and flower buds of capers (Capparis species) growing wild in Turkey. J Agric Food Chem 2002; 50(25): 7323-5.

[146] Eddouks M, Lemhadri A, Michel JB. Hypolipidemic activity of aqueous extract of Capparis spinosa L. in normal and diabetic rats. J Ethnopharmacol 2005; 98(3): 345-50.

[147] Daradka H, Almasad MM, Qazan W, El-Banna NM, Samara OH. Hypolipidaemic effects of Citrullus colocynthis L. in rabbits. Pak J Biol Sci 2007; 10(16): 2768-71.

[148] Abdel-Hassan IA, Abdel-Barry JA, Tariq Mohammeda S. The hypoglycaemic and antihyperglycaemic effect of citrullus colocynthis fruit aqueous extract in normal and alloxan diabetic rabbits. J Ethnopharmacol 2000; 71(1-2): 325-30.

[149] Al-Momani W, Abu-Basha E, Janakat S, Nicholas RA, Ayling RD. *In vitro* antimycoplasmal activity of six Jordanian medicinal plants against three Mycoplasma species. Trop Anim Health Prod 2007; 39(7): 515-9.

[150] Hadizadeh I, Peivastegan B, Kolahi M. Antifungal activity of nettle (Urtica dioica L.), colocynth (Citrullus colocynthis L. Schrad), oleander (Nerium oleander L.) and konar (Ziziphus spina-christi L.) extracts on plants pathogenic fungi. Pak J Biol Sci 2009; 12(1): 58-63.

[151] Memon U, Brohi AH, Ahmed SW, Azhar I, Bano H. Antibacterial screening of Citrullus colocynthis. Pak J Pharm Sci 2003; 16(1): 1-6.

[152] Tannin-Spitz T, Grossman S, Dovrat S, Gottlieb HE, Bergman M. Growth inhibitory activity of cucurbitacin glucosides isolated from Citrullus colocynthis on human breast cancer cells. Biochem pharmacol 2007; 73(1): 56-67.

[153] Banerjee SP, Dandiya PC. Smooth muscle and cardiovascular pharmacology of alpha-elaterin-2-D-glucopyranoside glycoside of Citrullus colocynthis. J Pharm Sci 1967; 56(12): 1665-7.

[154] Wynne PM, Vine JH, Amiet RG. Protopine alkaloids in horse urine. J Chromatogr B Analyt Technol Biomed Life Sci 2004; 811(1): 85-91.

[155] Brinkhaus B, Hentschel C, Von Keudell C, Schindler G, Lindner M, Stutzer H, Kohnen R, Willich SN, Lehmacher W, Hahn EG. Herbal medicine with curcuma and fumitory in the treatment of irritable bowel syndrome: a randomized, placebo-controlled, double-blind clinical trial. Scand J Gastroenterol 2005; 40(8): 936-43.

[156] Sturm S, Strasser EM, Stuppner H. Quantification of Fumaria officinalis isoquinoline alkaloids by nonaqueous capillary electrophoresis-electrospray ion trap mass spectrometry. J Chromatogr A 2006; 1112(1-2): 331-8.

[157] Petruczynik A, Waksmundzka-Hajnos M, Plech T, Tuzimski T, Hajnos ML, Jozwiak G, Gadzikowska M, Rompala A. TLC of alkaloids on cyanopropyl bonded stationary phases. Part II. Connection with RP18 and silica plates. J Chromatogr Sci 2008; 46(4): 291-7.

[158] Hentschel C, Dressler S, Hahn EG. Fumaria officinalis (fumitory)--clinical applications. Fortschr Med 1995; 113(19): 291-2.

[159] Sengul M, Yildiz H, Gungor N, Cetin B, Eser Z, Ercisli S. Total phenolic content, antioxidant and antimicrobial activities of some medicinal plants. Pak J Pharm Sci 2009; 22(1): 102-6.

[160] Suau R, Cabezudo B, Rico R, Najera F, Lopez-Romero JM. Direct determination of alkaloid contents in Fumaria species by GC-MS. Phytochem Anal 2002; 13(6): 363-7.

[161] Seger C, Sturm S, Strasser EM, Ellmerer E, Stuppner H. 1H and 13C NMR signal assignment of benzylisoquinoline alkaloids from Fumaria officinalis L. (Papaveraceae). Magn Reson Chem 2004; 42(10): 882-6.

[162] El Hilaly J, Israili ZH, Lyoussi B. Acute and chronic toxicological studies of Ajuga iva in experimental animals. J Ethnopharmacol 2004; 91(1): 43-50.

[163] El Hilaly J, Lyoussi B. Hypoglycaemic effect of the lyophilised aqueous extract of Ajuga iva in normal and streptozotocin diabetic rats. J Ethnopharmacol 2002; 80(2-3): 109-13.

[164] El-Hilaly J, Lyoussi B, Wibo M, Morel N. Vasorelaxant effect of the aqueous extract of Ajuga iva in rat aorta. J Ethnopharmacol 2004; 93(1): 69-74.

[165] El-Hilaly J, Tahraoui A, Israili ZH, Lyoussi B. Hypolipidemic effects of acute and sub-chronic administration of an aqueous extract of Ajuga iva L. whole plant in normal and diabetic rats. J Ethnopharmacol 2006; 105(3): 441-8.

[166] El-Hilaly J, Tahraoui A, Israili ZH, Lyoussi B. Acute hypoglycemic, hypocholesterolemic and hypotriglyceridemic effects of continuous intravenous infusion of a lyophilised aqueous extract of Ajuga iva L. Schreber whole plant in streptozotocin-induced diabetic rats. Pak J Pharm Sci 2007; 20(4): 261-8.

[167] Bennaghmouch L, Hajjaji N, Zellou A, Cherrah Y. Pharmacological study of Ajuga iva. Ann Pharm Fr 2001; 59(4): 284.

[168] Bondi ML, Al-Hillo MR, Lamara K, Ladjel S, Bruno M, Piozzi F, Simmonds MS. Occurrence of the antifeedant 14,15-dihydroajugapitin in the aerial parts of Ajuga iva from Algeria. Biochem Syst Ecol 2000; 28(10): 1023-5.

[169] Novaes AP, Rossi C, Poffo C, Pretti Junior E, Oliveira AE, Schlemper V, Niero R, Cechinel-Filho V, Burger C. Preliminary evaluation of the hypoglycemic effect of some Brazilian medicinal plants. Therapie 2001; 56(4): 427-30.

[170] Sahpaz S, Garbacki N, Tits M, Bailleul F. Isolation and pharmacological activity of phenylpropanoid esters from Marrubium vulgare. J Ethnopharmacol 2002; 79(3): 389-92.

[171] Herrera-Arellano A, Aguilar-Santamaria L, Garcia-Hernandez B, Nicasio-Torres P, Tortoriello J. Clinical trial of Cecropia obtusifolia and Marrubium vulgare leaf extracts on blood glucose and serum lipids in type 2 diabetics. Phytomedicine 2004; 11(7-8): 561-6.

[172] Knoss W, Reuter B, Zapp J. Biosynthesis of the labdane diterpene marrubiin in Marrubium vulgare *via* a non-mevalonate pathway. Biochem J 1997; 326 (Pt 2): 449-54.

[173] Meyre-Silva C, Yunes RA, Schlemper V, Campos-Buzzi F, Cechinel-Filho V. Analgesic potential of marrubiin derivatives, a bioactive diterpene present in Marrubium vulgare (Lamiaceae). Farmaco 2005; 60(4): 321-6.

[174] Roman Ramos R, Alarcon-Aguilar F, Lara-Lemus A, Flores-Saenz JL. Hypoglycemic effect of plants used in Mexico as antidiabetics. Arch Med Res 1992; 23(1): 59-64.

[175] El Bardai S, Lyoussi B, Wibo M, Morel N. Pharmacological evidence of hypotensive activity of Marrubium vulgare and Foeniculum vulgare in spontaneously hypertensive rat. Clin Exp Hypertens 2001; 23(4): 329-43.

[176] Gutierrez R, Alvarado JL, Presno M, Perez-Veyna O, Serrano CJ, Yahuaca P. Oxidative stress modulation by Rosmarinus officinalis in CCl(4)-induced liver cirrhosis. Phytother Res 2010; 24(4): 595-601.

[177] Harach T, Aprikian O, Monnard I, Moulin J, Membrez M, Beolor JC, Raab T, Mace K, Darimont C. Rosemary (Rosmarinus officinalis L.) Leaf Extract Limits Weight Gain and Liver Steatosis in Mice Fed a High-Fat Diet. Planta Med 2010; 76(6): 566-71.

[178] Khater HF, Ramadan MY, El-Madawy RS. Lousicidal, ovicidal and repellent efficacy of some essential oils against lice and flies infesting water buffaloes in Egypt. Vet Parasitol 2009; 164(2-4): 257-66.

[179] Klancnik A, Guzej B, Kolar MH, Abramovic H, Mozina SS. *In vitro* antimicrobial and antioxidant activity of commercial rosemary extract formulations. J Food Prot 2009; 72(8): 1744-52.

[180] Machado DG, Bettio LE, Cunha MP, Capra JC, Dalmarco JB, Pizzolatti MG, Rodrigues AL. Antidepressant-like effect of the extract of Rosmarinus officinalis in mice: involvement of the monoaminergic system. Prog Neuropsychopharmacol Biol Psychiatry 2009; 33(4): 642-50.

[181] Posadas SJ, Caz V, Largo C, De la Gandara B, Matallanas B, Reglero G, De Miguel E. Protective effect of supercritical fluid rosemary extract, Rosmarinus officinalis, on antioxidants of major organs of aged rats. Exp Gerontol 2009; 44(6-7): 383-9.

[182] Tada M, Ohkanda T, Kurabe J. Syntheses of carnosic acid and carnosol, anti-oxidants in Rosemary, from pisiferic acid, the major constituent of Sawara. Chem Pharm Bull (Tokyo) 2010; 58(1): 27-9.

[183] Ormeno E, Olivier R, Mevy JP, Baldy V, Fernandez C. Compost may affect volatile and semi-volatile plant emissions through nitrogen supply and chlorophyll fluorescence. Chemosphere 2009; 77(1): 94-104.

[184] Perez-Fons L, Garzon MT, Micol V. Relationship between the antioxidant capacity and effect of rosemary (Rosmarinus officinalis L.) polyphenols on membrane phospholipid order. J Agric Food Chem 2010; 58(1): 161-71.

[185] Topal U, Sasaki M, Goto M, Otles S. Chemical compositions and antioxidant properties of essential oils from nine species of Turkish plants obtained by supercritical carbon dioxide extraction and steam distillation. Int J Food Sci Nutr 2008; 59(7-8): 619-34.

[186] van Vuuren SF, Suliman S, Viljoen AM. The antimicrobial activity of four commercial essential oils in combination with conventional antimicrobials. Lett Appl Microbiol 2009; 48(4): 440-6.

[187] Rasooli I, Mirmostafa SA. Antibacterial properties of Thymus pubescens and Thymus serpyllum essential oils. Fitoterapia 2002; 73(3): 244-50.

[188] Sourgens H, Winterhoff H, Gumbinger HG, Kemper FH. Antihormonal effects of plant extracts. Planta Med 1982; 45(6): 78-86.

[189] Stahl-Biskup E, Laakso I. Essential Oil Polymorphism in Finnish Thymus Species. Planta Med 1990; 56(5): 464-8.

[190] Mihajlov M, Tucakov J. Pharmacognostic study of the medicinal flora in Southeast Bosnia. Thymus serpyllum L. IV. Glas Srp Akad Nauka Med 1969; (22): 43-58.

[191] Oh SY, Ko JW, Jeong SY, Hong J. Application and exploration of fast gas chromatography-surface acoustic wave sensor to the analysis of thymus species. J Chromatogr A 2008; 1205(1-2): 117-27.

[192] Paaver U, Orav A, Arak E, Maeorg U, Raal A. Phytochemical analysis of the essential oil of Thymus serpyllum L. growing wild in Estonia. Nat Prod Res 2008; 22(2): 108-15.

[193] Alzoreky NS, Nakahara K. Antibacterial activity of extracts from some edible plants commonly consumed in Asia. Int J Food Microbiol 2003; 80(3): 223-30.

[194] Arpadjan S, Celik G, Taskesen S, Gucer S. Arsenic, cadmium and lead in medicinal herbs and their fractionation. Food Chem Toxicol 2008; 46(8): 2871-5.

[195] Isman MB, Wan AJ, Passreiter CM. Insecticidal activity of essential oils to the tobacco cutworm, Spodoptera litura. Fitoterapia 2001; 72(1): 65-8.

[196] Jaric S, Popovic Z, Macukanovic-Jocic M, Djurdjevic L, Mijatovic M, Karadzic B, Mitrovic M, Pavlovic P. An ethno*botanical* study on the usage of wild medicinal herbs from Kopaonik Mountain (Central Serbia). J Ethnopharmacol 2007; 111(1): 160-75.

[197] Loziene K, Vaiciuniene J, Venskutonis PR. Chemical composition of the essential oil of creeping thyme (Thymus serpyllum s.l.) growing wild in Lithuania. Planta Med 1998; 64(8): 772-3.

[198] Raal A, Paaver U, Arak E, Orav A. Content and composition of the essential oil of Thymus serpyllum L. growing wild in Estonia. Medicina (Kaunas) 2004; 40(8): 795-800.

[199] Schratz E, Qedan S. Composition of the ethereal oil in the collective genus Thymus serpyllum. Thin-layer chromatographic proof of oil components. Pharmazie 1965; 20(11): 710-3.

[200] van den Berg LJ, Peters CJ, Ashmore MR, Roelofs JG. Reduced nitrogen has a greater effect than oxidised nitrogen on dry heathland vegetation. Environ Pollut 2008; 154(3): 359-69.

[201] Verma RS, Rahman L, Chanotiya CS, Verma RK, Singh A, Yadav A, Chauhan A, Yadav AK, Singh AK. Essential oil composition of Thymus serpyllum cultivated in the Kumaon region of western Himalaya, India. Nat Prod Commun 2009; 4(7): 987-8.

[202] Cavara S, Maksimovic M, Vidic D. The essential oil of Thymus aureopunctatus (Beck) K. Maly. Nat Prod Commun 2009; 4(3): 415-20.

[203] Haas LF. Thymus serpyllum (wild thyme). J Neurol Neurosurg Psychiatry 1996; 60(2): 224-9.

[204] Oral N, Gulmez M, Vatansever L, Guven A. Application of antimicrobial ice for extending shelf life of fish. J Food Prot 2008; 71(1): 218-22.

[205] Bang MA, Kim HA, Cho YJ. Alterations in the blood glucose, serum lipids and renal oxidative stress in diabetic rats by supplementation of onion (Allium cepa. Linn). Nutr Res Pract 2009; 3(3): 242-6.

[206] Kaiser P, Youssouf MS, Tasduq SA, Singh S, Sharma SC, Singh GD, Gupta VK, Gupta BD, Johri RK. Anti-allergic effects of herbal product from Allium cepa (bulb). J Med Food 2009; 12(2): 374-82.

[207] Khaki A, Fathiazad F, Nouri M, Khaki AA, Khamenehi HJ, Hamadeh M. Evaluation of androgenic activity of allium cepa on spermatogenesis in the rat. Folia Morphol (Warsz) 2009; 68(1): 45-51.

[208] Kitajima A, Asatsuma S, Okada H, Hamada Y, Kaneko K, Nanjo Y, Kawagoe Y, Toyooka K, Matsuoka K, Takeuchi M, Nakano A, Mitsui T. The rice alpha-amylase glycoprotein is targeted from the Golgi apparatus through the secretory pathway to the plastids. Plant Cell 2009; 21(9): 2844-58.

[209] Leme DM, Marin-Morales MA. Allium cepa test in environmental monitoring: a review on its application. Mutat Res 2009; 682(1): 71-81.

[210] Magdaleno A, Mendelson A, de Iorio AF, Rendina A, Moretton J. Genotoxicity of leachates from highly polluted lowland river sediments destined for disposal in landfill. Waste Manag 2008; 28(11): 2134-9.

[211] Rodriguez Galdon B, Rodriguez Rodriguez EM, Diaz Romero C. Flavonoids in onion cultivars (Allium cepa L.). J Food Sci 2008; 73(8): C599-605.

[212] Naseri MK, Arabian M, Badavi M, Ahangarpour A. Vasorelaxant and hypotensive effects of Allium cepa peel hydroalcoholic extract in rat. Pak J Biol Sci 2008; 11(12): 1569-75.

[213] Ola-Mudathir KF, Suru SM, Fafunso MA, Obioha UE, Faremi TY. Protective roles of onion and garlic extracts on cadmium-induced changes in sperm characteristics and testicular oxidative damage in rats. Food Chem Toxicol 2008; 46(12): 3604-11.

[214] Ali M, Thomson M, Afzal M. Garlic and onions: their effect on eicosanoid metabolism and its clinical relevance. Prostaglandins Leukot Essent Fatty Acids 2000; 62(2): 55-73.

[215] Haidari F, Rashidi MR, Eshraghian MR, Mahboob SA, Shahi MM, Keshavarz SA. Hypouricemic and antioxidant activities of Allium cepa Lilliaceae and quercetin in normal and hyperuricemic rats. Saudi Med J 2008; 29(11): 1573-9.

[216] Wiczkowski W, Romaszko J, Bucinski A, Szawara-Nowak D, Honke J, Zielinski H, Piskula MK. Quercetin from shallots (Allium cepa L. var. aggregatum) is more bioavailable than its glucosides. J Nutr 2008; 138(5): 885-8.

[217] Abdalla FH, Belle LP, De Bona KS, Bitencourt PE, Pigatto AS, Moretto MB. Allium sativum L. extract prevents methyl mercury-induced cytotoxicity in peripheral blood leukocytes (LS). Food Chem Toxicol 2010; 48(1): 417-21.

[218] Antioxidant properties of essential oils. Prikl Biokhim Mikrobiol 2009; 45(6): 710-6.

[219] El-Beshbishy HA. Aqueous garlic extract attenuates hepatitis and oxidative stress induced by galactosamine/lipoploysaccharide in rats. Phytother Res 2008; 22(10): 1372-9.

[220] Macias FA, Lacret R, Varela RM, Nogueiras C, Molinillo JM. Bioactive apocarotenoids from Tectona grandis. Phytochemistry 2008; 69(15): 2708-15.

[221] Iciek M, Kwiecien I, Wlodek L. Biological properties of garlic and garlic-derived organosulfur compounds. Environ Mol Mutagen 2009; 50(3): 247-65.

[222] Chakraborti D, Sarkar A, Mondal HA, Schuermann D, Hohn B, Sarmah BK, Das S. Cre/lox system to develop selectable marker free transgenic tobacco plants conferring resistance against sap sucking homopteran insect. Plant Cell Rep 2008; 27(10): 1623-33.

[223] Hui C, Jun W, Ya LN, Ming X. Effect of Allium sativum (garlic) diallyl disulfide (DADS) on human non-small cell lung carcinoma H1299 cells. Trop Biomed 2008; 25(1): 37-45.

[224] Das Gupta A, Das SN, Dhundasi SA, Das KK. Effect of garlic (Allium sativum) on heavy metal (nickel II and chromium VI) induced alteration of serum lipid profile in male albino rats. Int J Environ Res Public Health 2008; 5(3): 147-51.

[225] Koo HN, Um JY, Kim HM, Lee EH, Sung HJ, Kim IK, Jeong HJ, Hong SH. Effect of pilopool on forced swimming test in mice. Int J Neurosci 2008; 118(3): 365-74.

[226] Guarrera PM, Lucchese F, Medori S. Ethnophytotherapeutical research in the high Molise region (Central-Southern Italy). J Ethnobiol Ethnomed 2008; 4: 7-12.

[227] Lissiman E, Bhasale AL, Cohen M. Garlic for the common cold. Cochrane Database Syst Rev 2009(3): CD006206.

[228] Drobiova H, Thomson M, Al-Qattan K, Peltonen-Shalaby R, Al-Amin Z, Ali M. Garlic Increases Antioxidant Levels in Diabetic and Hypertensive Rats Determined by a Modified Peroxidase Method. Evid Based Complement Alternat. In Press.

[229] Kim JY, Kwon O. Garlic intake and cancer risk: an analysis using the Food and Drug Administration's evidence-based review system for the scientific evaluation of health claims. Am J Clin Nutr 2009; 89(1): 257-64.

[230] Butt MS, Sultan MT, Iqbal J. Garlic: nature's protection against physiological threats. Crit Rev Food Sci Nutr 2009; 49(6): 538-51.

[231] Kang MH, Park HM. Hypertension after Ingestion of Baked Garlic (Allium sativum) in a Dog. J Vet Med Sci 2010 ;72(4): 515-8.

[232] Dwivedi S, Aggarwal A. Indigenous drugs in ischemic heart disease in patients with diabetes. J Altern Complement Med 2009; 15(11): 1215-21.

[233] Hammami I, Nahdi A, Mauduit C, Benahmed M, Amri M, Ben Amar A, Zekri S, El May A, El May MV. The inhibitory effects on adult male reproductive functions of crude garlic (Allium sativum) feeding. Asian J Androl 2008; 10(4): 593-601.

[234] Lans C, Turner N, Khan T. Medicinal plant treatments for fleas and ear problems of cats and dogs in British Columbia, Canada. Parasitol Res 2008;103(4): 889-98.

[235] Khatoon H, Talat S, Younus H. Phospholipase D from Allium sativum bulbs: A highly active and thermal stable enzyme. Int J Biol Macromol 2008; 42(4): 380-5.

[236] Brunetti L, Menghini L, Orlando G, Recinella L, Leone S, Epifano F, Lazzarin F, Chiavaroli A, Ferrante C, Vacca M. Antioxidant effects of garlic in young and aged rat brain *in vitro*. J Med Food 2009; 12(5): 1166-9.

[237] Belle LP, De Bona KS, Abdalla FH, Pimentel VC, Pigatto AS, Moretto MB. Comparative evaluation of adenosine deaminase activity in cerebral cortex and hippocampus of young and adult rats: effect of garlic extract (Allium sativum L.) on their susceptibility to heavy metal exposure. Basic Clin Pharmacol Toxicol 2009; 104(5): 408-13.

[238] Rosa A, Deiana M, Casu V, Corona G, Appendino G, Bianchi F, Ballero M, Dessi MA. Antioxidant activity of oligomeric acylphloroglucinols from Myrtus communis L. Free Radic Res 2003; 37(9): 1013-9.

[239] Yadegarinia D, Gachkar L, Rezaei MB, Taghizadeh M, Astaneh SA, Rasooli I. Biochemical activities of Iranian Mentha piperita L. and Myrtus communis L. essential oils. Phytochemistry 2006; 67(12): 1249-55.

[240] Sepici A, Gurbuz I, Cevik C, Yesilada E. Hypoglycaemic effects of myrtle oil in normal and alloxan-diabetic rabbits. J Ethnopharmacol 2004; 93(2-3): 311-8.

[241] Deriu A, Branca G, Molicotti P, Pintore G, Chessa M, Tirillini B, Paglietti B, Mura A, Sechi LA, Fadda G, Zanetti S. *In vitro* activity of essential oil of Myrtus communis L. against Helicobacter pylori. Int J Antimicrob Agents 2007; 30(6): 562-3.

[242] Hayder N, Bouhlel I, Skandrani I, Kadri M, Steiman R, Guiraud P, Mariotte AM, Ghedira K, Dijoux-Franca MG, Chekir-Ghedira L. *In vitro* antioxidant and antigenotoxic potentials of myricetin-3-o-galactoside and myricetin-3-o-rhamnoside from Myrtus communis: modulation of expression of genes involved in cell defence system using cDNA microarray. Toxicol *In Vitro* 2008; 22(3): 567-81.

[243] Ruffoni B, Mascarello C, Savona M. *In vitro* propagation of ornamental myrtus (Myrtus communis). Methods Mol Biol 2010; 589: 257-69.

[244] Sacchetti G, Muzzoli M, Statti GA, Conforti F, Bianchi A, Agrimonti C, Ballero M, Poli F. Intra-specific biodiversity of Italian myrtle (Myrtus communis) through chemical markers profile and biological activities of leaf methanolic extracts. Nat Prod Res 2007; 21(2): 167-79.

[245] Tattini M, Remorini D, Pinelli P, Agati G, Saracini E, Traversi ML, Massai R. Morpho-anatomical, physiological and biochemical adjustments in response to root zone salinity stress and high solar radiation in two Mediterranean evergreen shrubs, Myrtus communis and Pistacia lentiscus. New Phytol 2006; 170(4): 779-94.

[246] Rossi A, Di Paola R, Mazzon E, Genovese T, Caminiti R, Bramanti P, Pergola C, Koeberle A, Werz O, Sautebin L, Cuzzocrea S. Myrtucommulone from Myrtus communis exhibits potent anti-inflammatory effectiveness *in vivo*. J Pharmacol Exp Ther 2009; 329(1): 76-86.

[247] Yoshimura M, Amakura Y, Tokuhara M, Yoshida T. Polyphenolic compounds isolated from the leaves of Myrtus communis. J Nat Med 2008; 62(3): 366-8.

[248] Rosa A, Melis MP, Deiana M, Atzeri A, Appendino G, Corona G, Incani A, Loru D, Dessi MA. Protective effect of the oligomeric acylphloroglucinols from Myrtus communis on cholesterol and human low density lipoprotein oxidation. Chem Phys Lipids 2008; 155(1): 16-23.

[249] Onal S, Timur S, Okutucu B, Zihnioglu F. Inhibition of alpha-glucosidase by aqueous extracts of some potent antidiabetic medicinal herbs. Prep Biochem Biotechnol 2005; 35(1): 29-36.

[250] Pinna W, Nieddu G, Moniello G, Cappai MG. Vegetable and animal food sorts found in the gastric content of Sardinian Wild Boar (Sus scrofa meridionalis). J Anim Physiol Anim Nutr (Berl) 2007; 91(5-6): 252-5.

[251] Bacles CF, Burczyk J, Lowe AJ, Ennos RA. Historical and contemporary mating patterns in remnant populations of the forest tree Fraxinus excelsior L. Evolution 2005; 59(5): 979-90.

[252] Bai N, He K, Ibarra A, Bily A, Roller M, Chen X, Ruhl R. Iridoids from Fraxinus excelsior with adipocyte differentiation-inhibitory and PPARalpha activation activity. J Nat Prod 2010; 73(1): 2-6.

[253] Eddouks M, Maghrani M. Phlorizin-like effect of Fraxinus excelsior in normal and diabetic rats. J Ethnopharmacol 2004; 94(1): 149-54.

[254] Hrabina M, Purohit A, Oster JP, Papanikolaou I, Jain K, Pascal P, Sicard H, Gouyon B, Moingeon P, Pauli G, Andre C. Standardization of an ash (Fraxinus excelsior) pollen allergen extract. Int Arch Allergy Immunol 2007; 142(1):11-8.

[255] Eddouks M, Maghrani M, Zeggwagh NA, Haloui M, Michel JB. Fraxinus excelsior L. evokes a hypotensive action in normal and spontaneously hypertensive rats. J Ethnopharmacol 2005; 99(1): 49-54.

[256] Weyens N, Taghavi S, Barac T, van der Lelie D, Boulet J, Artois T, Carleer R, Vangronsveld J. Bacteria associated with oak and ash on a TCE-contaminated site: characterization of isolates with potential to avoid evapotranspiration of TCE. Environ Sci Pollut Res Int 2009; 16(7): 830-43.

[257] Herbst M, Rosier PT, Morecroft MD, Gowing DJ. Comparative measurements of transpiration and canopy conductance in two mixed deciduous woodlands differing in structure and species composition. Tree Physiol 2008; 28(6): 959-70.

[258] Ridolfi M, Terenziani S, Patumi M, Fontanazza G. Characterization of the lipoxygenases in some olive cultivars and determination of their role in volatile compounds formation. J Agric Food Chem 2002; 50(4): 835-9.

[259] Barbouche N, Couillaud F, Girardie J, Ammar M, Ben Hammouda MH. [Effect of olive leaves (Olea europea) feeding on the *in vitro* JH III biosynthesis by the corpora allata in Schistocerca gregaria during vitellogenesis]. Arch Inst Pasteur Tunis 1996; 73(1-2): 9-12.

[260] Bennani-Kabchi N, Fdhil H, Cherrah Y, Kehel L, el Bouayadi F, Amarti A, Saidi M, Marquie G. Effects of Olea europea var. oleaster leaves in hypercholesterolemic insulin-resistant sand rats. Therapie 1999; 54(6): 717-23.

[261] Panzani RC, Mercier P, Delord Y, Riva G, Falagiani P, Reviron D, Auquier P. Prevalence of patent and latent atopy among a general normal adult population in the south east of France by RAST investigation and correlation with circulating total IgE levels. Allergol Immunopathol 1993; 21(6): 211-9.

[262] Reyes FJ, Centelles JJ, Lupianez JA, Cascante M. (2Alpha,3beta)-2,3-dihydroxyolean-12-en-28-oic acid, a new natural triterpene from Olea europea, induces caspase dependent apoptosis selectively in colon adenocarcinoma cells. FEBS Lett 2006; 580(27): 6302-10.

[263] Gilani AH, Khan AU, Shah AJ, Connor J, Jabeen Q. Blood pressure lowering effect of olive is mediated through calcium channel blockade. Int J Food Sci Nutr 2005; 56(8): 613-20.

[264] Shibli RA, Al-Juboory KH. Cryopreservation of 'Nabali' olive (Olea europea l.) somatic embryos by encapsulation-dehydration and encapsulation-vitrification. Cryo Letters 2000; 21(6): 357-66.

[265] Kontothanasi G, Moschovakis E, Tararas V, Delis A, Anagnostou E. Determination of sensitivity of inhalant allergens in patients with allergic rhinitis in West Athens. Rhinology 1995; 33(4): 234-5.

[266] Di Lorenzo G, Mansueto P, Pacor ML, Rizzo M, Castello F, Martinelli N, Ditta V, Lo Bianco C, Leto-Barone MS, D'Alcamo A, Di Fede G, Rini GB, Ditto AM. Evaluation of serum s-IgE/total IgE ratio in predicting clinical response to allergen-specific immunotherapy. J Allergy Clin Immunol 2009; 123(5): 1103-10.

[267]   Roman Perez F, Berlanga Cortes JA, Urquia M, Guerra Pasadas F, Pena Martinez J. [Human basophil degranulation test. Results of a modified technic (I)]. Allergol Immunopathol 1986; 14(4): 287-93.

[268]   Pereira JA, Casal S, Bento A, Oliveira MB. Influence of olive storage period on oil quality of three Portuguese cultivars of Olea europea, Cobrancosa, Madural, and Verdeal Transmontana. J Agric Food Chem 2002; 50(22): 6335-40.

[269]   Sensoz S, Demiral I, Ferdi Gercel H. Olive bagasse (Olea europea L.) pyrolysis. Bioresour Technol 2006; 97(3): 429-36.

[270]   Bello R, Moreno L, Primo-Yufera E, Esplugues J. Globularia alypum L. extracts reduced histamine and serotonin contraction *in vitro*. Phytother Res 2002; 16(4): 389-92.

[271]   Caldes G, Prescott B, King JR. A potential antileukemic substance present in Globularia alypum. Planta Med 1975; 27(1): 72-6.

[272]   Jouad H, Maghrani M, Eddouks M. Hypoglycaemic effect of Rubus fructicosis L. and Globularia alypum L. in normal and streptozotocin-induced diabetic rats. J Ethnopharmacol 2002; 81(3): 351-6.

[273]   Al Mofleh IA, Alhaider AA, Mossa JS, Al-Sohaibani MO, Al-Yahya MA, Rafatullah S, Shaik SA. Gastroprotective effect of an aqueous suspension of black cumin Nigella sativa on necrotizing agents-induced gastric injury in experimental animals. Saudi J Gastroenterol 2008; 14(3): 128-34.

[274]   Benhaddou-Andaloussi A, Martineau LC, Vallerand D, Haddad Y, Afshar A, Settaf A, Haddad PS. Multiple molecular targets underlie the antidiabetic effect of Nigella sativa seed extract in skeletal muscle, adipocyte and liver cells. Diabetes Obes Metab 2010; 12(2): 148-57.

[275]   Effenberger K, Breyer S, Schobert R. Terpene conjugates of the Nigella sativa seed-oil constituent thymoquinone with enhanced efficacy in cancer cells. Chem Biodivers 2010; 7(1): 129-39.

[276]   Goncagul G, Ayaz E. Antimicrobial Effect of Garlic (Allium sativum). Recent Pat Antiinfect Drug Discov 2010; 5(1): 91-3.

[277]   Hannan A, Saleem S, Chaudhary S, Barkaat M, Arshad MU. Anti bacterial activity of Nigella sativa against clinical isolates of methicillin resistant Staphylococcus aureus. J Ayub Med Coll Abbottabad 2008; 20(3): 72-4.

[278]   Keyhanmanesh R, Boskabady MH, Eslamizadeh MJ, Khamneh S, Ebrahimi MA. The Effect of Thymoquinone, the Main Constituent of Nigella sativa on Tracheal Responsiveness and White Blood Cell Count in Lung Lavage of Sensitized Guinea Pigs. Planta Med 2010; 76(3): 218-22.

[279]   Pari L, Sankaranarayanan C. Beneficial effects of thymoquinone on hepatic key enzymes in streptozotocin-nicotinamide induced diabetic rats. Life Sci 2009; 85(23-26): 830-4.

[280]   Ravindran J, Nair HB, Sung B, Prasad S, Tekmal RR, Aggarwal BB. Thymoquinone Poly(lactide-co-glycolide) Nanoparticles Exhibit Enhanced Anti-proliferative, Anti-inflammatory, and Chemosensitization Potential. Biochemical pharmacology 2010; 79(11): 1640-7

[281]   Xuan NT, Shumilina E, Qadri SM, Gotz F, Lang F. Effect of Thymoquinone on Mouse Dendritic Cells. Cell Physiol Biochem 2010; 25(2-3): 307-14.

[282]   Ali BH, Blunden G. Pharmacological and toxicological properties of Nigella sativa. Phytother Res 2003; 17(4): 299-305.

[283] Dehkordi FR, Kamkhah AF. Antihypertensive effect of Nigella sativa seed extract in patients with mild hypertension. Fundam Clin Pharmacol 2008; 22(4): 447-52.

[284] el Tahir KE, Ashour MM, al-Harbi MM. The cardiovascular actions of the volatile oil of the black seed (Nigella sativa) in rats: elucidation of the mechanism of action. Gen Pharmacol 1993; 24(5): 1123-31.

[285] Tennie C, Hedwig D, Call J, Tomasello M. An experimental study of nettle feeding in captive gorillas. Am J Primatol 2008; 70(6): 584-93.

[286] Turker AU, Usta C. Biological screening of some Turkish medicinal plant extracts for antimicrobial and toxicity activities. Nat Prod Res 2008; 22(2): 136-46.

[287] Lans C, Turner N, Khan T, Brauer G, Boepple W. Ethnoveterinary medicines used for ruminants in British Columbia, Canada. J Ethnobiol Ethnomed 2007; 3: 11.

[288] Otoom SA, Al-Safi SA, Kerem ZK, Alkofahi A. The use of medicinal herbs by diabetic Jordanian patients. J Herb Pharmacother 2006; 6(2): 31-41.

[289] Pacifico D, Alma A, Bagnoli B, Foissac X, Pasquini G, Tessitori M, Marzachi C. Characterization of Bois noir isolates by restriction fragment length polymorphism of a Stolbur-specific putative membrane protein gene. Phytopathology 2009; 99(6): 711-5.

[290] Rodriguez-Fragoso L, Reyes-Esparza J, Burchiel SW, Herrera-Ruiz D, Torres E. Risks and benefits of commonly used herbal medicines in Mexico. Toxicol Appl Pharmacol 2008; 227(1): 125-35.

[291] Tarhan O, Alacacioglu A, Somali I, Sipahi H, Zencir M, Oztop I, Dirioz M, Yilmaz U. Complementary-alternative medicine among cancer patients in the western region of Turkey. J BUON 2009; 14(2): 265-9.

[292] Criado PR, Criado RF, Valente NY, Queiroz LB, Martins JE, Vasconcellos C. The inflammatory response in drug-induced acute urticaria: ultrastructural study of the dermal microvascular unit. J Eur Acad Dermatol Venereol 2006; 20(9): 1095-9.

[293] Domola MS, Vu V, Robson-Doucette CA, Sweeney G, Wheeler MB. Insulin mimetics in Urtica dioica: structural and computational analyses of Urtica dioica extracts. Phytother Res 2010; 24: S175-82.

[294] Francois KO, Auwerx J, Schols D, Balzarini J. Simian immunodeficiency virus is susceptible to inhibition by carbohydrate-binding agents in a manner similar to that of HIV: implications for further preclinical drug development. Mol Pharmacol 2008; 74(2): 330-7.

[295] Doetkotte R, Opitz K, Kiianmaa K, Winterhoff H. Reduction of voluntary ethanol consumption in alcohol-preferring Alko alcohol (AA) rats by desoxypeganine and galanthamine. Eur J Pharmacol 2005; 522(1-3): 72-7.

[296] Fan B, Liang J, Men J, Gao F, Li G, Zhao S, Hu T, Dang P, Zhang L. Effect of total alkaloid of Peganum harmala L. in the treatment of experimental haemosporidian infections in cattle. Trop Anim Health Prod 1997; 29(4 Suppl): 77S-83S.

[297] Farouk L, Laroubi A, Aboufatima R, Benharref A, Chait A. Evaluation of the analgesic effect of alkaloid extract of Peganum harmala L.: possible mechanisms involved. J Ethnopharmacol 2008; 115(3): 449-54.

[298] Hamouda C, Amamou M, Thabet H, Yacoub M, Hedhili A, Bescharnia F, Ben Salah N, Zhioua M, Abdelmoumen S, El Mekki Ben Brahim N. Plant poisonings from herbal medication admitted to a Tunisian toxicologic intensive care unit, 1983-1998. Vet Hum Toxicol 2000; 42(3): 137-41.

[299] Harsh ML, Nag TN. Antimicrobial principles from *in vitro* tissue culture of Peganum harmala. J Nat Prod 1984; 47(2): 365-7.

[300] Im JH, Jin YR, Lee JJ, Yu JY, Han XH, Im SH, Hong JT, Yoo HS, Pyo MY, Yun YP. Antiplatelet activity of beta-carboline alkaloids from Perganum harmala: a possible mechanism through inhibiting PLCgamma2 phosphorylation. Vascul Pharmacol 2009; 50(5-6): 147-52.

[301] Kartal M, Altun ML, Kurucu S. HPLC method for the analysis of harmol, harmalol, harmine and harmaline in the seeds of Peganum harmala L. J Pharm Biomed Anal 2003; 31(2): 263-9.

[302] Khaliq T, Misra P, Gupta S, Reddy KP, Kant R, Maulik PR, Dube A, Narender T. Peganine hydrochloride dihydrate an orally active antileishmanial agent. Bioorg Med Chem Lett 2009; 19(9): 2585-6.

[303] Koko WS, Mesaik MA, Yousaf S, Galal M, Choudhary MI. *In vitro* immunomodulating properties of selected Sudanese medicinal plants. J Ethnopharmacol 2008; 118(1): 26-34.

[304] Lamchouri F, Settaf A, Cherrah Y, El Hamidi M, Tligui N, Lyoussi B, Hassar M. Experimental toxicity of Peganum harmala seeds. Ann Pharm Fr 2002; 60(2): 123-9.

[305] Lamchouri F, Settaf A, Cherrah Y, Zemzami M, Lyoussi B, Zaid A, Atif N, Hassar M. Antitumour principles from Peganum harmala seeds. Therapie 1999; 54(6): 753-8.

[306] Monsef HR, Ghobadi A, Iranshahi M, Abdollahi M. Antinociceptive effects of Peganum harmala L. alkaloid extract on mouse formalin test. J Pharm Pharm Sci 2004; 7(1): 65-9.

[307] Pieroni A, Muenz H, Akbulut M, Baser KH, Durmuskahya C. Traditional phytotherapy and trans-cultural pharmacy among Turkish migrants living in Cologne, Germany. J Ethnopharmacol 2005; 102(1): 69-88.

[308] Shahverdi AR, Monsef-Esfahani HR, Nickavar B, Bitarafan L, Khodaee S, Khoshakhlagh N. Antimicrobial activity and main chemical composition of two smoke condensates from Peganum harmala seeds. Z Naturforsch C2005; 60(9-10): 707-10.

[309] Sharaf M, el-Ansari MA, Matlin SA, Saleh NA. Four flavonoid glycosides from Peganum harmala. Phytochemistry 1997; 44(3): 533-6.

[310] Wang X, Geng Y, Wang D, Shi X, Liu J. Separation and purification of harmine and harmaline from Peganum harmala using pH-zone-refining counter-current chromatography. J Sep Sci 2008; 31(20): 3543-7.

[311] Berrougui H, Herrera-Gonzalez MD, Marhuenda E, Ettaib A, Hmamouchi M. Relaxant activity of methanolic extract from seeds of Peganum harmala on isolated rat aorta. Therapie 2002; 57(3): 236-41.

[312] Berrougui H, Martin-Cordero C, Khalil A, Hmamouchi M, Ettaib A, Marhuenda E, Herrera MD. Vasorelaxant effects of harmine and harmaline extracted from Peganum harmala L. seeds in isolated rat aorta. Pharmacol Res 2006; 54(2): 150-7.

[313] Cefalu WT, Ye J, Wang ZQ. Efficacy of dietary supplementation with *botanical*s on carbohydrate metabolism in humans. Endocr Metab Immune Disord Drug Targets 2008; 8(2): 78-81.

[314] Chandra A, Mahdi AA, Singh RK, Mahdi F, Chander R. Effect of Indian herbal hypoglycemic agents on antioxidant capacity and trace elements content in diabetic rats. J Med Food 2008; 11(3): 506-12.

Send Orders of Reprints at reprints@benthamscience.org

CHAPTER 7

Plants-Derived Natural Products and Drug Discovery

Mohamed Eddouks[*] and Naoufel Ali Zeggwagh

Moulay Ismail University, BP 21, Errachidia, 52000, Morocco

Abstract: Over the last decade, there has been a renewed interest in natural products research. The exceptional developments in the areas of separation science, spectroscopic techniques associated with microplate-based ultrasensitive *in vitro* assays provide a novel and interesting drug design from natural products. The various available chromatographic techniques have made possible the preisolation analyses of crude extracts or fractions from different natural sources. This chapter presents a general overview of the processes involved in natural product research, starting from extraction to determination of the structures of purified products.

Keywords: Natural products, extraction, identification, *in vitro*, drug, phytochemical, separation, isolation, analysis, molecules.

INTRODUCTION

In popular language, is not easy to clearly understand what is "Natural Product" (with capitalization), since all natural products are highly processed and redesigned by human before being presented to consumers. So, it is important to set the chapter with a definition of Natural Products. Globally, all products of natural origins can be called as "natural products". Natural Products include: (1) an entire organism (*e.g.*, a plant, an animal, or a microorganism) that has not been subjected to any kind of processing or treatment other than a simple process of preservation (*e.g.*, dying), (2) part of an organism (*e.g.*, different plant parts like leaves or flowers of a plant, an isolated animal organ), (3) extract of an organism or part of an organism and exudates, and (4) pure compounds (*e.g.*, alkaloids, coumarins, flavonoids, glycosides, lignans, phenolics, sugars, terpenoids, *etc.*) isolated form plants, animals, or microorganisms [1]. In most cases the term natural products refers to secondary metabolites, small molecules (mol wt <2000 Atomic Mass Unit (amu)) produced by an organism that are not strictly

*Address correspondence to Mohamed Eddouks: Moulay Ismail University, BP 21, 52000, Errachidia, Morocco; Tel: 00212535570024; Fax: 00212535573588; E-mail: mohamed.eddouks@laposte.net

Mohamed Eddouks and Debprasad Chattopadhyay (Eds)
All rights reserved-© 2012 Bentham Science Publishers

necessary for the survival of the organism [1]. Natural Products can also be from any terrestrial or marine source: plants (*e.g.* paclitaxel: Taxol from *Taxux brevifolia*), animals (*e.g.* vitamins A and D from cod liver oil), or microorganisms (*e.g.* doxorubicin from *Streptomyces peucetius*) [2-5]. Even if Natural Product definition is clear, the common uses of this word is ambiguous and is now more widely used to mean anything not manufactured. So, we have a situation where all Natural Products are products from natural sources but not all natural products are of natural origin [4-7]. Many scientists propose the use of secondary metabolites, produced by living organisms, indeed of Natural Products.

This chapter aims to review the main plant-derived Natural products and their importance in human healing and drug discovery throughout time.

NATURAL PRODUCTS AND MEDICINE: THE INCESSANT LOVE STORY

The use of Natural Products, especially plants, for healing is an ancient and universal practice as medicine itself. The therapeutic use of plants certainly goes back to the Sumerian civilization. Natural products played a prominent role in ancient traditional medicine systems of many civilizations like Chinese, Ayurveda and Egyptian. Over the last century, a number of top selling medicines have been developed from natural products (vinvristine from *Vinca rosea*, morphin from *Papaver somniferum*, Taxol® from *T. brevifolia*, *etc.*).

As per WHO estimates, 75% of people still rely on plant-based traditional medicine for primary healthcare. Actually, plant-derived natural products are subjects to a significant revival of interest. An average of 40% of the modern drugs in use has been developed from natural products. Between 1983 to 1993 about 39% of the 520 new approved drugs were from natural products or their derivatives, and 60-80% of antibacterial and anticancer drugs have their root in natural products [5, 8]. In 2000, approximately 60% of all drugs in clinical trials for the multiplicity of cancers had natural origins [9-12]. In 2001, eight (Simavastin, Pravastatin, Amoxicillin, Clavulanic acid, Azithromycin, Ceftriaxone, Cyclosporin and Paclitaxel) of the 30 top-selling medicine were from natural products or their derivatives, and these eight drugs together totaled $16 billion in sales [1, 3].

Arteether (trade name Artemotil®) is a potent anti-malarial drug derived from artemisinin, a sesquiterpene lactone isolated from *Artemisia annua* L. (Asteraceae) [7, 13, 14]. Galantamine (also known as galanthamine, trade name Reminyl®) is discovered through an ethnobotanical lead and first isolated from *Galanthus woronowii* Losinsk. (Amaryllidaceae) in Russia in the early 1950s, and approved for the treatment of Alzheimer's disease, as it can slow down the process of neurological degeneration by inhibiting acetylcholinesterase (AChE) as well as binding to and modulating the nicotinic acetylcholine receptor [15-19].

Nitisinone (trade name Orfadin®) is a newly released medicinal plant-derived drug that works on the rare inherited disease tyrosinaemia, demonstrating the usefulness of natural products as lead structures. Nitisinone is an analog of mesotrione, an herbicide based on the natural product leptospermone, a constituent of *Callistemon citrinus* Stapf. (Myrtaceae). Another drug Tiotropium (trade name Spiriva®) has recently been released to the United States for the treatment of chronic obstructive pulmonary disease (COPD). Tiotroprium is an inhaled anticholinergic bronchodilator, based on ipratropium, a derivative of atropine isolated from *Atropa belladonna* L. (Solanaceae) of the Solanaceae family.

The compound M6G or morphine-6-glucuronide is a metabolite of morphine from *Papaver somniferum* L. (Papaveraceae) is in Phase III clinical trials and registration. It is a subtle modification of drugs currently in clinical use and can be used as an alternate pain medication with fewer side effects than morphine [8, 17, 18, 20, 21]. Natural products can contribute to the search for new drugs in three different ways:

1. By acting as new drugs used in an unmodified state (*e.g.*, vincristine from *Catharanthus roseus*).

2. By providing chemical 'building blocks' used to synthesize more complex molecules (*e.g.*, diosgenin from *Dioscorea floribunda* for the synthesis of oral contraceptives).

3. By indicating new modes of pharmacological action that allow complete synthesis of novel analogs (*e.g.*, synthetic analogs of penicillin from *Penicillium notatum*).

Natural products will continue to be considered as one of the major sources of new drugs in the years to come because:

1.   They offer incomparable structure diversity.

2.   Many of them have relatively small molecular weight (<2000 Da).

3.   They have 'drug-like' properties.

ISOLATION AND IDENTIFICATION OF PLANT-DERIVED NATURAL PRODUCTS

The continuous development of chromatographic and spectrometric methods provided precious tools for the separation, identification and structure elucidation of various natural products. Furthermore, the use of highly sensitive chromatographic techniques in association with natural products library allowed fast screening of drug candidate of natural origins. In order to provide a common pathway in the search of new products from plants a generic protocol has been established and basic generic protocol has been effectively used to isolate and identify new natural products. However, it is important to remember that only small fraction of the world's biodiversity has been explored until today. For example, there are at least 250,000 species of higher plants that exist on this planet, but merely 5-10% of these have been investigated so far [7, 13, 15-18, 23-26].

The introduction and development of new highly specific *in vitro* bioassay techniques and nuclear magnetic resonance (NMR) have made it much easier to screen, isolate and identify potential drug lead compounds quickly and precisely.

The first step in the development of new natural product is the extraction. Natural products are especially localized in the inner of vegetal. In order to isolate the analytes from plant material, extraction with various solvents is used. The nature of the source material and the compounds to be isolated determine the choice of extraction procedure. Generally six extraction methods are used Maceration.

1.   Boiling.

2.   Soxhlet.

3. Supercritical fluid extraction.

4. Sublimation.

5. Steam distillation.

Various solvents can be used with different polarity:

- Polar solvents: water, ethanol, and methanol.

- Medium polarity solvents: ethyl acetate (EtOAc) and dichlomethane (DCM).

- Nonpolar solvents: n-hexane, pet-ether, Chloroform ($CHCl_3$).

A crude natural product extract contains a mixture of compounds and the application of one separation technique is difficult or impossible. Hence, it is important to achieve a separation of compounds according to their polarity or the molecular size. So, with the separation step the crude extract can be devised in fractions with different polarity or molecular size. These fractions may be obvious, physically discrete divisions such as the two phases of a liquid-liquid extraction or contiguous eluate from a chromatography column (vacuum liquid chromatography, column chromatography, size-exclusion chromatography, solid-phase extraction).

After transforming the crude extract to fractions, the isolation process can be performed. The key element in the separation process is the physico-chemical nature of the target compound such as: hydrophobicity, acid-base properties, charge, stability and molecular size. However, it is difficult to design an isolation protocol for a crude extract where the types of compounds present are totally unknown [5, 16]. Chromatographic techniques play an important role in the separation protocol, and can be broadly classified into two categories: classical or older, and modern:

Classical or older chromatographic techniques include:

- Thin layer chromatography (TLC).

- Preparative thin-layer chromatography (PTLC).

- Column chromatography (CC).

- Flash chromatography.

Modern chromatography techniques are:

- High-performance thin-layer chromatography (HPTLC).

- Multiflash chromatography (*e.g.*, Biotage®).

- Vacuum liquid chromatography (VLC).

- Chromatotron.

- Solid-phase extraction (*e.g.*, Sep-Pak®).

The aim of extraction and isolation of natural products is the identification of the compound or conclusive structure elucidation of the isolated compounds. This steep is generally time consuming, and sometimes can be the bottleneck in natural product research [17, 18, 27]. There are many useful spectroscopic methods of getting information about chemical structures, but the interpretation of these spectra normally requires specialists with detailed spectroscopic knowledge [28-30]. The following spectroscopic techniques are generally used for the structure determination of natural products:

1. Ultraviolet-visible spectroscopy (UV-Vis): Provides information on chromatophores present in the molecule.

2. Infrared spectrometry (IR): Determines different functional groups, *e.g.*, -C=O, -OH.

3. Mass spectrometry (MS): Gives information about the molecular mass, molecular formula, and fragmentation pattern.

4. Nuclear Magnetic Resonance (NMR) spectroscopy: Reveals information on the number and types of protons (and other elements like nitrogen, fluorine, *etc.*).

5. Present in the molecule, and the relationships among these atoms.

CHALLENGES IN DRUG DISCOVERY FROM MEDICINAL PLANTS

The process of drug development takes about an estimated period of ten years and cost more than 800 millions dollars [31-33]. Drug discovery form medicinal plants have traditionally been lengthier and more complicated than other drug discovery methods. Furthermore, drug discovery from medicinal plants has traditionally been so time-consuming. Thus, faster and better methodologies for plant collection, bioassay screening, compound isolation, and compound development must be employed. Hence, innovative strategies to improve the process of plant collection are needed, especially with the legal and political issues surrounding benefit-sharing agreements [1, 22, 34-37].

Compound development of drugs discovery from medicinal plants also faces unique challenges. Natural products are typically isolated in small quantities that are insufficient for lead optimization, lead development, and clinical trials [1, 22, 34-40]. Collaboration with synthetic and medicinal chemists is necessary to determine if synthesis or semi-synthesis might be possible [9, 41].

CONCLUSION

In conclusion, natural products discovered from medicinal plants have provided numerous clinically used medicines. In spite of all the challenges facing drug discovery from medicinal plants, natural products isolated from medicinal plants can be predicted to remain an essential component in the search for new medicines.

ACKNOWLEDGEMENTS

The authors extend their thanks to Bentham Science Publishers.

DECLARATION OF CONFLICT OF INTEREST

No conflict of interest was declared by the authors.

REFERENCES

[1]   Sarker SD, Latif Z, Gray AI. Natural products isolation. 2nd ed. Totowa, N.J.: Humana Press; 2005.
[2]   Do QT, Bernard P. Pharmacognosy and reverse pharmacognosy: a new concept for accelerating natural drug discovery. IDrugs 2004; 7(11): 1017-1027.

[3]   Phillipson JD. Phytochemistry and pharmacognosy. Phytochemistry. 2007; 68(22-24): 2960-2972.

[4]   Brower V. Back to nature: extinction of medicinal plants threatens drug discovery. J Natl Cancer Inst 2008; 100(12): 838-839.

[5]   Kinghorn AD. The discovery of drugs from higher plants. Biotechnology 1994; 26: 81-108.

[6]   Potterat O, Hamburger M. Drug discovery and development with plant-derived compounds. Prog Drug Res. 2008; 65: 47-118.

[7]   Balunas MJ, Kinghorn AD. Drug discovery from medicinal plants. Life Sci 2005; 78(5):431-441.

[8]   Kinghorn AD, Su BN, Jang DS, *et al.* Natural inhibitors of carcinogenesis. Planta Med 2004; 70(8): 691-705.

[9]   Littleton J, Rogers T, Falcone D. Novel approaches to plant drug discovery based on high throughput pharmacological screening and genetic manipulation. Life Sci 2005; 78(5): 467-475.

[10]   Mays TD, Mazan KD. Legal issues in sharing the benefits of biodiversity prospecting. J Ethnopharmacol 1996; 51(1-3): 93-102.

[11]   McLaughlin JL. Paw paw and cancer: annonaceous acetogenins from discovery to commercial products. J Nat Prod. 2008; 71(7): 1311-1321.

[12]   Patwardhan B. Ethnopharmacology and drug discovery. J Ethnopharmacol 2005; 100(1-2): 50-52.

[13]   Bedoya LM, Alvarez A, Bermejo M, *et al.* Guatemalan plants extracts as virucides against HIV-1 infection. Phytomedicine. 2008; 15(6-7): 520-524.

[14]   Bertha SL. Academic research: policies and practice. J Ethnopharmacol 1996; 51(1-3): 59-73.

[15]   Calixto JB, Beirith A, Ferreira J, Santos AR, Filho VC, Yunes RA. Naturally occurring antinociceptive substances from plants. Phytother Res 2000;14(6): 401-418.

[16]   Cannell RJP. Natural products isolation. Totowa, N.J: Humana Press; 1998.

[17]   Chatterjee SS, Bhattacharya SK, Wonnemann M, Singer A, Muller WE. Hyperforin as a possible antidepressant component of hypericum extracts. Life Sci 1998; 63(6): 499-510.

[18]   Chen X, Ung CY, Chen Y. Can an *in silico* drug-target search method be used to probe potential mechanisms of medicinal plant ingredients? Nat Prod Rep 2003; 20(4): 432-444.

[19]   Cordell GA, Quinn-Beattie ML, Farnsworth NR. The potential of alkaloids in drug discovery. Phytother Res 2001; 15(3): 183-205.

[20]   Cragg GM, Newman DJ, Snader KM. Natural products in drug discovery and development. J Nat Prod 1997; 60(1): 52-60.

[21]   Elisabetsky E, Costa-Campos L. Medicinal plant genetic resources and international cooperation: the Brazilian perspective. J Ethnopharmacol 1996; 51: 1-3.

[22]   Schmidt B, Ribnicky DM, Poulev A, Logendra S, Cefalu WT, Raskin I. A natural history of botanical therapeutics. Metabolism 2008; 57(7 Suppl 1): S3-9.

[23]   Slish DF, Ueda H, Arvigo R, Balick MJ. Ethnobotany in the search for vasoactive herbal medicines. J Ethnopharmacol 1999; 66(2): 159-165.

[24]   Alviano DS, Alviano CS. Plant extracts: search for new alternatives to treat microbial diseases. Curr Pharm Biotechnol 2009; 10(1): 106-121.

[25]   Butler MS, Newman DJ. Mother Nature's gifts to diseases of man: the impact of natural products on anti-infective, anticholestemics and anticancer drug discovery. Prog Drug Res 2008; 65: 3-44.

[26] Cheng Y, Wang Y, Wang X. A causal relationship discovery-based approach to identifying active components of herbal medicine. Comput Biol Chem 2006; 30(2): 148-154.

[27] Romanik G, Gilgenast E, Przyjazny A, Kaminski M. Techniques of preparing plant material for chromatographic separation and analysis. J Biochem Biophys Methods. 2007; 70(2): 253-261.

[28] Cox PA, Balick MJ. The ethnobotanical approach to drug discovery. Sci Am. 1994; 270(6): 82-87.

[29] Cragg GM. Natural product drug discovery and development: the United States National Cancer Institute role. P R Health Sci J 2002; 21(2): 97-111.

[30] Elisabetsky E, Costa-Campos L. The alkaloid alstonine: a review of its pharmacological properties. Evid Based Complement Alternat Med 2006; 3(1): 39-48.

[31] Firn RD, Jones CG. Avenues of discovery in bioprospecting. Nature 1998; 392(6676): 535-7.

[32] Fisar Z. Phytocannabinoids and endocannabinoids. Curr Drug Abuse Rev 2009; 2(1): 51-75.

[33] Jung M, Lee S, Kim H. Recent studies on natural products as anti-HIV agents. Curr Med Chem 2000; 7(6): 649-661.

[34] Grzanna R, Lindmark L, Frondoza CG. Ginger--an herbal medicinal product with broad anti-inflammatory actions. J Med Food 2005; 8(2): 125-132.

[35] Ramasamy K, Lim SM, Abu Bakar H, *et al.* Antimicrobial and cytotoxic activities of Malaysian endophytes. Phytother Res 2010; 24(5): 640-643.

[36] Rollinger JM, Langer T, Stuppner H. Integrated *in silico* tools for exploiting the natural products' bioactivity. Planta Med 2006; 72(8): 671-678.

[37] Saxena M, Faridi U, Mishra R, *et al.* Cytotoxic agents from Terminalia arjuna. Planta Med 2007; 73(14): 1486-1490.

[38] Soejarto DD, Zhang HJ, Fong HH, *et al.* Studies on biodiversity of Vietnam and Laos 1998-2005: examining the impact. J Nat Prod 2006; 69(3): 473-481.

[39] Stepp JR. The role of weeds as sources of pharmaceuticals. J Ethnopharmacol 2004; 92(2-3): 163-166.

[40] Xue T, Zhang L. Avenues of discovery in bioprospecting. Nature 1998; 392(6676): 535-7.

[41] Phillipson JD. Natural products as drugs. Trans R Soc Trop Med Hyg 1994; 88(1): S17-19.

Index

Mohamed Eddouks and Debprasad Chattopadhyay (Eds)
All rights reserved-© 2012 Bentham Science Publishers

www.ingramcontent.com/pod-product-compliance
Lightning Source LLC
Chambersburg PA
CBHW050823220326
41598CB00006B/300